WILLIAM F. MAAG LIBRARY
YOUNGSTOWN STATE UNIVERSITY

BODY FLUID BALANCE
Exercise and Sport

NUTRITION in EXERCISE and SPORT

Editors, Ira Wolinsky and James F. Hickson, Jr.

Published Titles

Nutrients as Ergogenic Aids for Sports and Exercise
Luke Bucci

Nutrition in Exercise and Sport, 2nd Edition
Ira Wolinsky and James F. Hickson, Jr.

Exercise and Disease
Ronald R. Watson and Marianne Eisinger

Nutrition Applied to Injury Rehabilitation and Sports Medicine
Luke Bucci

Nutrition for the Recreational Athlete
Catherine G.R. Jackson

NUTRITION in EXERCISE and SPORT

Editor, Ira Wolinsky

Published Titles

Nutrition, Physical Activity, and Health in Early Life
Jana Pařízková

Exercise and Immune Function
Laurie Hoffman-Goetz

Sports Nutrition: Minerals and Electrolytes
Constance Kies and Judy Driskell

Forthcoming Titles

Nutrition and the Female Athlete
Jaime S. Rudd

Biochemical Methods for Exercise Assessment
Jon Karl Linderman

Handbook of Sports Nutrition: Vitamins and Trace Minerals
Ira Wolinsky and Judy Driskell

BODY FLUID BALANCE
Exercise and Sport

Edited by

ELSWORTH R. BUSKIRK, Ph. D.
Professor of Applied Physiology, Emeritus
The Pennsylvania State University
University Park, Pennsylvania

SUSAN M. PUHL, Ph. D.
Associate Professor of Physical Education
State University of New York at Cortland
Cortland, New York

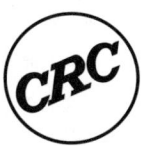

CRC Press
Boca Raton   New York   London   Tokyo

Library of Congress Cataloging-in-Publication Data

Body fluid balance: exercise and sport / edited by Elsworth R. Buskirk and Susan M. Puhl
    p. cm.—(Nutrition in exercise and sport)
   Includes bibliographical references and index.
   ISBN 0-8493-7918-0
   1. Body fluids—Regulation. 2. Exercise—Physiological aspects.
 I. Buskirk, (Elsworth R.) II. Puhl, Susan M.
 III. Series.
 QP90.5.B63 1996
 612.3'9—dc20
                                                                    95-53970
                                                                         CIP

This book contains information obtained from authentic and highly regarded sources. Reprinted material is quoted with permission, and sources are indicated. A wide variety of references are listed. Reasonable efforts have been made to publish reliable data and information, but the author and the publisher cannot assume responsibility for the validity of all materials or for the consequences of their use.

Neither this book nor any part may be reproduced or transmitted in any form or by any means, electronic or mechanical, including photocopying, microfilming, and recording, or by any information storage or retrieval system, without prior permission in writing from the publisher.

All rights reserved. Authorization to photocopy items for internal or personal use, or the personal or internal use of specific clients, may be granted by CRC Press, Inc., provided that $.50 per page photocopied is paid directly to Copyright Clearance Center, 27 Congress Street, Salem, MA 01970 USA. The fee code for users of the Transactional Reporting Service is ISBN 0-8493-7918-0/96/$0.00+$.50. The fee is subject to change without notice. For organizations that have been granted a photocopy license by the CCC, a separate system of payment has been arranged.

The consent of CRC Press does not extend to copying for general distribution, for promotion, for creating new works, or for resale. Specific permission must be obtained in writing from CRC Press for such copying.

Direct all inquiries to CRC Press, Inc., 2000 Corporate Blvd., N.W., Boca Raton, Florida 33431.

© 1996 by CRC Press, Inc.

No claim to original U.S. Government works
International Standard Book Number 0-8493-7918-0
Library of Congress Card Number 95-53970
Printed in the United States of America 1 2 3 4 5 6 7 8 9 0
Printed on acid-free paper

SERIES PREFACE

The CRC series on *Nutrition in Exercise and Sport* provides a setting for in-depth exploration of the many and varied aspects of nutrition and exercise, including sports. The topic of exercise and sports nutrition has been a focus of research among scientists since the 1960s, and the healthful benefits of good nutrition and exercise have been appreciated. As our knowledge expands, it will be necessary to remember that there must be a range of diets and exercise regimens that will support excellent physical condition and performance. There is not a single diet-exercise treatment that can be the common denominator, or the single formula for health, or panacea for performance.

This series is dedicated to providing a stage to explore these issues. Each volume provides a detailed and scholarly examination of some aspect of the topic.

Contributors from any bona fide area of nutrition and physical activity, including sports and the controversial, are welcome.

We welcome to the series the timely contribution, *Body Fluid Balance: Exercise and Sport,* edited by Elsworth R. Buskirk and Susan M. Puhl.

Ira Wolinsky, Ph.D.
Series Editor

PREFACE

An update of the topic of body fluid balance and exercise was deemed necessary to provide a current compendium of the thinking of active investigators in the field. Although some overlap in coverage is provided by the several contributors, each brings a unique perspective that should not only provide ideas for other investigators, but also supply independent analyses for practitioners and educators who will undoubtedly use this volume. A variety of topics are covered including: the mechanisms for controlling fluid ingestions (thirst); the gastrointestinal handling of fluids; the role of specific systems in regulating fluid balance (hormonal, neural, renal, sweat glands, and the lung); environmental influences (heat, cold, altitude, immersion); other influences (age, gender, types of exercise); fluid replacement considerations; clinical complications; and the integrated control of body fluid balance during exercise. Not only is the historical perspective presented, but critical experiments are also described, appropriate analyses set forth, and pertinent conclusions drawn. Although the authors have provided a comprehensive review of the topics, there are numerous gaps in our knowledge and hopefully some of the thought-provoking ideas expressed will encourage others to build on the presented background and advance the field.

Elsworth R. Buskirk
Susan M. Puhl

THE EDITORS

Elsworth R. Buskirk, Ph.D., is the founder and past Director of the Laboratory for Human Performance Research at The Pennsylvania State University. He is also past chairman of the Physiology Program. His academic titles have been Professor of Applied Physiology and Marie Underhill Noll Professor of Human Performance.

Dr. Buskirk obtained his training in physiology at the University of Minnesota, Minneapolis where he received an M.A. in 1951 and a Ph.D. in 1954. His principal laboratory affiliation at Minnesota was with the Laboratory of Physiological Hygiene. In 1954 he assumed a position with the Environmental Physiology Section of the Quartermaster Research and Development Center, Natick, MA. Following his tenure at Natick, he joined the faculty of the National Institute of Arthritis and Metabolic Diseases, National Institutes of Health in 1957. He worked as the physiologist in charge of the metabolic chamber facility from 1957 until 1963 when he assumed a professorship and directorship at The Pennsylvania State University. In 1988 he was honored with a named professorship. Dr. Buskirk retired and was granted emeritus status in 1992.

Dr. Buskirk has retained membership or fellowship in The American Academy of Physical Education; American Association for Health, Physical Education, and Recreation; American Association for the Advancement of Science; American Association of Cardiovascular and Pulmonary Rehabilitation; American College of Sports Medicine; American Heart Association; American Society of Clinical Nutrition; American Institute of Nutrition; American Physiological Society; Sigma Xi and the Gerontology Society of America. Over the years he was also a member of the Aerospace Medical Association; American Society of Heating, Refrigeration and Air Conditioning Engineers; Association of Chairmen of Departments of Physiology; National Institutes of Health Alumni Association; New York Academy of Sciences; North American Association for the Study of Obesity and the International Society of Biometeorology. He has held offices in several of these organizations and has been honored both by the American College of Sports Medicine and the American Physiological Society as well as by his undergraduate school, St. Olaf College and The Pennysylvania State University. His investigations have been supported by the NIH and other federal, state and private organizations for 30 years.

Dr. Buskirk has served in several editorial capacities and is the author or coauthor of well over 200 papers in the open physiological literature. His current major research interests reside in several aspects of exercise physiology including body fluid balance.

Susan M. Puhl, Ph.D., is an Associate Professor of Physical Education and Coordinator of the program in Adult Fitness at the State University of New York College at Cortland. Prior to coming to Cortland, she was at The Pennsylvania State University, where she conducted research in both metabolism and thermoregulation.

Dr. Puhl has presented over 100 papers on topics related to exercise physiology and physical fitness development. Her written work appears in both peer-reviewed journals and lay publications. She has co-authored chapters in books targeted to the scientific community and to the lay population.

Dr. Puhl received her Ph.D. in exercise physiology from the Pennsylvania State University in 1986. Her professional affiliations include the American College of Sports Medicine and the American Alliance for Health, Physical Education, Recreation and Dance.

CONTRIBUTORS

Lawrence E. Armstrong, Ph.D.
Human Performance Laboratory, University of Connecticut, Storrs, Connecticut

Eric K. Birks, D.V.M., Ph.D.
Cardiovascular Research Center, Medical College of Wisconsin, Milwaukee, Wisconsin

Richard A. Boileau, Ph.D.
Department of Kinesiology, University of Illinois, Urbana, Illinois

E.R. Buskirk, Ph.D.
Noll Physiological Research Center, Penn State University, University Park, Pennsylvania

Richard M. Effros, M.D.
Chief, Pulmonary and Critical Care Medicine, MCW Clinic at Froedtert Hospital, Milwaukee, Wisconsin

Murray Epstein, M.D.
Department of Medicine, Division of Nephrology, University of Miami Medical School, Miami, Florida

Suzanne M. Fortney, Ph.D.
NASA Johnson Space Center, Houston, Texas

Ralph P. Francesconi, Ph.D.
Comparative Physiological Division, U.S. Army Research Institute of Environmental Medicine, Natick, Massachusetts

Beau J. Freund, Ph.D.
Thermal Physiology and Medicine Division, U.S. Army Research Institute of Environmental Medicine, Natick, Massachusetts

Carl V. Gisolfi, Ph.D.
Department of Physiology and Biophysics/Exercise Science, University of Iowa, Iowa City, Iowa

John E. Greenleaf, Ph.D.
Life Sciences Division, Laboratory for Human Environmental Physiology, NASA-Ames Research Center, Moffett Field, California

Arnold Honig, M.D., Ph.D.
Institute of Physiology, Ernst-Moritz-Arndt University of Greifswald, Greifswald, Germany

Reed W. Hoyt, Ph.D.
Altitude Physiology and Medicine Division, U.S. Army Research Institute of Environmental Medicine, Natick, Massachusetts

Roger W. Hubbard, Ph.D.
Environmental Pathophysiology Directorate, U.S. Army Research Institute of Environmental Medicine, Natick, Massachusetts

James P. Knochel, M.D.
Department of Internal Medicine, Presbyterian Hospital of Dallas, Dallas, Texas

William A. Latzka, D.Sc.
Thermal Physiology and Medicine Division, U.S. Army Research Institute of Environmental Medicine, Natick, Massachusetts

Carl M. Maresh, Ph.D.
Human Performance Laboratory, University of Connecticut, Storrs, Connecticut

Scott Montain, Ph.D.
Thermal Physiology and Medicine Division, U.S. Army Research Institute of Environmental Medicine, Natick, Massachusetts

Taketoshi Morimoto, M.D.
Department of Physiology, Kyoto Prefectural University of Medicine, Kyoto, Japan

Susan N. Puhl, Ph.D.
Department of Physical Education, SUNY College at Cortland, Cortland, New York

Alan J. Ryan, Ph.D.
Department of Internal Medicine, University of Iowa, Iowa City, Iowa

Michael N. Sawka, Ph.D.
Thermal Physiology and Medicine Division, U.S. Army Research Institute of Environmental Medicine, Natick, Massachusetts

Patricia C. Szlyk-Modrow, Ph.D.
Comparative Physiology Division, U.S. Army Research Institute of Environmental Medicine, Natick, Massachusetts

Marta D. Van Loan, Ph.D.
Western Human Nutrition Research Center, USDA, San Francisco, California

Charles E. Wade, Ph.D.
Life Sciences Division, NASA Ames Research Center, Moffett Field, California

Andrew J. Young, Ph.D.
Thermal Physiology and Medicine Division, U.S. Army Research Institute of Environmental Medicine, Natick, Massachusetts

Edward J. Zambraski, Ph.D.
Department of Biological Sciences, Nelson Biological Laboratories, Rutgers University, Piscataway, New Jersey

CONTENTS

I. Control of Body Fluid Balance During Exercise

Chapter 1   Mechanisms Controlling Fluid Ingestion: Thirst and Drinking 3
John E. Greenleaf and Taketoshi Morimoto

Chapter 2   Gastrointestinal Physiology During Exercise 19
Carl V. Gisolfi and Alan J. Ryan

Chapter 3   Hormonal Control of Body Fluid Volume 53
Charles E. Wade

Chapter 4   The Kidney and Body Fluid Balance During Exercise 75
Edward J. Zambraski

Chapter 5   Fluid and Electrolyte Balance of the Lung During Exercise 97
E. K. Birks and Richard M. Effros

Chapter 6   Integrated Control of Body Fluid Balance During Exercise 117
Patricia C. Szlyk-Modrow, Ralph P. Francesconi, and Roger W. Hubbard

II. Environmental Influences on Body Fluid Balance During Exercise

Chapter 7   Body Fluid Balance During Exercise–Heat Exposure 139
Michael N. Sawka, Scott J. Montain, and William A. Latzka

Chapter 8   Environmental Influences on Body Fluid Balance During Exercise: Cold Exposure 159
Beau J. Freund and Andrew J. Young

Chapter 9   Environmental Influences on Body Fluid Balance During Exercise: Altitude 183
Reed W. Hoyt and Arnold Honig

Chapter 10   Renal, Endocrine, and Hemodynamic Effects of Water Immersion in Humans 197
Murray Epstein

III. Special Considerations with Regard to Body Fluid Balance During Exercise

Chapter 11 Age, Gender, and Fluid Balance 215
Marta D. Van Loan and Richard A. Boileau

Chapter 12 Hormonal Control of Fluid Balance in Women During Exercise 231
Suzanne M. Fortney

Chapter 13 Fluid Replacement During Exercise and Recovery from Exercise 259
Lawrence E. Armstrong and Carl M. Maresh

Chapter 14 Effects of Acute Body Weight Loss in Weight-Controlling Athletes 283
E. R. Buskirk and Susan M. Puhl

Chapter 15 Clinical Complications of Body Fluid and Electrolyte Imbalance 297
James P. Knochel

Index 319

Part I

CONTROL OF BODY FLUID BALANCE DURING EXERCISE

Chapter 1

MECHANISMS CONTROLLING FLUID INGESTION: THIRST AND DRINKING

John E. Greenleaf
Taketoshi Morimoto

CONTENTS

I. Introduction...3
   A. Historical Milestones 4

II. Body Water and Electrolytes 6
   A. Body Fluid Compartments 6
   B. Change in Body Fluid Compartment Volumes During
      Exercise and Heat Stress..6

III. Cellular Dehydration Drinking (Osmoreceptors)..................7
   A. Cerebral Osmoreceptors 7
   B. Extracerebral Osmoreceptors 8

IV. Extracellular Dehydration Drinking (Volume Receptors) 9

V. Mechanism of Involuntary Dehydration 10

VI. Summary...12

References 13

I. INTRODUCTION

Water, comprising about two thirds of body weight, is probably the most important chemical compound in mammals. It is the critical component of the internal milieu that engenders and facilitates homeostasis by means of its power as a solvent, its dielectric constant and related ionizing potential, its high thermal conductivity facilitating temperature equilibrium within and between cells, its high latent heat of evaporation, and its high specific heat allowing for transfer of a relatively large amount of heat with relatively small change in cell or body temperature.[36] Plasma proteins (via their oncotic pressure), and sodium and its most closely regulated anions[73] (via their osmotic pressure), play important roles in maintaining body fluid homeostasis.

Thirst, "a desire for potable liquids or to drink,"[29] is a subjective sensation that, at this time, can only be expressed by humans; whether animals become thirsty is conjectural. Thus, emphasis here will be on measured fluid consumption.

A. HISTORICAL MILESTONES

Excellent historical treatises on thirst and its satiation have been published by Wolf,[90] Fitzsimons,[23] de Caro et al.,[20] and Ramsey and Booth.[64] Although most humans experience some moderate thirst on a day-to-day basis, apparently some do not and are capable of living normally without significant dehydration.[90] This wide variability in drinking may be the result of variability (10-fold) in the setpoint and sensitivity of the vasopressin–osmoregulatory system that is determined genetically.[95] Because thirst is often associated with a dry feeling in the mouth and throat, cause and effect (drinking) was assumed — rightly so in some but not all cases. Deneufbourg,[21] in 1813, differentiated the dry mouth and throat sensation that stimulates drinking from the general body state resulting from dehydration. These two factors, mouth dryness and total body dehydration, are often associated but can act independently to initiate drinking. Haller,[35] in 1764, provided the first clear description of the "dry-mouth" (peripheral) theory of thirst, which was reemphasized by Cannon[16] in 1918; the stimuli were purported to be in the tongue, mouth, esophagus, and stomach. However, men with congenital absence of salivary glands, when tested for salivary function by response to pilocarpine and amylotic enzymes, apparently have normal thirst and fluid intake.[78] These observations strengthen the hypothesis of a general origin of thirst from sensation or response of unspecified deeper tissues; that is, general-body cellular dehydration. In 1881, Nothnagel[60] first referred to a thirst center, which he located in the pons or medulla, that induced drinking in a man with head injury. In 1900, Mayer[48] reported an association between increased serum osmotic concentration and drinking in dogs, and also postulated a center in the brainstem that stimulated drinking. A year later, in 1901, Wettendorff[88] concluded that blood homeostasis in dehydrated dogs was maintained by shift of water from tissue cells into the vascular system; it was loss of cellular water and not increase in serum osmolality that caused drinking. Greater specificity of the drinking mechanism was elucidated in the late 1920s by Gamble[26] and in the 1930s by Arden[8] and Gilman,[28] who found that consumption or intravenous (i.v.) infusion of sodium chloride instigated drinking, while similar intake of potassium chloride or urea did not. These findings focused attention on the sodium ion as the dipsogenic agent; it does not readily cross cell membranes and acts to withdraw water from cells osmotically. In the next two decades, Verney and associates[42,87] reported their classic findings that intracarotid infusion of nonpenetrating solutes (sodium chloride and sucrose) caused cellular dehydration of "osmoreceptors," which in turn released a "post-pituitary antidiuretic substance" that attenuated diuresis[87]; and that the osmoreceptors were located in the anterior hypothalamic or preoptic areas of the brain.[42] These findings were questioned by Anderson[5,6] who proposed that sodium-sensitive receptors, located in the anterior area of the third cerebral ventricle of the goat, may act as solute-receptors that stimulate drinking. The finding that intracarotid and i.v. infusion of hyperosmolar NaCl solutions into water-diuresing dogs[12,14] and into hydrated goats[61] which resulted in similar or increased urinary excretion rates of sodium and potassium, and similar renal clearances of inulin and p-aminohippuric acid, led Bie[13] to question the exclusive role of the classic osmoreceptor hypothesis of Verney. There is increasing evidence that localizes at least some cerebral osmoreceptors on the blood side of the blood–brain barrier— that is, in the anterio-ventral area of the third cerebral ventricle near the supraoptic nucleus (SON) and in a circumventricular organ such as the organum vasculosum laminae terminalis.[67,85] These cerebral osmoreceptors and those located elsewhere will be discussed later.

In 1954, Adolph and colleagues[3] proposed their classic multiple-factor theory of thirst, which states that no single mechanism can account for all drinking behavior and that multiple (perhaps redundant) mechanisms must be functioning. This theory has not been refuted[2,65,66,82] and seems reasonable considering the importance of maintaining body fluid–electrolyte homeostasis. An example of multiple factors (cellular, extracellular, volume) involved in drinking are those in a stepwise linear regression equation[32] for predicting actual water intake ($r = 0.79$, $p<0.01$) in 87 young Army trainees in field conditions: Water intake (mL/day) = $-11,502 + 45.8$ (serum Osm) + 1.2 (mean daily urinary vol.) $- 18.9$ (mean daily urinary K$^+$) + 4.4 (mean daily urinary Cl$^-$) $- 18.7$ (lying pulse rate) + 1.8 (daily sweat rate).

Stimuli for control of drinking and its satiation have been allocated into cellular osmoreceptor factors (cerebral and extracerebral) and extracellular volume factors, probably more for ease of study and conceptualization than for physiological integration. It appears that osmotic factors contribute about 70% and volemic factors contribute about 25% to moderate dehydration-induced drinking in resting rats[65] and dogs.[66] This ratio could change with intense heat-exercise stress, which would result in greater hypovolemia. Brain osmoreceptors within or outside the blood–brain barrier might be better protected from systemic volume[58] and osmotic fluctuations.[55] Thus, volemic factors could play a relatively greater role for controlling drinking with greater perturbations in extracelluar fluid volume.[25] Strange[80] concludes that cells can detect more than just change in their volume; they may have multiple volume detectors and regulatory mechanisms that respond to the magnitude of change in volume.

II. BODY WATER AND ELECTROLYTES

A. BODY FLUID COMPARTMENTS

The total body water, which accounts for 50–70% of the body weight, is arbitrarily divided by cell membranes into intracellular fluid (ICF) and extracellular fluid (ECF) compartments; ICF (~45% of body weight) sustains cell integrity and function, while the ECF (~20% of body weight) provides the constant internal environment necessary to support cell function. ECF is further subdivided into interstitial fluid (ISF, ~15% of body weight) and plasma volume (PV, ~5% of body weight) by the capillary endothelium.

The major cation of the ECF is Na^+ (~140 meq/l), and its attendant anions are Cl^- (~110 meq/l) and HCO_3^- (~27 meq/l). Thus, the osmolality of the ECF can be approximated by doubling plasma Na^+ concentration. Although water is in osmotic equilibrium between body fluid compartments, water molecules move freely among the compartments in response to change in hydrostatic and osmotic pressure. Both exercise and heat exposure influence circulation and body fluid osmolality, which shift water between body fluid compartments and modify thirst and drinking.[31]

B. CHANGE IN BODY FLUID COMPARTMENT VOLUMES DURING EXERCISE AND HEAT STRESS

Plasma volume decreases proportionately with exercise intensity.[18,89] Because sweat is hypotonic when compared to plasma, sweating causes hyperosmolality of body fluid, which results in fluid shift between fluid compartments.

Figure 1 shows the reduction of body fluid and distribution within body fluid compartments in 8 men after 2 h of exercise in heat and after 3 h of recovery with or without fluid replacement.[52,53] The subjects lost ~27 ml/kg body weight, and 23–26% of this loss (~7.0 ml/kg) came from plasma with each treatment. There was further reduction of body weight during 3 h of recovery due to residual sweating and urine output. Reduction of PV (hypovolemia) with dehydration recovered to 8% (2.7 ml/kg) after 3 h of recovery even though no water was consumed, while loss of ICF volume increased from 20% to 44% (6.1 to 14.8 ml/kg), indicating mobilization of ICF into the ISF and plasma compartments. Rehydration with tap water or saline solution modifies the recovery of each fluid compartment: showing higher recovery of PV according to the degree of rehydration, and the recovery of ICF varies considerably between the groups, while the difference in ISF was less. Hyperosmolality of the ECF from heat-induced sweating is the major cause of the ICF shift.[56] Reduction of ICF (cellular dehydration) stimulates osmoreceptors, and reduction of PV (extracellular dehydration) stimulates volume receptors; both influence thirst and drinking behavior.

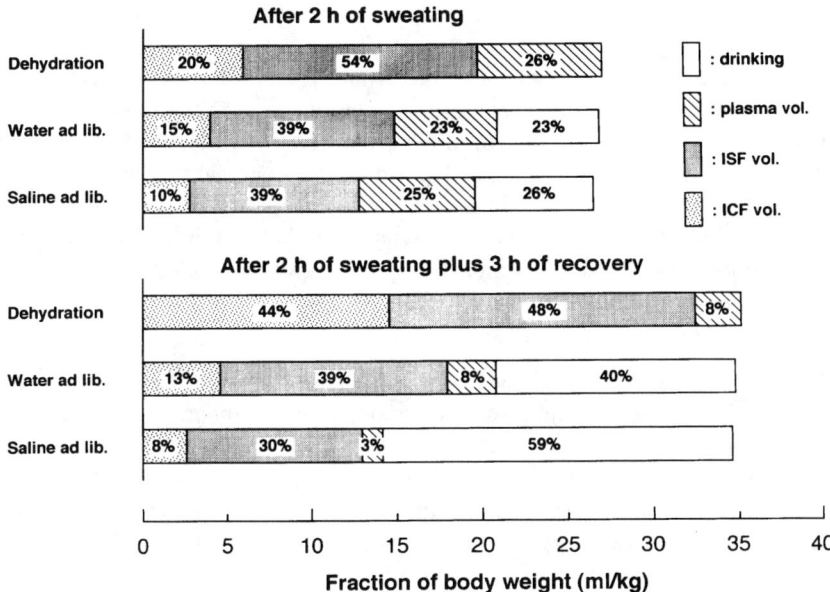

FIGURE 1 Loss of body weight in 8 subjects due to sweating, reduction of body fluid compartments, and amount of fluid replacement. Values were obtained after 2 h of sweating (heat-exercise stress) and after 3 h of recovery with no drinking (dehydration), or with water or saline solution ad libitum. (Based on data from Reference 52).

III. CELLULAR DEHYDRATION DRINKING (OSMORECEPTORS)

A. CEREBRAL OSMORECEPTORS

Most body cells respond to extracellular fluid osmotic stimuli, but Verney's "osmoreceptors" are specialized cells in the hypothalamic region that somehow transduce change in their osmotic state to neuronal and hormonal stimuli that may be involved with arginine vasopressin (AVP) release and drinking. For example, angiotensin II (AII) stimulates AVP[63] and also drinking directly,[24] while intracerebroventricular (i.c.v.) injection of brain natriuretic peptide (BNP) into conscious rats suppresses water and salt intake[40] and the AVP secretion[91] evoked by AII stimulation. The AVP suppression by BNP occurs by inhibition of anteroventral third ventricle (AV3V) neurons and the SON.[93] In addition, i.c.v. administration of atrial natriuretic peptide (ANP) also blocks AII-induced drinking[92] as well as dehydration and hemorrhage-induced AVP secretion.[72] Thus, an ever-increasing number of activation and inhibitory neuronal and hormonal factors and interactions that control drinking are being elucidated.

The sodium receptor–osmotic receptor dichotomy has not been resolved satisfactorily. However, the convergence of thermal and osmotic stimuli on preoptic-anterior hypothalamic neurons,[37] and the similar increase in rectal temperature of exercising dogs during i.v. infusion of hypertonic mannitol (which depresses plasma [Na⁺]) or of hypertonic NaCl (which increases plasma [Na⁺]),[46] as well as the unchanged plasma AVP–osmolality relationship in resting humans also during similar i.v. infusion of hypertonic mannitol or NaCl,[96] substantially strengthens the hypothesis that osmoreceptors are generally more important than sodium receptors for control of drinking as well as for thermoregulation.

B. EXTRACEREBRAL OSMORECEPTORS

There is some evidence for the existence of peripheral (extracerebral) osmoreceptors in the oropharyngeal and gastrointestinal tracts, but more solid evidence for their existence in the liver–portal system. Most of the latter studies involved oral or portal vein fluid administration of various composition on vasopressin response or renal function. In 1980 Bie[13] concluded, from the sparse literature, that solutes injected into the portal vein of mainly rat and guinea pig may influence fluid–electrolyte homeostasis, and that infusion of hypo- and hyperosmolar solutions and AII into the renal artery of dogs increased plasma renin secretion and vasopressin concentration, indicating the kidney can influence vasopressin secretion by osmotic stimuli effecting renin-induced AII.

Existence of oropharyngeal receptors for stimulating and modulating drinking were associated years ago with the dry-mouth theory of thirst, and for the rapid rehydration of dehydrated dogs.[1] More recently, Thrasher et al.[86] observed suppression of dehydration-induced elevation of plasma AVP in dogs immediately (within 3 min) after drinking that preceded postabsorptive change in plasma volume or osmolality. This suppression was confirmed in humans where the decreasing plasma AVP reached the control water-replete level 9 min after drinking when plasma potassium increased significantly, suggesting cellular fluid loss.[27] This AVP suppression is not associated with concomitant change in plasma sodium,[25,27,71] osmolality,[27,71,84] renin activity or aldosterone,[25,27] ANP,[25] volume,[19,25,27,86] gastric distention,[9,86] hepatoportal or cerebral osmoreceptors,[84,86] drink taste,[7] temperature,[7] or ion–osmotic composition.[7,19,71,74] But the AVP suppression may be associated with the act of drinking itself,[7] extracerebral osmoreceptor activity,[84] cold-sensitive oropharyngeal receptors,[71] or level of physical fitness.[25] Shingai et al.[77] reported water-sensitive pharyngolaryngeal receptors that initiate the swallowing reflex. These data suggest stimulation of oropharyngeal receptors by the act of drinking (muscular action and/or fluid flow during swallowing) may effect AVP suppression.

Postulated oropharyngeal-receptor stimulation (fluid metering) alone is not sufficient for control of drinking or its termination. Gastric[50] and duodenal[22] osmoreceptors generally act to control emptying of intestinal contents[75] and thus influence drinking by reverse mass action; that is, drinking slows or ceases via stimulation of mechanoreceptors[49] as the stomach and small intestine fill. Maddison et al.[47] have concluded that receptor action beyond mid-duodenum is required for control of drinking. A direct effect of gastrointestinal osmoreceptor function on control of drinking or its termination is unproved.

There is more solid evidence from rats and humans that osmoreceptors within the vascular bed of the liver influence drinking,[15,45] increase vasopressin secretion,[10,17] increase renal nerve activity,[38] and influence urinary excretion of sodium and water.[34,62] Portal vein osmotic afferent stimuli to the hypothalamus appear to be calcium-mediated via cholinergic neurotransmission in the vagus nerve.[17,79] The function of portal-bed osmoreception is to modulate the effect of gastrointestinal osmols and water on the systemic circulatory fluid–electrolyte homeostasis.

IV. EXTRACELLULAR DEHYDRATION DRINKING (VOLUME RECEPTORS)

Osmoreceptor stimulation is the more powerful stimulus for drinking, although in some conditions hypovolemia can stimulate and modify drinking behavior independently of osmoreceptor action. Reduction of plasma volume due to hemorrhage causes drinking in the absence of cellular dehydration (osmoreceptor stimulation), and water intake in rats is proportional to the amount of blood removed.[69] Stricker[81] used subcutaneous injection of concentrated colloid that sequesters plasma and observed a dose-dependent relation between drinking and sodium appetite. Sagawa et al.[70] measured voluntary water intake of dehydrated men (~3.6% body weight) during 3 h of sitting in air and immersed to the neck in thermoneutral water. Water intake at the beginning of water immersion was suppressed by 50% compared to that when the subjects were dehydrated in air, which indicates that the fluid shifted from the lower extremities to the central circulation inhibits drinking when dehydrated. A fall in blood volume and pressure modulates activity of stretch and pressure receptors in the low-pressure chambers of the heart that exert tonic influence on brain ADH secretion. Inflation of balloons implanted into the junction of the superior vena cava and right atrium of the rat heart decreases ad libitum as well as deprivation-induced water intake.[43] From the finding that drinking in dogs occurs when central venous pressure (CVP) falls to a fixed level,[41] it is clear that receptors in the low-pressure system transmit signals to the brain that activate mechanisms that stimulate extracellular thirst and drinking.

Extracellular dehydration stimulates the renin–angiotensin system, another volume receptor–dipsogenic mechanism,[24] but data on the effect of AII on drinking during exercise are not available.

V. MECHANISM OF INVOLUNTARY DEHYDRATION

Drinking behavior in humans is divided into homeostatic (primary or regulatory) drinking and nonhomeostatic (secondary or nonregulatory) drinking.[68] When nonregulatory fluid consumption exceeds the homeostatic volume, body fluid balance is maintained by increased urination, while regulatory drinking becomes more important in dehydrated subjects when osmoregulation precedes volume regulation. As mentioned above, dehydration due to water deprivation or sweating increases osmolality of extracellular fluid, which causes cellular (osmoreceptor) dehydration, which leads to thirst and drinking. Concomitant hypovolemia would activate fluid shifts between body fluid compartments that stimulate volume receptors via change in CVP. Under extreme conditions, such as exercise under heat stress, the homeostatic demands to maintain circulatory function, body fluid balance, and temperature regulation compete.[51]

Involuntary dehydration (defined as the delay in rehydration by spontaneous drinking after dehydration induced by exercise, fluid restriction, and environmental heat and cold,[30]) is the result of interaction between homeostatic demands. Loss of solutes in sweat had been suggested as the cause of involuntary dehydration,[4,39] but it took until 1981 for Morimoto et al.[52] to confirm this hypothesis. Eight men were exposed to heat and exercise for 2 h to obtain their maximal sweat rate (Figure 1). The exposure was repeated with free intake of tap water and with free intake of saline solution (23 meq/l Na^+, 5 meq/l K^+, and 7g/dl glucose). Sweat (body weight) loss was similar (about 0.8 l/h) in each group. Voluntary fluid intake during the 2 h of heat and exercise exposure was 23% of sweat loss with tap water and 26% with saline solution (Figure 1, upper panel). When fluid consumed during 5 h (2 h of heat and exercise plus 3 h of recovery in 25°C ambient temperature) was compared, subjects replaced only 40% of fluid loss by drinking water but replaced 59% by drinking saline[52] (Figure 1, lower panel). The 5-h result showed a moderate but significant correlation ($r = -0.51$, $p<0.05$) between the degree of involuntary dehydration and sweat osmolality.[53] In this experiment a glucose–electrolyte solution was provided, and the difference from the supplementation of tap water was compared. To eliminate the influence of taste, Nose et al.[57] provided capsules containing either placebo or 0.45 g NaCl/100 ml water during recovery from thermal dehydration in 6 men and confirmed suppression of involuntary dehydration with ingestion of NaCl. They suggested that the lower sweat Na^+ concentration in heat-acclimated subjects is likely to elevate ECF Na^+ concentration, causing water to shift from the ICF to ECF, which would stimulate drinking and reduce the fluid deficit as reported by Greenleaf et al.[33] More recently Bar-Or et al.[11] found that the level of involuntary dehydration in cystic fibrosis patients was much higher than in healthy patients and suggested that the high salt loss in sweat of the former prevented ECF hyperosmolality, thereby depriving the patients of a stimulus for thirst and drinking.

The effect of salt loss on regulatory drinking was studied in thermally dehydrated rats who spread saliva (containing salt) on their fur for heat dissipation and who also exhibited involuntary dehydration.[44,59,83,94] When only water was provided to rats dehydrated by ~7–8% of their initial body weight, their fluid balance reached a subnormal steady state when only half the fluid lost during heat exposure was regained by means of reduction in fluid intake and increase in urine output. Complete rehydration was achieved in about 8 h when the rats drank either 0.45 or 0.9% NaCl solutions.[59] When dehydrated rats were given a choice of tap water, and 0.9 or 1.8% NaCl solutions, they consumed more water than saline for the first 2 h but consumed more saline than water thereafter; the average NaCl concentration ingested was about 55 mmol for the initial 2 h and then increased to about 125 mmol thereafter.[94] The concentrations were almost identical in rats provided 0.9 or 1.8% NaCl, suggesting that the fluid selection was a regulated response. The change in salt intake occurred when about 90% of Na^+ loss and 60% of fluid loss were regained. This phase shift of salt appetite was observed in rats dehydrated by 6 and 8%, but not in rats dehydrated by 3% of their initial body weight,[44] suggesting a threshold between 3 and 6% of body weight loss for regulation of salt ingestion.

Change in blood volume and plasma Na^+ concentration during rehydration following thermal dehydration were measured in rats with continuous analysis of these parameters.[83] After dehydration of ~6% body weight, the rats consumed 1.1 ml/100 g body weight of tap water but no 1.8% saline within the first 45 min (Figure 2). Thereafter, the rats consumed both water and the NaCl solution alternately. The plasma Na^+ concentration decreased to the pre-dehydration level rapidly with the initial consumption of water at time zero and regulated to within the normal range after about 60 min; blood volume increased continuously during the 240 min. Urinary excretion began only when blood volume approached normal.

These collective results indicate that during the initial stage of rehydration, rats chose tap water and then a dilute NaCl solution to decrease their plasma Na^+ concentration and to restore lost sodium; that is, blood volume was expanded with drinking of almost isotonic saline, and final blood volume homeostasis was achieved by kidney function. Thus, in this context osmoregulation precedes volume regulation.

Regulation of vascular compliance may be involved in the mechanism of the time delay to recover blood volume during rehydration.[51] Change in blood volume is sensed mainly by cardiac volume receptors from change in CVP, while CVP may be modified from change in venous vascular compliance or distensibility of the vascular bed, which is controlled by sympathetic tone.[76] Thus, because neither hypovolemia nor hypervolemia within certain limits causes changes in CVP, extracellular fluid hyperosmolality becomes the more important stimulus for water intake.

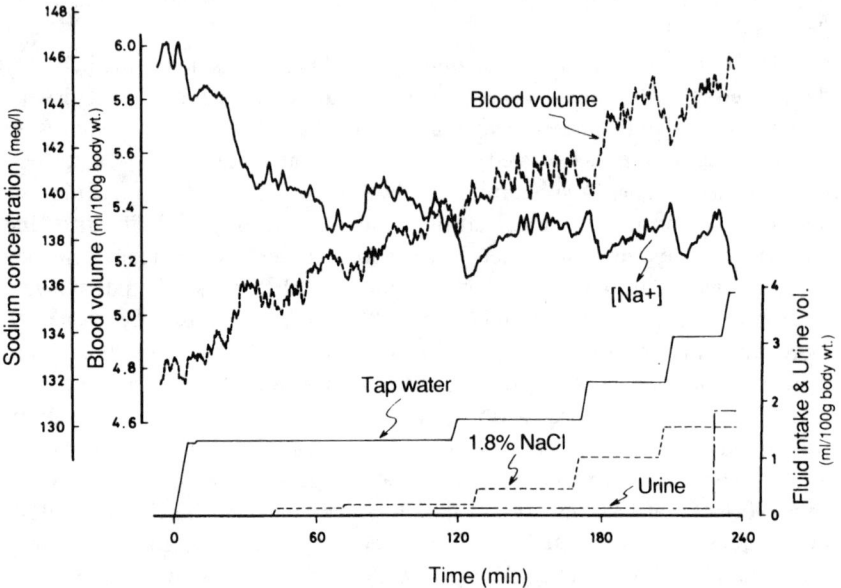

FIGURE 2 Change in blood volume and Na+ concentration measured continuously during recovery from thermal dehydration (6% body weight) in a rat that was allowed free access to tap water and 1.8% NaCl solution at time 0. Urine volume and cumulative intake of tap water and 1.8% NaCl solution are also shown. (From Morimoto et al., *Seventh Symposium on Salt*, Vol. 2, Kakihana, H. et al., Eds., Elsevier, Amsterdam, 1993. With permission.)

It is clear that the early termination of water intake (involuntary dehydration) observed after thermal dehydration is due to initial hemodilution, and sodium (perhaps osmotic) intake is required to restore plasma volume and body hydration.

VI. SUMMARY

Heat exposure and exercise stress cause loss of body fluid mainly from thermoregulatory sweating, which results in body dehydration. Cellular and extracellular dehydration induce many regulatory responses such as splanchnic vasoconstriction, shift of body fluid from extravascular to intravascular space, increase in heart rate, etc., but recovery from dehydration is possible only with fluid intake.

Thirst and drinking are controlled by integration of signals from osmoreceptors and volume receptors, as well as palatability of fluid available. Osmoreceptors are activated by cellular dehydration of hypothalamic and circumventricular organs with probable contribution from peripheral osmoreceptors in the oropharyngeal, hepatoportal, and renal regions. Extracellular dehydration of the interstitium and plasma volume (hypovolemia) is mainly sensed by cardiac receptors from a decrease in CVP; CVP is controlled by circulatory responses to maintain cardiac output which causes delay in volume regulation.

Because dehydration impairs thermoregulation and work capacity, it is important to drink in order to correct the osmotic and volume changes resulting from exercise, especially when combined with imposed heat stress.

ACKNOWLEDGMENT

The authors thank Ms. R. Looft-Wilson for manuscript preparation.

REFERENCES

1. Adolph, E.F., Thirst and its inhibition in the stomach, *Am. J. Physiol.,* 161: 374–386, 1950.
2. Adolph, E.F., Termination of drinking: Satiation, *Fed. Proc.,* 41: 2533–2535, 1982.
3. Adolph, E.F., Barker, J.P., and Hoy, P.A., Multiple factors in thirst, *Am. J. Physiol.,* 178: 538–562, 1954.
4. Adolph, E.F. and Dill, D.B., Observations on water metabolism in the desert, *Am. J. Physiol.,* 123: 369–378, 1938.
5. Andersson, B., The effect of injections of hypertonic NaCl solutions into different parts of the hypothalamus of goats, *Acta Physiol. Scand.,* 28: 188–201, 1953.
6. Andersson, B., Regulation of water intake, *Physiol. Rev.,* 58: 582–603, 1978.
7. Appelgren, B.H., Thrasher, T.N., Keil, L.C., and Ramsay, D.J., Mechanism of drinking-induced inhibition of vasopressin secretion in dehydrated dogs, *Am. J. Physiol.,* 261: R1226–R1233, 1991.
8. Arden, F., Experimental observations upon thirst and on potassium overdosage, *Aust. J. Exp. Biol. Med. Sci.,* 12: 111–120, 1934.
9. Arnauld, E. and DuPont, J., Vasopressin release and firing of supraoptic neurosecretory neurons during drinking in the dehydrated monkey, *Pfluegers Arch.,* 394: 195–201, 1982.
10. Baertschi, A.J. and Vallet, P.G., Osmosensitivity of the hepatic portal vein area and vasopressin release in rats, *J. Physiol. London,* 315: 217–230, 1981.
11. Bar-Or, O., Blimkie, C.J.R., Hay, J.A., MacDougall, J.D., Ward, D.S., and Wilson, W.M., Voluntary dehydration and heat intolerance in cystic fibrosis, *Lancet,* 339: 696–699, 1992.
12. Bie, P., Sustained water diuresis in anesthetized dogs: Antidiuresis in response to intravenous and bilateral intracarotid infusion of hyperosmolar solutions of sodium chloride, *Acta Physiol. Scand.,* 101: 446–457, 1977.
13. Bie, P., Osmoreceptors, vasopressin, and control of renal water excretion, *Physiol. Rev.,* 60: 961–1048, 1980.
14. Bie, P., Studies of cerebral osmoreceptors in anesthetized dogs: The effect of intravenous and intracarotid infusion of hyper-osmolar sodium chloride solutions during sustained water diuresis, *Acta Physiol. Scand.,* 96: 306–318, 1976.
15. Blake, W.D. and Lin, K.K., Hepatic portal vein infusion of glucose and sodium solutions on the control of saline drinking in the rat, *J. Physiol. London,* 274: 129–139, 1978.
16. Cannon, W.B., The physiological basis of thirst, *Proc. R. Soc. London Ser. B.,* 90: 283–301, 1918.
17. Chwalbinska-Moneta, J., Role of hepatic portal osmoreception in the control of ADH release, *Am. J. Physiol.,* 236: E603–E609, 1979.

18. Convertino, V.A., Keil, L.C., Bernauer, E.M., and Greenleaf, J.E., Plasma volume, osmolality, vasopressin, and renin activity during graded exercise in man, *J. Appl. Physiol.,* 50: 123–128, 1981.
19. Cotter, T.P., Gerbruers, E.M., Hall, W.J., and O'Sullivan, M.F., Plasma expansion does not precipitate the fall in plasma vasopressin in humans drinking isotonic fluids, *J. Physiol. London,* 376: 429–438, 1986.
20. de Caro, G., Epstein, A.N., and Massi, M., *The Physiology of Thirst and Sodium Appetite,* Plenum Press, New York, 1986.
21. Deneufbourg, E.-F., Quelques considerations sur la soif. Paris: Theses No. 117, 1813, 39 (from Ref. 89).
22. Dooley, C.P. and Valenzuela, J.E., Duodenal volume and osmoreceptors in the stimulation of human pancreatic secretion, *Gastroenterology,* 86: 23–27, 1984.
23. Fitzsimons, J.T., Historical perspectives in the physiology of thirst, in *The Physiology of Thirst and Sodium Appetite,* Cambridge University Press, Cambridge, 1979, chap. 1.
24. Fitzsimons, J.T. and Simons, B.J., The effect on drinking in the rat of intravenous angiotensin, given alone or in combination with other stimuli of thirst. *J Physiol. London,* 203: 45–57, 1969.
25. Freund, B.J., Claybaugh, J.R., Hashiro, G.M, and Dice, M.S., Hormonal and renal responses to water drinking in moderately trained and untrained humans, *Am. J. Physiol.,* 254: R417–R423, 1988.
26. Gamble, J.L., Putnam, M.C., and McKhann, C.F., The optimal water requirement in renal function; measurements of water drinking by rats according to increments of urea and of several salts in food, *Am. J. Physiol.,* 88: 571–580, 1929.
27. Geelen, G., Keil, L.C., Kravik, S.E., Wade, C.E., Thrasher, T.N., Barnes, P.R., Pyka, G., Nesvig, C., and Greenleaf, J.E., Inhibition of plasma vasopressin after drinking in dehydrated humans, *Am. J. Physiol.,* 247: R968–R971, 1984.
28. Gilman, A., The relation between blood osmotic pressure, fluid distribution and voluntary water intake, *Am. J. Physiol.,* 120: 323–328, 1937.
29. Gove, P.B. (Ed.), *Webster's Third New International Dictionary of the English Language Unabridged,* Merriam-Webster, Springfield, MA, 1986, 2378.
30. Greenleaf, J.E., Dehydration-induced drinking in humans, *Fed. Proc.,* 41: 2509–2514, 1982.
31. Greenleaf, J.E., Importance of fluid homeostasis for optimal adaptation to exercise and environmental stress: Acceleration, in *Perspectives in Exercise Science and Sports Medicine,* Vol. 3, *Fluid Homeostasis During Exercise,* Gisolfi, C.V. and Lamb, D.R., Eds., Benchmark Press, Indianapolis, IN, 1990, chap. 9.
32. Greenleaf, J.E., Averkin, E.G., and Sargent, F., II, Water consumption by man in a warm environment: A statistical analysis, *J. Appl. Physiol.,* 21: 93–98, 1966.
33. Greenleaf, J.E., Brock, P.J., Keil, L.C., and Morse, J.T., Drinking and water balance during exercise and heat acclimation, *J. Appl. Physiol.,* 54: 414–419, 1983.
34. Haberich, F.J., Osmoreception in the portal circulation, *Fed. Proc.,* 27: 1137–1141, 1968.
35. Haller, A. von, Fames et sitis, in *Elementa Physiologiae Corporis Humani,* Vol. 6, Sumptibus Societatis Typographicae, Berne, 1764, 164-187 (from Ref. 23).
36. Henderson, L.J., *The Fitness of the Environment,* Beacon Press, Boston, 1958.
37. Hori, T., Nakashima, T., Koga, H., Kiyohara, T., and Inoue, T., Convergence of thermal, osmotic and cardiovascular signals on preoptic and anterior hypothalamic neurons in the rat, *Brain Res. Bull.,* 20: 879–885, 1988.
38. Ishiki, K., Morita, H., and Hosomi, H., Reflex control of renal nerve activity originating from the osmoreceptors in the hepatoportal region, *J. Auton. Nerv. Syst.,* 36: 139–148, 1991.
39. Itoh, S., The water loss and blood changes by prolonged sweating without intake of food and drink, *Jpn. J. Physiol.,* 3: 148–156, 1953.

40. Itoh, H., Nakao, K., Yamada, T., Shirakami, G., Kangawa, K., Minamino, N., Matsuo, H., and Imura, H., Antidipsogenic action of a novel peptide, brain natriuretic peptide in rats, *Eur. J. Pharmacol.,* 150: 193–196, 1989.
41. Itoh, T., Oda, Y., Asaeda, H., Sohma, A., Shigemi, K., and Morimoto, T., Central venous pressure and plasma Na concentration during drinking behavior in the dehydrated dog, *Jpn. J. Physiol.,* 38: 101–108, 1988.
42. Jewell, P.A. and Verney, E.B., An experimental attempt to determine the site of the neurohypophysial osmoreceptors in the dog, *Philos. Trans. R. Soc. London Ser. B.,* 240: 197–324, 1957.
43. Kaufmann, S., Role of right atrial receptors in the control of drinking in the rat, *J. Physiol. London,* 349: 389–396, 1984.
44. Kawabata, T., Okuno, T., and Morimoto, T., The effect of dehydration level on the NaCl concentration chosen by rats, *Physiol. Behav.,* 53: 731–736, 1993.
45. Kozlowski, S. and Drzewiecki, K., The role of osmoreception in portal circulation in control of water intake in dogs, *Acta Physiol. Pol.,* 24: 325–330, 1973.
46. Kozlowski, S., Greenleaf, J.E., Terlejska, E., and Nazar, K., Extracelluar hyperosmolality and body temperature during physical exercise in dogs, *Am. J. Physiol.,* 239: R180–R183, 1980.
47. Maddison, S., Wood, R.J., Rolls, E.T., Rolls, B.J., and Gibbs, J., Drinking in the Rhesus monkey: Peripheral factors, *J. Comp. Physiol. Psychol.,* 94: 365–374, 1980.
48. Mayer, A., Variations de la tension osmotique du sang chez les animaux privés de liquides, *C. R. Soc. Biol. Paris,* 52: 153–155, 1900.
49. Mei, N., Recent studies of intestinal vagal afferent innervation. Functional implications, *J. Auton. Nerv. Syst.,* 9: 199–206, 1983.
50. Minami, H. and McCallum, R.W., The physiology and pathophysiology of gastric emptying in humans, *Gastroenterology,* 86: 1592–1610, 1984.
51. Morimoto, T., Thermoregulation and body fluids: Role of blood volume and central venous pressure, *Jpn. J. Physiol.,* 40: 165–179, 1990.
52. Morimoto, T., Miki, K., Nose, H., Yamada, S., Hirakawa, K., and Matsubara, C., Changes in body fluid volume and its composition during heavy sweating and the effect of fluid and electrolyte replacement, *Jpn. J. Biometeorol.,* 18: 31–39, 1981.
53. Morimoto, T. and Nose, H., Regulatory responses to thermal dehydration, in *Man in Stressful Environments, Thermal and Work Physiology,* Shiraki, K. and Yousef, M.K., Eds., C.C. Thomas, Springfield, IL, 1987, chap. 9.
54. Morimoto, T., Nose, H., Sugimoto, E., Yawata, T., and Okuno, T., Role of sodium chloride in rehydration from thermal dehydration. *Seventh Symposium on Salt,* Vol. 2, Kakihana, H., Hardy, H.R., Jr., Hoshi, T., and Toyokura, K., Eds., Elsevier, Amsterdam, 1993, 389–393.
55. Nose, H., Doi, Y., Usui, S., Kubota, T., Fujimoto, M., and Morimoto, T., Continuous measurement of Na concentration in CSF during gastric water infusion in dehydrated rats, *J. Appl. Physiol.,* 73: 1419–1424, 1992.
56. Nose, H., Mack, G.W., Shi, X., and Nadel, E.R., Shift in body fluid compartments after dehydration in humans, *J. Appl. Physiol.,* 65, 318–324, 1988.
57. Nose, H., Mack, G.W., Shi, X., and Nadel, E.R., Role of osmolality and plasma volume during rehydration in humans, *J. Appl. Physiol.,* 65: 325–331, 1988.
58. Nose, H., Morimoto, T., and Ogura, K., Distribution of water losses among fluid compartments of tissues under thermal dehydration in the rat, *Jpn. J. Physiol.,* 33: 1019–1029, 1983.
59. Nose, H., Yawata, T., and Morimoto, T., Osmotic factors in restitution from thermal dehydration in rats, *Am. J. Physiol.,* 249: R166–R171, 1985.
60. Nothnagel, H., Durst und Polydipsie, *Arch. Path. Anat. Physiol.,* 86: 435–447, 1881.
61. Olsson, K., Further evidence for the importance of CSF Na^+ concentration in central control of fluid balance, *Acta Physiol. Scand.,* 88: 183–188, 1973.

62. Passo, S.S., Thornborough, J.R., and Rothballer, A.B., Hepatic receptors in control of sodium excretion in anaesthetized cats, *Am. J. Physiol.*, 224: 373–375, 1973.
63. Phillips, M.I., Angiotensin in the brain, *Neuroendocrinology*, 25: 354–377, 1978.
64. Ramsay, D.J. and Booth, D., *Thirst: Physiological and Psychological Aspects*, Springer-Verlag, Berlin, 1991.
65. Ramsay, D.J., Rolls, B.J., and Wood, R.J., Body fluid changes which influence drinking in the water deprived rat, *J. Physiol. London*, 266: 453–469, 1977.
66. Ramsay, D.J., Rolls, B.J., and Wood, R.J., Thirst following water deprivation in dogs, *Am. J. Physiol.*, 232: R93–R100, 1977.
67. Ramsay, D.J. and Thrasher, T.N., Thirst and water balance, in *Handbook of Behavioral Neurobiology*, Vol. 10, *Neurobiology of Food and Fluid Intake*, Stricker, E.M., Ed., Plenum Press, New York, 1990, chap. 14.
68. Rolls, B.J. and Rolls, E.T., *Thirst*, Cambridge University Press, Cambridge, 1982, 5.
69. Russell, P.J.D., Abdelaal, A.E., and Mogenson, G.J., Graded levels of hemorrhage, thirst and angiotensin II in the rat, *Physiol. Behav.*, 15: 117–119, 1975.
70. Sagawa, S., Miki, K., Tajima, F., Tanaka, H., Choi, J.K., Keil, L.C., Shiraki, K., and Greenleaf, J.E., Effect of dehydration on thirst and drinking during immersion in men, *J. Appl. Physiol.*, 72: 128–134, 1992.
71. Salata, R.A., Verbalis, J.G., and Robinson, A.G., Cold water stimulation of oropharyngeal receptors in man inhibits release of vasopressin, *J. Clin. Endocrinol. Metab.*, 65: 561–567, 1987.
72. Samson, W.K., Atrial natriuretic factor inhibits dehydration and hemorrhage-induced vasopressin release, *Neuroendocrinology*, 40: 277–279, 1985.
73. Sargent, F., II, and Weinman, K., Physiological variability in young men, in *Physiological Measurements of Metabolic Functions in Man*, Consolazio, C.F., Johnson, R.E., and Pecorea, L.J., McGraw-Hill, New York, 1963, section 14.
74. Seckl, J.R., Williams, T.D.M., and Lightman, S.L., Oral hypertonic saline causes transient fall of vasopressin in humans, *Am. J. Physiol.*, 251: R214–R217, 1986.
75. Shi, X., Summers, R.W., Schedl, H.P., Chang, R.T., Lambert, G.P., and Gisolfi, C.V., Effects of solution osmolality on absorption of select fluid replacement solutions in human duodenojejunum, *J. Appl. Physiol.*, 77: 1178–1184, 1994.
76. Shigemi, K., Morimoto, T., Itoh, T., Natsuyama, T., Hashimoto, S., and Tanaka, Y., Regulation of vascular compliance and stress relaxation by the sympathetic nervous system, *Jpn. J. Physiol.*, 41: 577–588, 1991.
77. Shingai, T., Miyaoka, Y., Ikarashi, R., and Shimada, K., Swallowing reflex elicited by water and taste solutions in humans, *Am. J. Physiol.*, 256: R822–R826, 1989.
78. Steggerda, F.R., Observations on the water intake in an adult man with dysfunctioning salivary glands, *Am. J. Physiol.*, 132: 517–521, 1941.
79. Stoppini, L. and Baertschi, A.J., Activation of portal-hepatic osmoreceptors in rats: Role of calcium, acetylcholine and cyclic AMP, *J. Auton. Nerv. Syst.*, 11: 297–308, 1984.
80. Strange, K., Are all cell volume changes the same?, *NIPS*, 9: 223–228, 1994.
81. Stricker, E.M., Thirst and sodium appetite after colloid treatment in rats, *J. Comp. Physiol. Psychol.*, 95: 1–25, 1981.
82. Stricker, E.M. and Verbalis, J.G., Sodium appetite, in *Handbook of Behavioral Neurobiology*, Vol. 10, *Neurobiology of Food and Fluid Intake*, Stricker, E.M., Ed., Plenum Press, New York, 1990, chap. 15.
83. Sugimoto, E., Analysis of salt and water intake by continuous determination of blood volume and plasma sodium concentration, *Jpn. J. Physiol.*, 38: 519–529, 1988.
84. Thompson, C.J., Burd, J.M., and Baylis, P.H., Acute suppression of plasma vasopressin and thirst after drinking in hypernatremic humans, *Am. J. Physiol.*, 252: R1138–R1142, 1987.
85. Thrasher, T.N., Osmoreceptor mediation of thirst and vasopressin secretion in the dog, *Fed. Proc.*, 41: 2528–2532, 1982.

86. Thrasher, T.N., Nistal-Herrera, J.F., Keil, L.C., and Ramsay, D.J., Satiety and inhibition of vasopressin after drinking in dehydrated dogs, *Am. J. Physiol.*, 240: E394–E401, 1981.
87. Verney, E.B., The antidiuretic hormone and the factors which determine its release, *Proc. R. Soc. London Ser. B.*, 135: 25–106, 1947.
88. Wettendorff, H., Modifications du sang sous l'influence de la privation d'eau. Contribution a l'etude de la soif, *Travaux Lab. Physiol. Inst. Solvay,* 4: 353–484, 1901.
89. Wilkerson, J.E., Gutin, B., and Horvath, S.M., Exercise-induced changes in blood, red cell, and plasma volumes in man, *Med. Sci. Sports,* 9: 155–158, 1977.
90. Wolf, A.V., Thirst and drinking, in *Thirst,* C.C. Thomas, Springfield, IL, 1958, chap. 2.
91. Yamada, T., Nakao, K., Itoh, H., Shirakami, G., Kangawa, K., Minamino, N., Matsuo, H., and Imura, H., Intracerebroventricular injection of brain natriuretic peptide inhibits vasopressin secretion in conscious rats, *Neurosci. Lett.,* 95: 223–228, 1988.
92. Yamada, T., Nakao, K., Morii, N., Itoh, H., Shiono, S., Sakamoto, M., Sugawara, A., Saito, Y., Ohno, H., Kanai, A., Katsuura, G., Eigyo, M., Matsushita, A., and Imura, H., Central effect of atrial natriuretic polypeptide on angiotensin II–stimulated vasopressin secretion in conscious rats, *Eur. J. Pharmacol.,* 125: 453–456, 1986.
93. Yamamoto, S., Inenaga, K., and Yamashita, H., Inhibition by brain natriuretic peptide of vasopressin neurons in the supraoptic nucleus and neurons in the region of the anteroventral third ventricle in rat hypothalamic slice preparations, *J. Neuroendocrinol.,* 3: 45–49, 1991.
94. Yawata, T., Okuno, T., Nose, H., and Morimoto, T., Change in salt appetite due to rehydration level in rats, *Physiol. Behav.,* 40: 363–368, 1987.
95. Zerbe, R.L., Miller, J.Z., and Robertson, G.L., The reproducibility and heritability of individual differences in osmoregulatory function in normal human subjects, *J. Lab. Clin. Med.,* 117: 51–59, 1991.
96. Zerbe, R.L. and Robertson, G.L., Osmoregulation of thirst and vasopressin secretion in human subjects: Effect of various solutes, *Am. J. Physiol.,* 244: E607–E614, 1983.

Chapter 2

GASTROINTESTINAL PHYSIOLOGY DURING EXERCISE

Carl V. Gisolfi
Alan J. Ryan

CONTENTS

I. Introduction..20

II. Gastric Emptying 20
   A. Effect of Volume.....................................21
   B. Effect of Osmolality and Carbohydrate Type and
      Concentration 23
   C. Effect of Acute and Chronic Exercise 24
   D. Effect of Environment and Hydration State................24

III. Control of Gastric Emptying 25

IV. Gastric Sensations...26

V. Intestinal Absorption......................................27
   A. Water Absorption 28
   B. Carbohydrate - Electrolyte Absorption....................32
   C. Effects of Exercise 34
   D. Role of Motility 36

VI. Neural and Hormonal Control 38
   A. Gastrointestinal Peptides and Nitric Oxide 39

VII. Gastrointestinal Adaptation 42

VIII. Gastrointestinal Bleeding and Barrier Function 44

IX. Summary..45

References 46

I. INTRODUCTION

During exercise, sweat rate can exceed 3 l/h,[2] and the oxidation of exogenous carbohydrate (CHO) approximates 1 g/min.[20] If exercise is prolonged and/or performed in the heat, sweat losses can exceed 10 l, Na^+ losses can reach 300 mEq, glycogen stores become depleted, plasma volume contracts, plasma osmolality increases, and the exerciser is at risk for thermal injury and hyponatremia. In fact, heat stroke may result from gastrointestinal dysfunction leading to endotoxemia and circulatory failure.[69] Although not often considered in discussions of fluid homeostasis, gastrointestinal (GI) function is crucial to fuel, electrolyte and fluid replenishment. Because CHO, Na^+, and water are key ingredients required to sustain prolonged exercise, this chapter will focus on gastric and intestinal functions that relate to their provision. It will also focus primarily on human studies, although animal data will be presented to elucidate mechanisms or to point out species differences. The specific questions that will be addressed include the following: How do maximal rates of gastric emptying and intestinal absorption relate to maximal sweat rate? Are these maximal rates influenced by the concentration and type of CHO used to formulate a rehydration beverage? Can the stomach and intestine adapt to heat, exercise, and the greater energy intake of the chronic exerciser? Does dehydration influence gastric and intestinal function? What role does motility play in the absorption of water, electrolytes, and CHO? For the reader interested in pursuing this topic in greater depth or in pursuing different aspects of GI function, there are several excellent recent reviews of this area.[12,18,31,55,63,71,93]

Discussion of GI physiology and digestive/absorptive processes usually begins with the mouth and ends with the colon. The mouth produces as much as 1.5 l of saliva per day and the colon can absorb as much as 5 l of water per day before diarrhea occurs. Although little is known about these two ends of the system during exercise, drinking has its first effect on fluid homeostasis by stimulating the oropharyngeal reflex in the mouth. Initiation of this reflex enhances ongoing sweating and can result in a significant increase in sweat output.[104] Strenuous exercise also relaxes the lower esophogeal sphincter leading to gastric reflux.[100]

II. GASTRIC EMPTYING

Gastric emptying (GE) follows an exponential time course that varies markedly among individuals[36]; women empty more slowly than men.[75] The primary stimulus is gastric distention, not the weight of chyme in the stomach (see Marabaix).[18] The most common method of measuring GE is gastric aspiration and calculating the difference between volume consumed and gastric residue corrected for gastric secretions. This method assumes a linear rate of emptying; however, radiographic and repeated sampling techniques confirm that GE follows an exponential time course. Thus, much of the disparity in the literature may be explained by the techniques employed and precisely when GE is measured following beverage ingestion.

The major factors influencing GE of fluids are volume and substrate concentration. CHO is the primary substrate included in sport drinks, although protein and fat are consumed in both liquid and solid form during ultraendurance competition. Solids retard GE and should be avoided under most circumstances.[13] CHO has the least inhibitory effect on GE, followed by protein, then fat. The importance of osmolality is secondary to substrate concentration. These factors and others that contribute to the determination of GE rate are illustrated in Figure 1. Detailed explanations of how they influence GE can be found elsewhere.[12,13,18,55,63,71] Because most oral rehydration beverages are CHO-electrolyte (CHO-E) solutions and because liquids are the most appropriate forms of replenishing water and nutrients during exercise, the present discussion will be limited to the GE of fluids with and without CHO. The volume ingested should be adjusted for body weight.

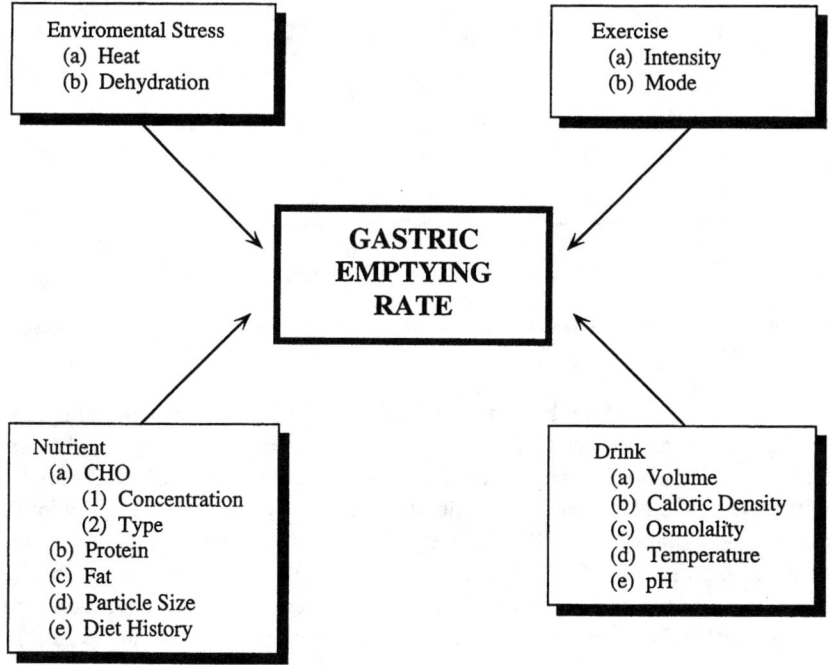

FIGURE 1 Factors contributing to the determination of gastric emptying.

A. EFFECT OF VOLUME

The larger the volume ingested, up to approximately 700 ml, the greater the GE rate.[19,74] Thus, it is advantageous to maintain as high a gastric volume as possible during exercise to sustain a high GE rate. This can be achieved by ingesting 150–200 ml of fluid every 10–15 min during competition. Figure 2 shows the emptying rates for water and a CHO-E beverage at rest. Note that the periodic ingestion of fluid increases gastric volume and helps to maintain a relatively high mean emptying rate. Mean values for water and 10% solutions were 40 and 25 ml/min, respectively.[27] These values translate to 2.4 and 1.5 l/h, which compare favorably with reported sweat rates of 1.5–2.0 l/h in most endurance athletes.[2] Rehrer et al.[83] also reported high (>30 ml/min) GE rates following ingestion of a 7% CHO-E beverage.

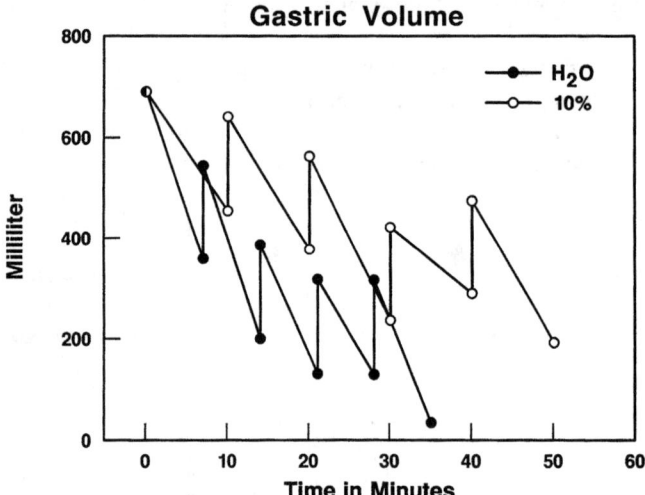

FIGURE 2 Effect of repeated drinking of water and a 10% CHO solution on gastric emptying rate over time.

Thus, GE should not be considered a limiting factor in maintaining hydration during exercise for most endurance athletes. According to Coyle and Montain,[21] a 68 kg exerciser should be able to provide the fluid and CHO (30–60 g/h) needed to sustain prolonged endurance exercise by ingesting 625–1250 ml/h of beverages containing 4–8% CHO. Ryan et al.[91] demonstrated that during 3 h of cycle exercise at 60% $\dot{V}O_2$ max in the heat (33°C), subjects were able to ingest 350 ml every 20 min of placebo or different 5% CHO beverages and empty greater than 90% of this volume to approximate a sweat rate of 1.2 l/h. In rare cases, such as Alberto Salazar, who sweats in excess of 3 l/h,[2] consuming 3 l of fluid and emptying it from the stomach may be difficult to achieve and likely to impair rehydration and performance.

B. EFFECT OF OSMOLALITY AND CARBOHYDRATE TYPE AND CONCENTRATION

In the mid-1970s, it was generally believed that sport drinks containing more than 2.5% CHO delayed GE and promoted gastric secretion leading to impaired thermal and circulatory functions.[1] This concept was based on GE measures using the aspiration technique 10–20 min after ingesting approximately 400 ml of fluid containing increasing amounts of glucose. Subsequent research in which GE was measured using the repeated sampling technique or aspiration following intermittent drinking over 1–2 h showed little difference between the GE of water and of beverages containing as much as 10% CHO.[18,78] This discrepancy is attributed in part to (1) the exponential time course of GE, (2) the rise in gastric volume and thus GE following intermittent drinking, which leaves a small gastric residue to which the next drink is added, and (3) the possible stimulatory effect of exercise on GE.

Despite these observations, there is considerable evidence showing that increasing the concentration of "glucose" in a beverage reduces GE.[19,49,63,72] Interestingly, this is not true for fructose, which has repeatedly been shown to exert less of an inhibitory influence than glucose on GE.[13,29,68] This may be explained by a glucose receptor located in the duodenum that elicits a strong inhibitory feedback control over GE.[61] Maltodextrins (which have a lower osmolality for a given energy density) have less of an inhibitory effect on GE because they must be hydrolyzed before they can exert such an influence. Dissaccharides, which also require hydrolysis, act similarly to maltodextrins, but to a lesser extent. In a recent study we found that a hypotonic solution with an initial osmolality of 186 mOsm/kg rose to 329 mOsm/kg within 50 cm of intestine as a result of hydrolysis, whereas a hypertonic solution with an initial osmolality of 403 mOsm/kg fell to 279 mOsm/kg over the same distance of intestine.[96] In the end, duodenal feedback control of GE will be determined by the concentration and type of CHO ingested, its rate of hydro-lysis, rate of absorption within the intestine, and the change in osmolality that it produces.

Osmolality is negatively correlated with GE.[18] It plays a secondary role to CHO concentration. The rationale for this interpretation is based on evidence showing that isocaloric solutions of glucose and maltodextrins empty from the stomach equally well despite significant differences in osmolality. Moreover, isoosmolar solutions with markedly different CHO concentrations empty at different rates, the more concentrated beverages emptying more slowly.[18,63,72]

These osmolar data have been interpreted to support the concept that GE is controlled by caloric density. For example, Brener et al.[9] found that solutions of 5.0, 12.5, and 25 g/100 ml glucose all delivered 2.13 kcal/min, but that GE rate was inversely related to solution concentration. This concept is supported by some investigators but not others and can be overridden by increasing the volume ingested or the energy content of the beverage.[18,71]

Taken together, data over the last two decades support the notion that solutions containing 4–8% CHO, regardless of CHO type (glucose, sucrose, maltodextrins, combinations), do not empty significantly slower than water and do not impair thermal or circulatory functions.[55,63,71]

C. EFFECT OF ACUTE AND CHRONIC EXERCISE

Although exercise has been reported to increase, decrease, or not change GE rate, recent studies in the last decade show that mild to moderate exercise either enhances or does not affect GE. Discrepancies in the literature are attributed in part to differences in the technique employed, lack of control data, time of the measurement following ingestion, and volume and composition of the solution consumed. Only when exercise intensity reaches 65–80% $\dot{V}O_2$ max is GE delayed.

The duration of exercise does not seem to affect GE. Costill and Saltin[19] found that even fatiguing exercise lasting 2 h did not reduce GE rate. On the other hand, mode of exercise may influence GE. Running produces greater GE rates compared with rest or cycling exercise.[18] Cycling has not consistently been shown to enhance GE above resting values. Data on other modes of exercise does not exist. Continuous and intermittent exercise produce similar GE rates. The effects of training are controversial. Two studies show that training enhances GE[14,15] while another shows no effect.[83]

D. EFFECT OF ENVIRONMENT AND HYDRATION STATE

The tendency for exercise (65% $\dot{V}O_2$ max) in the heat (35°C) to reduce GE was first shown by Owen et al.[79] Neufer et al.[73] reported similar results and further demonstrated that heat acclimation had no effect on GE. Neufer et al.[73] and Rehrer et al.[85] also demonstrated that dehydration can reduce GE; however, Neufer's subjects were markedly hyperthermic with heart rates above 190 bpm, and Rehrer's subjects showed only a modest decline in GE rate when her subjects were dehydrated by 4% body weight. In a recent study we found that hypohydration to approximately 3% of body weight had no effect on GE of 6–9% CHO-E solutions during 90 min of cycle exercise at 65% $\dot{V}O_2$ max in a cool (22°C) environment.[90] Core temperature in these subjects did not exceed 39°C. Because the dehydrated subjects in the studies above were hyperthermic and had high heart rates, both of which show significant negative correlations with GE, one cannot conclude that dehydration per se reduces GE.

Taken together, we suggest from these results that the stomach functions extremely well during exercise and under adverse environmental conditions. Even following mild hypohydration and fatiguing exercise up to 2 h in duration, GE was not delayed. Gastric function is impaired and GI symptoms emerge only when subjects become severely hyperthermic and dehydrated beyond 4.0% body weight. Although the gut may not be an athletic organ in the sense that it adapts to an exercise stimulus with a structural or functional change,[12] it is able to maintain its emptying function during mild to severe exercise (25–75% $\dot{V}O_2$ max for up to 2 h).

III. CONTROL OF GASTRIC EMPTYING

Adequate control of GE is important to prevent large fluctuations in nutrient flow, and to ensure that nutrient delivery is matched with intestinal digestion and absorption. GE of liquids occurs when proximal gastric contractions elevate intragastric pressure to levels that exceed pyloric sphincter resistance. To a considerable extent, gastric functions are controlled by feedback inhibition, whereby nutrients and other products of food digestion are sensed by either sensory nerves or endocrine cells located within the intestinal mucosa. Control of GE by intestinal sensory nerves is considered below; hormonal control is presented under section VI.A.

The "duodenal brake" is the first of several feedback loops whereby the quantity or quality of digested nutrients is monitored such that gastric delivery can be adjusted to ensure adequate intestinal digestion and absorption. The importance of duodenal sensory receptors in the regulation of GE was highlighted by Hunt,[48] who stated that the major question regarding control of GE should be, "How is the emptying of the duodenum controlled?" Hunt[48] postulated that diverse stimuli such as carbohydrates, proteins, fats, and acids slow gastric emptying by stimulating a signal transducer located within the duodenal mucosa. The generated signal is then carried by vagal afferent nerves and/or hormones to slow GE. The duodenal brake is thought to slow GE via an integrated response that may include relaxation of the gastric fundus, suppression of antral motility, enhanced pyloric tone, and a switch in duodenal motility from a propulsive to a mixing pattern.

The "ileal brake," another well-known feedback loop, describes the potent effect of ileal lipid infusion on inhibiting GE, jejunal motility, and flow rate. Attempts to activate the ileal brake by ileal infusion of CHO have been thwarted in humans by nausea and abdominal pain.[102] However, infusion of either lipid or hyperosmotic glucose into the jejunum or ileum slows GE in experimental animals. The neural or hormonal mediators of the ileal brake are unknown; potential pathways include neural or endocrine release of neurotensin, enteroglucagon, and peptide YY.[102]

As described above, sensory nerves located throughout the small intestine (duodenum, jejunum, and ileum) are thought to assume a primary role in feedback control of GE. Recently, Mei[65] summarized three decades of electrophysiological studies that identify and characterize different types of intestinal sensory receptors. To briefly summarize, nerve recordings obtained from experimental animals show that both vagal and sympathetic afferent nerves have sensory receptors located within the intestinal mucosa. These sensory receptors respond to a variety of chemical stimuli, exhibit a variable degree of stimuli specificity, and may include specific receptors for glucose (carbohydrate), amino acids, acids, and possibly osmolality. Activation of these intestinal mucosal receptors may initiate an "enterogastric inhibitory reflex" whereby the rate of GE is altered according to the nature of intestinal contents. Mei[65] postulated that these intestinal chemoreceptors may also participate in regulation of endocrine secretions, gastrointestinal motility and secretion, intestinal circulation and absorption, and food and water intake.

Recent studies suggest that intestinal chemoreceptor control of GE may be altered by acute changes in dietary CHO[23] and fat intake.[22] These findings are important for exercise physiologists for at least three reasons. First, they suggest that prior dietary history may contribute to the relatively large inter- and intraindividual variability in GE. Second, they suggest that the intestinal tract can rapidly adapt to acute alterations in dietary CHO intake. Intestinal adaptations (see Section VII) to a high CHO diet, for example, may enhance absorption of glucose, resulting in reduced intestinal chemoreceptor feedback and improved GE. And third, these findings could be evaluated in view of the current debate on the relative importance of gastric delivery of fluids vs. CHOs during prolonged exercise in a hot environment.[21] By altering their dietary habits, can athletes improve gastric delivery of both fluids and CHO's, and thereby reduce the risks associated with exercise in the heat (dehydration, hyperthermia, and glycogen depletion)?

IV. GASTRIC SENSATIONS

Knowledge of GI sensations is important because GI distress will likely alter both feeding behavior and GI function. Briefly, sensations from the stomach and small intestine are mediated through both vagal and sympathetic afferent nerve fibers.[16] Sensory receptors of the vagal afferents include smooth muscle tension receptors that respond to changes in stomach distension, and gastric mucosal receptors that respond to mechanical, chemical, and thermal stimuli. The healthy stomach appears to be relatively insensitive to thermal and chemical stimuli, but may readily respond to changes in intragastric pressure. The small intestine also appears to be relatively insensitive to thermal and traumatic (cutting or clamping) stimuli, but is sensitive to mechanical events such as distension and intense peristaltic contractions. GI pain is thought to be mediated by sympathetic afferent nerves, whereas vagal afferent nerves may contribute to sensations associated with vomiting (malaise or nausea).

Gastric distension enhances GE and gastric secretions, and may evoke sensations of fullness, bloating, and pain.[16] Sensations of bloated or full stomachs have been reported by athletes, especially runners,[13] who consume fluid replacement drinks at high rates.[66] GI complaints are relatively common in athletes engaged in training and competition[13] and are important to consider because they may discourage the consumption of needed fluids and nutrients.

Recent investigations have provided some information on the sensory perceptions to gastric distension in humans.

Using healthy volunteers, Khan et al.[52] obtained perceptions of gastric sensations elicited by inflation of an intragastric balloon. Increasing the rate of gastric distension not only reduced gastric motor activity, but also caused sensations of fullness and discomfort to occur at higher volumes and higher intragastric pressures. When the stomach was distended at rates of 20 and 200 ml/min, perceptions of fullness (discomfort) were found to occur at balloon volumes of ~190 ml (~410 ml) and ~450 ml (~670 ml), respectively. In contrast, very rapid gastric distension (75 ml/s) produced fullness and discomfort at much lower balloon volumes, ~145 ml and ~190 ml, respectively, but these sensations were transient in nature.

Moragas et al.[67] provided evidence that high intragastric pressure elicits gastric symptoms without significantly altering GE. In this study, both gastric sensations and emptying of a 300-ml mixed meal were monitored in healthy volunteers fitted with a gastric barostat set at either a slightly (low) or markedly (high) elevated intragastric pressure. While liquid GE was enhanced to a similar extent by elevations in intragastric pressure, only the high pressure level produced symptomatic sensations (pressure, fullness, nausea). Gastric accommodation to the 300-ml meals was large; the stomach expanded an additional volume of 285 and 327 ml under the low and high pressure conditions, respectively. Notably, other investigators[85] have also documented large gastric accommodation to ingested meals. Mean (±SE) values for gastric accommodation to a 200-, 400-, and 600-ml volume of a liquid (1 kcal/ml) meal were 466 ± 105, 354 ± 109, and 364 ± 85 ml, respectively.

Together, these findings suggest that gastric accommodation to ingested fluids may limit increments in wall tension, and perhaps gastric sensations, over a relatively large range of meal volumes. Questions relevant to the exercising athlete include: What are the effects of repeated ingestion of large volumes of fluid repacement drinks on gastric accommodation and gastric sensations? and, Can gastric accommodation be enhanced or gastric sensations reduced by habitual repeated consumption of fluid replacement drinks during exercise?

V. INTESTINAL ABSORPTION

Virtually no absorption occurs in the stomach[95]; thus, we depend on the intestine for CHO, electrolyte, and fluid absorption. Much of this occurs in the proximal small intestine or duodenum and jejunum. The standard technique for measuring intestinal absorption of water and solute is "segmental perfusion."[37] This is a steady-state luminal perfusion technique in which the perfusion solution is infused at a constant rate through a multilumen tube positioned in the small intestine (Figure 3). It provides a precise measurement of water and solute transport at the specific intestinal site occupied by the "test segment" of the multilumen tube. The perfusion solution mixes with intestinal secretions and forms a homogeneous solution before entering the test segment (Figure 4). Thus, the composition of the solution evaluated in the test segment is not the composition of the fluid perfused, but the composition sampled at the proximal sampling site (Figure 4). Net transport of electrolytes or CHO is the difference between their concentrations at the beginning and end of the test segment, adjusted for net water movement. Thus, net fluid movement must also be measured in the test segment. This is accomplished by including a nonabsorbable marker in the test solution whose concentration increases with absorption and decreases with secretion. Polyethylene glycol (PEG 4000) is such a marker. It is absorbed very slowly from the normal gut and reliably measures fluid transport in the test segment.[93]

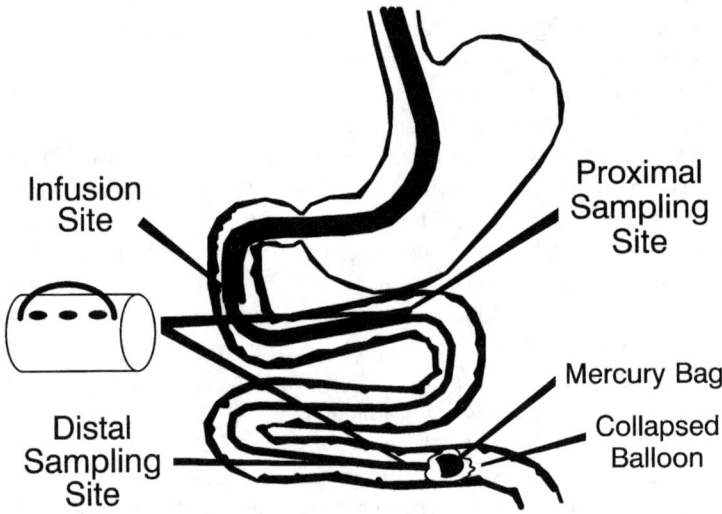

FIGURE 3 Diagram illustrating placement of a multi-lumen tube into the small intestine.

A. WATER ABSORPTION
1. Enterosystemic Water Cycle

Before discussing water absorption per se, it is instructional to consider the enterosystemic water cycle (Figure 5). In addition to ingesting about 2 l of fluid per day, saliva (1.5 l/d), gastric secretions (2.0 l/d), bile (0.5 l/d), pancreatic and intestinal secretions (3.0 l/d) add another 7.0 l/d making a total of 9 l presented to the intestine for reabsorption. Importantly, 6.5 l, or 72% of this total, is absorbed from the proximal (duodenojejunum) small intestine, 1.8 l or 20% from the distal intestine, and only 0.5 l or 5.6% from the colon. The epithelial lining of the duodenojejunum is relatively leaky and fluid is absorbed isotonically. In contrast, the colon has a relatively tight epithelial

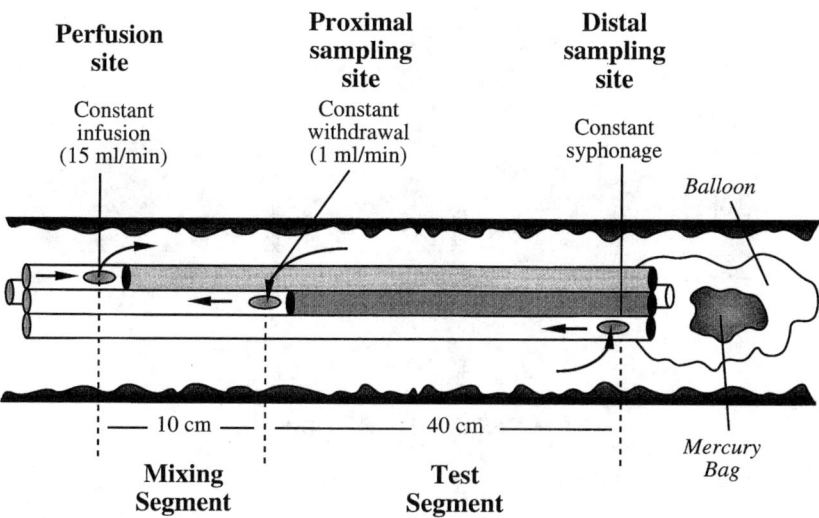

FIGURE 4 Illustration of the segmental perfusion technique using a triple-lumen tube with attached balloon and mercury bag. (From *Perspectives in Exercise and Sports Medicine: Fluid Homeostasis During Exercise,* Grisolfi, C. and Lamb, D.R., Eds., 1990. With permission.)

lining; it absorbs relatively little fluid, but does so very efficiently. Of the 9 l presented to the intestines, only 0.2–0.3 l appear in the stool.

2. Role of Osmolality and Solute Transport

Water absorption is a passive process dependent upon net solute movement and the osmolality of the chyme passing through the intestinal lumen. In general, hypotonic CHO solutions promote more water absorption than isotonic solutions, whereas hypertonic solutions produce net water secretion.[46,47] Animal studies show a significant inverse correlation between solution osmolality and jejunal water absorption,[107] and more than 40% of net water absorption has been attributed to solution osmolality.[108] However, it is not true that the lower the osmolality, the greater the water absorption. Humans ingesting spring water (10 ± 5 mOsm/kg) did not produce more water absorption than an isotonic glucose–electrolyte solution,[57] and ingesting an oral rehydration solution (ORS) containing 210 mOsm/kg did not produce greater water absorption than an ORS containing 240 mOsm/kg.[46]

In a recent study we found that the relationship between intestinal water absorption and solution osmolality depended upon the number of transportable substrates in the solution.[97] This is illustrated in Figure 6 by the significant difference in y-intercepts for solutions formulated with one transportable CHO and solutions formulated with two or more different transportable CHOs. Thus, at any given osmolality of a solution perfusing the intestine, significantly more water is absorbed from a solution containing two or more transportable CHOs

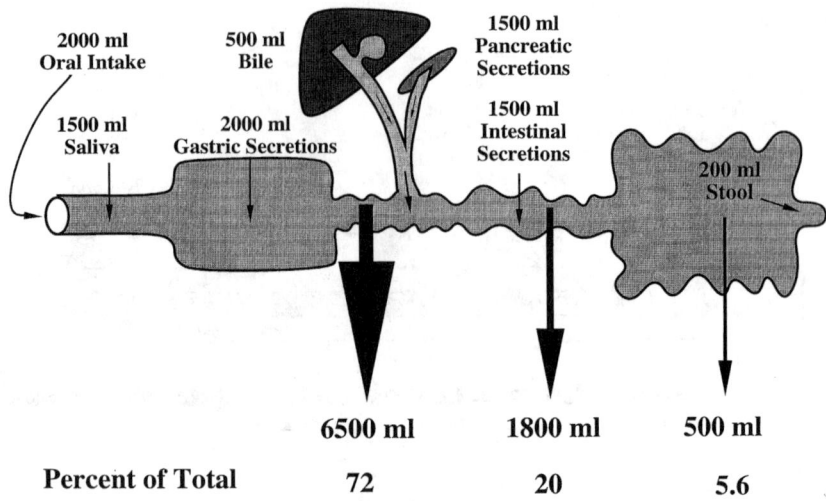

FIGURE 5 Approximate values for the water load entering the intestines each day and the volumes absorbed by the small and large intestine. (From *Perspectives in Exercise and Sports Medicine: Fluid Homeostasis During Exercise,* Grisolfi, C. and Lamb, D.R., Eds., 1990. With permission.)

than a solution containing only one CHO. This observation emphasizes the importance of solute absorption to water absorption. Even hypertonic solutions formulated with multiple transportable CHOs produced more water absorption than hypotonic solutions with only one transportable CHO. All of the solutions containing more than one CHO contained fructose, either in free or combined form (sucrose) in addition to glucose. Glucose is transported by the Na^+-glucose cotransporter and fructose is transported by GLUT5. In addition, both are transported by the disaccharidase-related transport system and both may use the paracellular pathway. Furthermore, both glucose and fructose share the same exit mechanism (GLUT2) from the enterocyte at the basolateral membrane.[17] Multiple regression analysis of water absorption, total solute absorption, and osmolality in the test segment revealed a partial correlation coefficient (r) of 0.69 for solute absorption, and 0.33 for osmolality, respectively. This analysis further revealed that total solute transport accounted for 48% and osmolality only 11% of the total variance in water absorption. Water flux significantly correlated with Na^+ (r = 0.81), and CHO flux (r = 0.42), but not K^+ flux. Thus, water absorption was primarily associated with Na^+ and CHO transport. Regardless of solution CHO concentration or osmolality, solutions containing two or three transportable CHOs produced more solute and water absorption than solutions containing only one CHO.

3. Pathways of Water Transport

In the intestine, water crosses from the lumen into the blood either through the cell (transcellular) or around the cell (paracellular). The rate of water

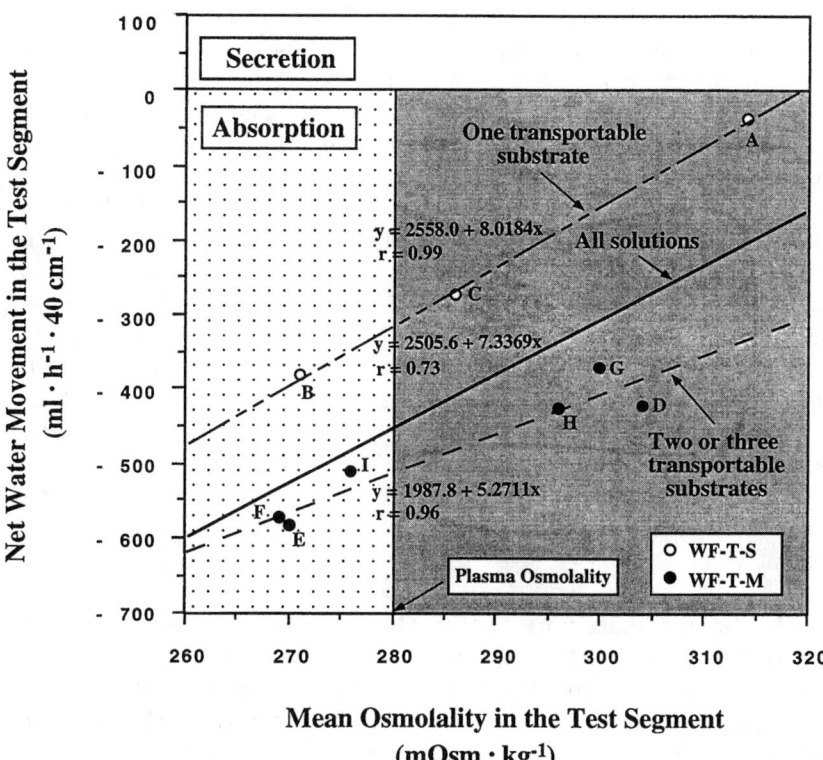

FIGURE 6 Net water movement in relation to mean osmolality in the test segment. Absorption is shown by negative and secretion by positive values. Data points are means from 6–8 subjects. The upper line shows the correlation among the 3 solutions containing one transportable substrate (○), the bottom regression line is from 6 solutions containing two or three transportable substrates (●). The middle solid line represents the correlation among all 9 solutions. Net water movement increases as osmolality decreases, but correlates with the number of transportable substrates and is greater with solutions containing more than one. WF = Water flux; T = Test segment; S = Single substrate; and M = Multiple substrates. (From Shi et al., *Med. Sci. Sports*, 27(12), 1607, 1995. With permission.)

movement depends upon brush border surface area and the intestinal site under observation. Although specific water channel proteins that insert into the cell membrane have been identified in renal tubules,[92] they have not been shown to exist in the small intestine. Moreover, D-glucose transporters do not function as water channels in the intestine.[26]

Movement of water between cells—that is, across the tight junctions—is called "solvent drag" and depends upon the number and size of these pathways. In animal models, there is evidence that D-glucose and amino acids, cotransported with sodium, open tight junctions by causing the contraction of cytoskeleton actomyosin. This actomyosin is connected to the cytoplasmic face of the tight junction so that when it contracts the tight junction opens.[79] This opening of the tight junctions presumably allows bulk absorption of luminal fluid (solvent drag) and provides the pathway for maximal absorption of substrate and water. The proportion of water moving transcellular as opposed to paracellular is not known. Persson and Spring[80] suggest that transcellular water movement is sufficient to account for reported water flow, but Pappenheimer and his colleagues[79] believe that paracellular transport is the primary pathway for glucose, and therefore water, in the presence of high luminal glucose concentrations. At a luminal glucose concentration of 200 mmol, Pappenheimer[79] suggests that as much as half of D-glucose transport occurs paracellularly. Other investigators suggest that 50–70% of solute movement occurs paracellularly.[50] There is also evidence that tight junctions open in humans,[35] but this concept is not supported by others.[32,33] Ferraris et al.[32] showed that luminal glucose concentration of normal fed animals ranged from 0.2 to 48 mmol, well within the K_m for the brush border Na-glucose cotransporter. Moreover, they demonstrated that the Na-glucose cotransporter was reversibly and specifically regulated by dietary levels of their substrate.[31] Both the number and the activity of transporters can be increased by dietary manipulation.

4. Maximal Capacity for Water Absorption

As indicated above, gastric emptying can reach 30–40 ml/min or 1.8–2.4 l/h. Can the intestine absorb fluid at this rate? Maximal absorptive capacity of the gut has been measured by steady-state total gut perfusion.[94] In the study reported, 30 ml/min were infused into the stomach for 8 h. The difference between the amount infused and the rectal effluent was the amount absorbed. When a solution containing 100 mmol D-glucose and 100 mmol NaCl was perfused, water absorption was 1.4 l/h.

In another study in which GE of a 6% glucose solution was 21 ml/min, intestinal perfusion at a flow rate of 36 ml/min did not produce diarrhea or GI distress.[27] This amounts to an absorption rate of 2.16 l/h, which certainly equals or exceeds the sweating rate of most endurance athletes. Thus, results from total gut and segmental perfusion studies suggest that the absorptive capacity of the normal human small intestine is unlikely to limit the effectiveness of an oral rehydration solution.

B. CARBOHYDRATE–ELECTROLYTE ABSORPTION

Water transport is directly proportional to solute transport, so it is imperative to discuss CHO–electrolyte absorption. Glucose is the dominant CHO and Na^+ is the dominant cation to be transported from the intestinal lumen. Evidence suggests that both are transported transcellularly and paracellularly. Quantitatively, which pathway dominates? This is a difficult question and beyond the scope of this chapter, but the answer will vary with the composition of the fluid consumed and the segment of the intestine under study. Entry of Na^+ into the enterocyte (Figure 7) involves electrochemical diffusion (Figure

7A), cotransport (symport) (Figure 7B) or exchange (antiport) with another ion (Figure 7C), and coupled transport with an organic nonelectrolyte (sugars, amino acids) (Figure 7D). Here we will focus on Na^+-glucose cotransport. A more complete discussion of the different pathways and mechanisms involved can be found elsewhere.[38]

The observation that glucose stimulates intestinal Na^+ absorption formed the basis for developing sport drinks and ORS to treat diarrhea (Figure 7). Glucose and two Na^+ molecules form an obligatory ternary complex with a membrane protein carrier in the brush border. Na^+ is transported down its electrochemical gradient, providing the energy for glucose movement into the mucosal cell. The Na^+ gradient across the mucosal membrane is conserved by active Na^+ transport across the basolateral membrane via the Na^+/K^+ pump. Glucose is transported out of the cell via another membrane carrier (Glut 2).

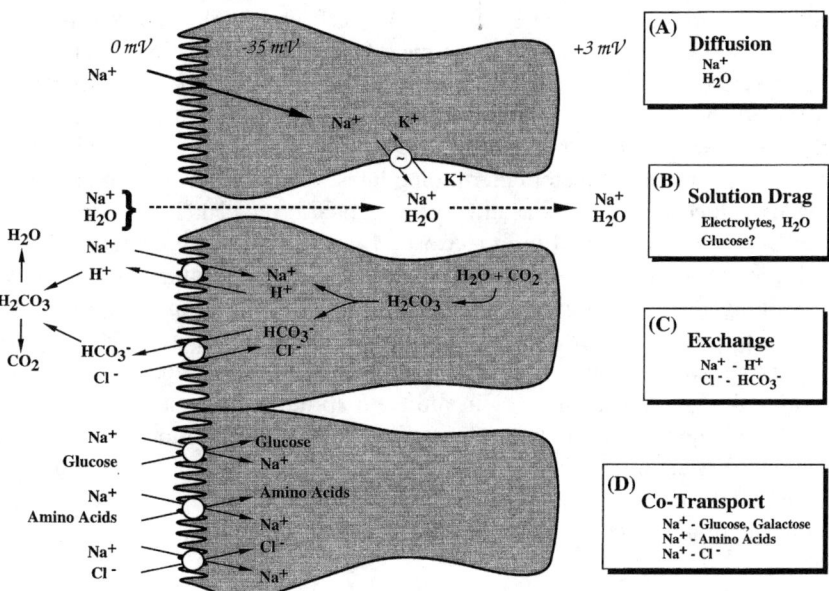

FIGURE 7 Mechanisms of Na^+ transport in the small intestine. See text for explanation. (From *Perspectives in Exercise and Sports Medicine: Fluid Homeostasis During Exercise*, Grisolfi, C. and Lamb, D.R., Eds., 1990. With permission.)

1. Na^+-Glucose Ratio

How much CHO and Na^+ is necessary to optimize water absorption? Although the optimal glucose/Na^+ ratio to maximize water absorption has been reported to be 2:1, this is controversial and may depend upon the number of different transportable CHOs used to formulate the beverage. Sladen and Dawson[99] showed that adding 56 mmol glucose to saline increased water absorption tenfold. Lifshitz and Wapnir,[6D] using an *in vivo* intestinal perfusion system in rats, found that optimal net water absorption was produced by a solution containing 111 mmol glucose and 60 mmol Na^+ and had a glucose-to-Na^+ concentration ratio of slightly less than 2:1. In a subsequent study, they found that hypotonic (155–220 mOsm/kg) solutions were even more effective in promoting water absorption and concluded that an ORS with an osmolality of ~200 mOsm/kg, a glucose-to-Na^+ ratio of 1:2, and a glucose concentration not exceeding 60 mmol optimized water absorption from the rat jejunum. In a recent human study of isotonic solutions containing 2, 4, 6, or 8% glucose, sucrose, maltodextrin, or corn syrup solids, we found that net water absorption was independent of glucose-to-Na^+ ratios in the test solution, ranging from 1.2:1 up to 8.5:1.[96] We attributed this to the speed with which the intestine can change luminal [Na^+] and to a certain extent to the changes that occur in luminal glucose concentration. The glucose-to-Na^+ ratios in the test segment for the 2, 4, and 6% glucose solutions, which did not produce significant differences in water absorption, were 0.4:1, 2:1, and 3.5:1, respectively.

In another study we investigated the effects of increasing [Na^+] in a CHO-electrolyte solution on intestinal absorption. We found that [Na^+]s of 0, 25, or 50 meq/l in a 6% CHO solution had similar effects on water, Na^+, K^+, and glucose absorption from the duodenojejunum. Glucose in the infusion solution was a more important factor determining intestinal water absorption than Na^+, because glucose alone was as effective as glucose plus Na^+.

Does the amount and form (hexose, disaccharide, maltodextrin) of CHO influence water absorption? In the discussion of GE, we found that beverages containing up to 8% CHO, regardless of form, did not significantly affect emptying rate. Is the same true for intestinal absorption? In a recent study we found that isotonic solutions up to 6% glucose, sucrose, maltodextrin, or corn syrup solids were similar in their ability to stimulate water absorption from the duodenojejunum;[39] however, increasing CHO concentration to 8% significantly reduced water absorption for solutions containing glucose and corn syrup solids, but not maltodextrins or sucrose. Thus, CHO form seems to be more important in governing intestinal absorption than GE.

C. EFFECTS OF EXERCISE

Despite a marked rise in cardiac output and a moderate elevation in mean arterial pressure, splanchnic blood flow (which includes flow to the stomach, spleen, liver, and intestines) decreases linearly with increasing exercise intensity.[88] This decrease depends upon circulatory capacity—that is, the decline is less for highly trained individuals at a given absolute $\dot{V}O_2$.[88] During maximal exercise, splanchnic blood flow is reduced to 80% of its resting value in both trained and untrained subjects. Recent studies using Doppler flowmetry of the portal vein showed that cycle exercise at 70% $\dot{V}O_2$ max reduced portal flow to 80% of its initial value in 30 min and that flow remained at this level until exercise stopped at 60 min.[82]

Does this decline in splanchnic blood flow during exercise reduce intestinal absorption? The answer is controversial. In dogs, intestinal absorption of glucose and xylose is significantly reduced when mesenteric blood flow is diminished by 50%.[109] In isolated surviving intestine, sugar absorption is reduced when mucosal cells are made hypoxic.[25] However, splanchnic nerve stimulation reduces blood flow to the muscularis and crypts of the intestinal wall without affecting blood flow to the villi, the site of absorption. Thus, intense exercise may reduce splanchnic blood flow without affecting intestinal absorption.

Experimental evidence from human experiments is also conflicting. Williams et al.[109] had 6 heat-acclimated men ingest D-xylose (a passively absorbed sugar) and 3-O-methyl-D-glucose (3MG, sodium-coupled carrier mediated absorption, but not metabolized) during 4.5 h (50 min exercise, 10 min rest/h) of treadmill exercise at 3 mph in the heat (38°C dry bulb, 27°C wet bulb). They found significant reductions in 3MG concentration in the blood and excretion in the urine, but no changes in xylose. These data provide indirect evidence for a reduction in active absorption during exercise; however, because these experiments were performed in the heat, the decline in 3MG absorption may be attributed to the combined effect of heat and exercise rather than exercise alone. Maughan et al.[64] also concluded that exercise reduces intestinal absorption, although they were unable to distinguish between GE and intestinal absorption. They had 6 men perform cycle exercise at 42, 61, and 80% $\dot{V}O_2$ max for 30 min after ingesting 200 ml of a CHO-electrolyte beverage containing deuterium oxide (D_2O). They found that the accumulation of D_2O in the plasma was significantly greater at rest than during exercise at 61 or 80% $\dot{V}O_2$ max. The advantage of this technique is that it evaluates both gastric emptying and intestinal absorption and takes the entire intestine into account. The disadvantage is that it does not evaluate intestinal absorption per se. The tracer technique is also unable to distinguish between substances that cause absorption from those that cause secretion.[40]

The advantage of segmental perfusion is that it provides a quantitative measure of net water and solute flux. Three studies used this technique to evaluate the effect of exercise on intestinal absorption. One evaluated only a saline solution; the other two evaluated CHO-E solutions. Barclay and Turnberg[4] had 5 women and 2 men perform mild cycle exercise for 1 h at 15 km/h (about 40 rpm). Load varied with the level of fitness of the subject and elicited a mean HR of 103 ± 7 bpm. They perfused (10 ml/min) the jejunum with isotonic saline and found that exercise significantly reduced water, sodium, chloride, and potassium absorption. However, the values for water and solute absorption were extremely low. Water absorption was only 1–2 ml/cm/h. Adding 2–6% CHO to an electrolyte solution increases water absorption to 10–13 ml/cm/h, a six- to tenfold increase.[37] Thus, removing CHO from the perfusion solution unmasked an inhibitory effect of exercise on absorption, but this reduction is probably of little biological importance.

The next two studies both show no effect of exercise on intestinal absorption. Fordtran and Saltin[34] studied carrier-mediated and passive absorption during treadmill exercise for 1 h at 64–78% $\dot{V}O_2$ max in 4 men and 1 woman. They perfused (12 or 16 ml/min) the jejunum with four different CHO-E solutions, but only 1 or 2 subjects were perfused with a given solution. They found no consistent effect of exercise on glucose, water, electrolyte, or urea absorption, and concluded that exercise had no effect on intestinal permeability, active transport, or passive transport. Gisolfi et al.[37] also used segmental perfusion (15 ml/min) during 1-h bouts of cycle exercise at 30, 50, and 70% $\dot{V}O_2$ max to study absorption in 6 trained male cyclists (Figure 8). They found no significant effect of exercise on water absorption, but fluid absorption was significantly greater from a 6% CHO-E solution than from water when the data were pooled over rest, exercise, and recovery periods. When exercise was extended to 90 min at 70% $\dot{V}O_2$ max, the results were the same.

Although segmental perfusion provides the most precise measurement of water and solute transport, the disadvantage of this technique is that it only evaluates a segment of the intestine and one must be careful in trying to extrapolate these data to what would occur if these solutions were ingested orally. Another consideration is that the latter studies usually evaluate the proximal small intestine, which is rather leaky compared with more distal portions of the gut. The question arises as to how much of the fluid perfused is actually reabsorbed. In the study by Gisolfi et al.,[37] absorption from the 40-cm test segment accounted for ~50% of the volume infused. In a recent paper it was emphasized that if the main objective of the study is to evaluate the effects of a particular solution on water absorption, then net fluid movement across the mixing segment as well as the test segment should be considered.[98] When the entire multilumen tube (mixing + test segments) is taken into account, greater than 60% of the total amount of fluid infused can be accounted for.

D. ROLE OF MOTILITY

The effect of gut motility on intestinal absorption has not been clearly defined. The pattern of intestinal contraction is more important than the frequency or amplitude of contraction in determining the flow of chyme through the intestinal lumen. What occurs in the "fed" condition may vary markedly from what occurs in the "unfed" condition. There are three phases of intestinal contraction. Phase I represents the fasted state when there are no contractions and flow is slow or absent. Phase II represents intermittent contractions and phase III represents regular contractions. The later represents the fed pattern and is characterized by rapid flow and maximal absorption. Nutrients also influence contractions, with CHO producing more contractions than proteins or fats. Unabsorbed CHO accelerates transit probably by inducing secretion, creating distension, and stimulating migrating contractions.[93] In dogs, jejunal myoelectric recordings showed that

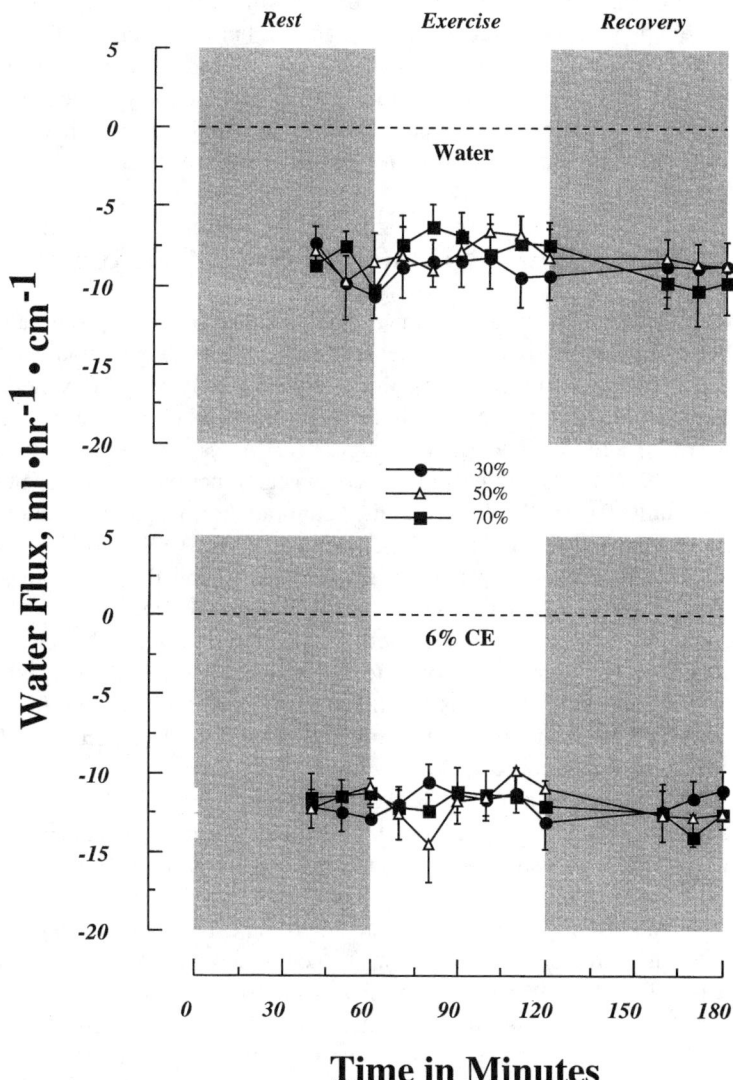

FIGURE 8 Design II net water flux during perfusion of water or 6% carbohydrate-electrolyte (CHO-E) solution (means ± SE) at rest, during 60 min of exercise at 30, 50, and 70% maximal O_2 uptake ($\dot{V}O_2$ max), and during 60 min of recovery. Infusion began at time 0. Negative values indicate absorption. Note that net water flux values were all greater (more negative) during perfusion of 6% CE solution than during perfusion of water. (From Grisolfi et al., *J. Appl. Physiol.*, 71(6), 2518, 1991. With permission.)

intense exercise (80% of heart rate max) interrupted the fed pattern by an activity front.[51] In humans, intestinal motility is difficult to study for technical reasons. We studied duodenal and jejunal motility in the fed state at 60, 70, and 80% $\dot{V}O_2$ max. Although exercise did not alter the duration of the fed pattern, this pattern was interrupted by rhythmic bursts of activity that were propagated from the duodenum to the jejunum. Moreover, the induction of these fronts occurred more frequently as exercise intensity increased, but transit time was unaffected.[101] Others have found that small intestinal transit decreases, but that caloric transit increases with exercise.[12]

VI. NEURAL AND HORMONAL CONTROL

Neural control of gastrointestinal function is provided by the central, autonomic, and enteric nervous systems. Briefly, the central nervous system (CNS) regulates gastrointestinal function either directly via sympathetic or parasympathetic pathways (ANS) or indirectly via modulating enteric nervous system (ENS) activity. The ENS is large. It contains 10^8 neurons, located within the wall of the gastrointestinal tract, and can function as an independent integrative unit. The ENS is known as the "gut brain" for its ability to integrate sensory information from a variety of sources (CNS, ANS, and ENS), and then coordinate and regulate gut function. Fibers within the vagus, sympathetic, and enteric nerves release a variety of neuropeptides that not only demonstrate diverse physiological responses (see Section VI.A), but may also act in a neurotransmitter, neuromodulator, paracrine, and/or endocrine fashion. In addition, some sensory nerves are thought to demonstrate efferent function where neuropeptides are released from sensory nerves in response to alterations in intraluminal contents.[62]

In short, nerves from the CNS, ANS, and ENS form a complex communication network whereby they function to: (1) monitor the presence and quality (nutrient type, osmolality, pH, etc.) of chyme at different gut locations, (2) provide pathways to integrate sensory information arriving in both the CNS and ENS, and (3) provide pathways to coordinate and regulate numerous gastrointestinal effector functions. How this neural network regulates gut function in response to the diverse stimuli presented by fluid and carbohydrate ingestion during strenuous exercise remains unknown.

Feedback control by the ENS may be important in an athlete who consumes fluids and nutrients (luminal stimuli) during strenuous exercise (high sympathetic tone). Neural control of intestinal ion and water transport was thought to be primarily influenced by the balance between sympathetic and parasympathetic tone. Today, the ENS is recognized to "fine-tune" ion transport by responding to luminal thermal, mechanical and chemical stimuli in a negative feedback fashion.[105] The type and number of neurotransmittors associated with feedback regulation are numerous, and may include autocoids and neuropeptides.[105]

Strenuous exercise enhances sympathetic tone and activates the renin–angiotensin–aldosterone system. Enhanced sympathetic tone may stimulate small intestinal absorption and inhibit intestinal secretion.[98] Norepinephrine released from sympathetic nerves may act to stimulate Na+ and water absorption in both the small and large intestine.[58] Angiotensin II is also thought to stimulate small intestinal Na+ and water absorption through its stimulatory effects on both central sympathetic outflow and norepinephrine release from enteric sympathetic nerves. Aldosterone, released in response to angiotensin II, may promote Na+ and water absorption in the large, but not the small, intestine. Thus, extracellular volume depletion resulting from hemorrhage, dehydration, or salt depletion may stimulate intestinal Na+ and water absorption via mechanisms involving both the sympathetic and renin–angiotensin–aldosterone systems. Available evidence suggests that, despite marked elevations in circulating catecholamines and reductions in plasma volume, strenuous (90 min at 70% $\dot{V}O_2$ max) cycling exercise will not alter intestinal absorption of either water or a 6% CHO-E solution.[37]

A. GASTROINTESTINAL PEPTIDES AND NITRIC OXIDE

More than 30 different peptides have been identified in the mammalian gastrointestinal tract.[41] These peptides can be located in nerves within the brain and gut, and in single endocrine cells dispersed throughout the gastrointestinal tract. Regulation of gastrointestinal function by these peptides is complex, and may occur in an autocrine, paracrine, endocrine, neurotransmittor, or neuromodulator fashion. As a group, these peptides act to regulate gut function by modulating appetite (food intake) and gut secretion, absorption, motility, and tissue growth. The following brief review focuses on selected peptides, their role in regulating gastrointestinal function, and their response to acute exercise. Questions regarding the potential role of nitric oxide (NO) in modulating GI function are also presented. The following information highlights the fact that little is known about the physiological roles of either GI peptides or NO in regulating fluid and nutrient absorption during exercise.

Cholecystokinin (CCK) is contained in neurons of the brain and intestinal tract, and in endocrine cells of the small intestine.[41] Release of CCK is stimulated primarily by ingestion of proteins, amino acids, and fats, but not by glucose. Stimulation of gallbladder contractions and pancreatic secretions are well-known actions of CCK. Less appreciated are the roles of CCK in regulation of GE[59] and food intake.[45] CCK enhances contraction of the gastroduodenal junction, inhibits proximal gastric contractions, reduces intragastric pressure, and slows gastric emptying. Presently, the CCK response to exercise alone or to food ingestion during or immediately following exercise is unknown. A recent study showed that female long-distance runners at rest demonstrate a reduced CCK response to a mixed meal compared to values obtained in age- and weight-matched sedentary women.[45] The investigators attributed the reduced CCK response to the larger caloric intakes of the athletes.

Gastrin endocrine cells are located in the gastric antrum, and to a lesser extent, in the duodenal mucosa.[41] Gastrin release is stimulated by food ingestion, bile salts within the antral lumen, intravenous infusions of adrenaline, and performance of prolonged exercise. Release of gastrin can be inhibited by numerous stimuli including low antral pH (below 3), starvation, and several gut hormones (somatostatin, secretin, glucagon, and vasoactive intestinal peptide). Gastrin acts on the stomach to stimulate mucosal blood flow and the secretion of hydrochloric acid, pepsin and intrinsic factor. Increases in circulating gastrin during either prolonged (30-km run) running or intravenous infusion of adrenaline tend to parallel increases in circulating adrenaline,[8,103] suggesting that the β-adrenergic system may stimulate gastrin release. Gastrin release in response to a meal is also reported to increase following exhaustive (70% $\dot{V}O_2$ max) running[8] or 3 days of combat training with caloric and sleep deprivation.[76] The physiological effects of elevated gastrin during and following exercise remain unknown.

Secretin is contained in mucosal endocrine cells of the duodenum (highest), jejunum, and ileum (lowest). The release of secretin in response to a meal is directly related to the acid load presented to the duodenum. Secretin acts on the pancreas and stomach to either neutralize meal-induced duodenal acidification or reduce the acid load originating from the stomach. Physiological actions of secretin include stimulation of pancreatic bicarbonate secretion, and inhibition of gastric acid secretion, gastric emptying, and meal-induced gastrin release. Hilsted et al.[44] reported that plasma secretin increases in response to prolonged (3 h) cycling at 40% $\dot{V}O_2$ max. These investigators noted that neither the stimuli for release of gastrointestinal peptides nor their physiological roles during exercise are known.

Motilin is located in endocrine cells distributed throughout the intestinal tract, from the esophagus to the colon.[41] Motilin release is stimulated by ingestion of fat, but not by ingestion of a mixed meal, and may be inhibited by ingestion of glucose. Physiological actions of motilin include enhanced gastric emptying, and stimulation of small intestinal and colonic motility. Sullivan et al.[103] observed elevated plasma motilin concentrations in male marathoners during the final 20 km of a 30-km run. These[103] and other[13] investigators have speculated that elevated motilin may contribute to enhanced gut transit of food associated with endurance exercise. However, as noted above, the effect of exercise on transit time is unclear.

Vasoactive intestinal peptide (VIP) can be located in neurons of the central nervous system, cardiovascular system, lungs and gastrointestinal tract. VIP release can be stimulated via intraduodenal infusion of fat or hypertonic solutions, ingestion of a meal, or electrical stimulation of the vagus nerve.[41] Prolonged cycling (3 h at 40% $\dot{V}O_2$ max) or running (30 km) may also stimulate VIP release.[44,103] VIP, as its name suggests, is a potent vasodilatory agent, and is well known for its ability to alter intestinal motility and increase intestinal ion and water secretion. Brouns and Beckers[12] suggest that, during exhaustive exercise, VIP release may act with other factors, such as reduced gut blood flow, to reduce intestinal absorption and enhance secretion.

Neurotensin is contained in neurons of the brain, and in endocrine cells of the distal small intestine. Ingestion of fat or rapid movement of fat or glucose to the ileum may stimulate neurotensin release. Physiological actions of neurotensin include mesenteric vasodilation, enhanced intestinal motility, reduced gastric mucosal blood flow, and inhibition of gastric emptying. Available evidence shows that plasma neurotensin may not increase during a marathon or 30-km run.[12,103] One may postulate that, if it occurs during strenuous exercise, malabsorption of ingested fat or glucose may elicit neurotensin release with a consequent slowing of gastric emptying.

Opiate peptides, enkephalins and endorphins, are widely distributed in neurons of the brain and gut, and in endocrine cells of the intestinal tract.[53] A variety of stresses can stimulate opioid release, including fasting and strenuous exercise.[106] Endogenous opioids are thought to be involved in the regulation of blood pressure, body temperature, pain perception, and elevation of mood. Opioids also demonstrate diverse effects on GI function; these peptides can alter gastric and intestinal motility, inhibit GE and intestinal transit, and reduce meal-induced CCK and secretin release.[53] The physiological effects of opioid release on GI function during strenuous exercise, with or without food ingestion, remain unknown. Prior investigators have speculated that opioid release may impair GE in response to the mental stress of competition[12] and the thermal strain associated with strenuous exercise in the heat.[73,78]

Substance P is located in neurons of the CNS, ANS, and ENS, and a few endocrine cells of the intestinal tract. It is thought to act primarily in a neurotransmittor or paracrine fashion; however, its roles in regulating GI function are largely unknown. In rats, intravenous infusion of Substance P reduces fluid secretion in the duodenum and increases fluid absorption in the jejunum and proximal ileum. Recent evidence suggests that endogenous Substance P can be released in response to thermal stimuli applied to the GI tract.[89] Specifically, application of warm (45°C) saline to the stomach, jejunum, or ileum was shown to provoke rapid arterial hypotension, tachycardia, and reductions in intestinal blood flow. Although the relevance to the hyperthermic athlete is unclear, these findings do highlight the possibility that a variety of GI stimuli can exert diverse and profound physiological effects.

Nitric oxide (NO) can be produced within numerous tissues of the GI tract, most notably the endothleium, epithelium, smooth muscle, and some nerves. Within these tissues, NO production and release may be activated during stimulation of enteric nerves and/or exposure to cytokines, endotoxins, bacteria, and some irritants (bile acids, acids). The release of NO has been implicated in mediating numerous GI functions including receptive relaxation of the stomach, inhibition of GE, inhibition of GI motor activity, and enhancement of GI mucosal blood flow.[42] NO release may also elicit the phenomenon known as adaptive cytoprotection, in which the stomach, and possibly the intestines, become resistant to the injurious effects of nonsteroidal antiinflammatory drugs and other irritants.[54] Because NO elicits such diverse physiological effects, future studies may be required to evaluate the potential role of

NO in modulating GI function during and following strenuous exercise. Are the GI disturbances (impaired GE, gut barrier failure) associated with exhaustive exercise in the heat related to enhanced NO release?

VII. GASTROINTESTINAL ADAPTATION

It has been suggested that the gastrointestinal tract does not adapt to the physiological stresses imposed by exercise—that is, it does not respond to chronic exercise with enhanced function or structural changes.[12] On the other hand, the GI tract of an endurance athlete may demonstrate structural and functional adaptations associated with high caloric and carbohydrate intake that are not present in sedentary individuals.

Two recent studies suggest that physically active individuals may demonstrate enhanced GI function. First, Carrio et al.[15] reported that marathon runners demonstrate enhanced GE of a mixed meal compared to sedentary subjects. Enhanced parasympathetic tone associated with physical training was cited as a possible explanation. More recently, Harris et al.[43] found a significant negative correlation ($r = -0.69$) between orocecal transit time and daily energy intake in 20 men who demonstrated a wide range in daily physical activity and food intake. Orocecal transit time of a liquid meal ranged from ~200 min to below 50 min for two individuals with daily energy intakes of ~1300 and ~4500 kcal/d, respectively. The investigators postulated that high daily caloric intakes associated with chronic physical activity may promote adaptations within the small intestine. Presumably, these intestinal adaptations could enhance intestinal absorptive capacity, reduce intestinal chemoreceptor feedback to the stomach and intestines, and thereby enhance food transit through the gut.

Recent studies have also shown that GE of either mixed meals, high-fat meals, or hypertonic glucose solutions can be enhanced by acute alterations in dietary intake. For example, when maintained on low daily caloric intakes, patients with anorexia nervosa demonstrate normal GE of saline, but delayed emptying of a mixed meal or a hypertonic glucose solution.[86] Placing patients on a 2-week refeeding diet normalized GE of these meals. Cunningham et al.[22] showed, in healthy volunteers, that consumption of a high-fat diet for 14 days enhanced both GE and orocecal transit of a high-fat test meal. Total fat intake for the low-fat and high-fat diets was 12 and 270 g/day, respectively. The investigators emphasized the possibility that prior dietary history may contribute to the relatively large inter- and intraindividual variability of GE measurement. In a similar study, these investigators showed that GE of a hypertonic glucose solution, but not a protein drink, could be enhanced by supplementation of a standard diet with 400 g glucose/day for 3 days.[23] Total carbohydrate intake for the standard diet and the supplemented diet was 287 and 687 g/day. Together, these findings indicate that the GI tract can rapidly adapt to increased daily intake of dietary fats and carbohydrates.

The nature of these adaptations remain undefined, but could include reductions in intestinal chemoreceptor sensitivity and/or elevations in intestinal absorptive capacity.

Can endurance athletes, who demonstrate relatively large energy and carbohydrate intakes, improve their intestinal absorptive capacity by altering their diets? If so, will this enhanced intestinal absorptive capacity be associated with enhanced GE of carbohydrate fluid replacement drinks? The absorptive capacity of mammalian intestine is closely matched to dietary intake.[31] Furthermore, alterations in either the quality or quantity of dietary intake, if sufficient in magnitude and duration, may induce intestinal adaptations to accommodate these dietary changes. The magnitude of dietary change required to produce alterations in GI structure and function in humans is not well known.

Evidence from experimental animals shows that intestinal adaptations can be associated with conditions that increase both caloric intake and energy expenditure, such as pregnancy and lactation. In such conditions, adaptations that increase intestinal surface area can be prominent, and may include increases in total intestinal length, and mucosal hypertrophy with increases in villi length and number.[10] These intestinal adaptations, presumably responding to chronic elevations in luminal nutrients, are observable within several weeks of hyperphagia, and may provide enhanced intestinal absorptive capacity. It seems reasonable to postulate that endurance athletes, who consume two to four times more calories than sedentary individuals, may demonstrate some form of intestinal adaptation.

Compared to the nonspecific adaptations associated with hyperphagia, more rapid and nutrient-specific intestinal adaptions can occur in response to alterations in dietary carbohydrate intake. In humans and animals, high dietary intakes of sucrose or fructose, but not glucose, can increase jejunal sucrase and maltase activities.[87] Jejunal glycolytic enzyme activities may also be increased by glucose, fructose, and galactose feedings. These diet-induced changes are rapid. Alterations in enterocyte glycolytic enzyme activities and brush border disaccharidase activities can occur within several hours and 2–5 days, respectively, following the initiation or cessation of sugar feedings. Recent studies in rodents also show that switching from a low- to a high-carbohydrate diet can rapidly (1–7 days) increase carrier-mediated glucose uptake in the proximal small intestine.[31] The rapid increase in glucose uptake is thought to be due to increases in the number and/or intrinsic activity of the glucose transporter located within both the enterocyte brush border and basolateral membrane.

From these observations, it seems reasonable to postulate that endurance athletes, who consume two to four times more calories than sedentary individuals, may demonstrate some form of intestinal adaptation. Although currently undefined, these intestinal adaptations may allow for rapid GE and enhanced intestinal absorption of needed fluids and nutrients during exercise.

VIII. GASTROINTESTINAL BLEEDING AND BARRIER FUNCTION

Bleeding from the GI tract is a common untoward effect of intense and prolonged running. The incidence of visible and occult bleeding in marathoners is estimated to be ~2% and 8–30%, respectively.[28] Perhaps reflecting the severity of stress, a much higher percentage of ultramarathoners, up to 85%, may demonstrate guaic positive stools following a 100-km race.[5] Although GI bleeding appears to be mild in most runners, it can be dramatic, causing hemetemesis, melena, iron-deficient anemia or death.[28] The most commonly reported sites of bleeding are the stomach and proximal colon, although this may vary from athlete to athlete. The etiology of bleeding is unknown, but is frequently attributed to gut ischemia, repetitive mechanical trauma, and use of nonsteroidal antiinflammatory drugs (NSAIDs). The fact that GI bleeding commonly occurs in runners not only suggests that the gut is uniquely susceptible to injury during strenuous running, but also suggests that runners may frequently experience some degree of impairment in their GI barrier function.

For all practical purposes, substances within the GI tract lie outside the body. In addition to its digestive and absorptive functions, it provides an important barrier function that acts to exclude numerous luminal aggressive factors (gastric and pancreatic juices, bile acids, bacteria, and food antigens) from reaching the body interior. The GI barrier consists of both immunological (gut-associated lympoid tissue) and nonimmunological (gastric acidity, peristalsis, epithelial cells, and a mucus coat) processes.[56] Failure of the gut barrier may initiate a local or systemic inflammatory response by allowing toxic subtances to enter the intestinal mucosa and systemic circulation.

At least four lines of evidence suggest that strenuous exercise may impair gut barrier function. First, as cited above, GI bleeding in runners can be viewed as an example of impaired barrier function. The significance of mild bleeding (impaired barrier function) is unclear; however, in ultramarathon runners and perhaps other athletes, the appearance of bleeding may be associated with GI symptoms such as nausea, diarrhea, and abdominal cramps.[5] These symptoms, presumably related to gut barrier breakdown, are likely to be associated with both impaired gut function and reduced consumption of needed fluids and nutrients. Second, recent endoscopic studies of competitive endurance runners show that mucosal lesions, such as hemorrhagic gastritis and ischemic colitis, can be observed following strenuous exercise.[70] These lesions, thought to be transient (<72 h) in nature, may also be associated with the development of GI symptoms, impaired gut function, and reduced feeding during and immediately following exercise.

Third, recent evidence suggests that intestinal permeability to ^{51}Cr-labeled ethylenediaminetetracetic acid is markedly enhanced by performance of a half or full marathon run.[77] From this observation, it can be speculated that enhanced permeability to macromolecules and/or bacteria could activate the gut-associated lymphoid tissue, trigger a local inflammatory response, and perhaps contribute to the development of abdominal cramps during exercise.[77] Possibly related to this scenario are the observations that NSAIDs can produce significant GI bleeding, and can enhance intestinal permeability,[6] markedly impair intestinal absorption of glucose and water,[3] and may contribute to GI disturbances during exercise.[70] Little is known about the effect of NSAIDs on GI function during exercise, in spite of the fact that NSAIDs are widely used by athletes during training and competition.

The last and perhaps most serious example of gut barrier failure in athletes is the development of endotoxemia. Recent studies show that triathletes[7] and ultramarathon runners[11] may exhibit significant endotoxemia following completion of their respective events. The study of ultramarathoners[11] deserves further comment. The investigators studied 89 ultramarathon runners who collasped during 90-km runs and required medical attention. Eighty-one percent of the collapsed runners showed endotoxemia, and 2% had plasma endotoxin concentrations (1 ng/ml) thought to be lethal for humans. These collapsed, endotoxemic runners also required fluid replacement therapy, exhibited vomiting and diarrhea, and required several days to recover.

Can ingestion of fluids and/or nutrients during exercise help to maintain GI barrier function? The answer is unknown. Ingestion of fluids during exercise may attenuate numerous physiological responses such as hyperthermia, dehydration, reductions in splanchnic blood flow,[81] and the development of GI distress.[84] On the other hand, ingestion of nutrients during exercise may attenuate reductions in splanchnic blood flow,[81] and provide needed substrates to the gut-associated lymphoid tissue and the metabolically stressed intestinal epithelial barrier.[30] Thus, it seems reasonable to suggest that fluid and nutrient ingestion during exercise may benefit the athlete's gut barrier function by reducing thermal and ischemic damage to the GI tract and/or by providing intestinal fuels. Benefits to the athlete may include reduction of GI distress and bleeding, prevention of endotoxemia, and the ability to continue consumption of fluids and nutrients.

IX. SUMMARY

From the evidence presented, the stomach and small intestine function extremely well under conditions of exercise and environmental stress, despite a reduction in splanchnic blood flow. Neither GE nor intestinal absorption are delayed or impaired during exercise ranging from 30–70% $\dot{V}O_2$ max, even when exercise is prolonged and causes fatigue. Moreover, the GI system has the capacity to meet the nutrient and fluid needs of prolonged exercise. If gastric volume is maintained relatively high (200–400 ml), GE of sport drinks containing 4–8% CHO can exceed 30 ml/min or 1800 ml/h, which is sufficient to keep pace with evaporative cooling of the vast majority of exercisers. Maximal estimates of intestinal absorption range from 1.4–2.2 l/h indicating that the intestine can readily handle the gastric volume that it receives and that intestinal absorption does not limit rehydration. Even when subjected to conditions of 3–4% hypohydration, the GI system operates within the normal range. Heat acclimation and training seem to have little effect on GI function, but the system adapts structurally and functionally to high caloric and CHO intake. Orocecal transit time correlates negatively with daily energy intake and placing subjects on high energy and CHO intakes improves intestinal absorptive capacity. Thus, there is evidence that the GI system of the endurance athlete responds well to high energy and CHO intake.

On the other hand, there is considerable evidence that the GI system can be the "canary of the body"[24] — that is, if there is an underlying GI disorder at rest, exercise will exacerbate the problem and elicit GI symptoms. At exercise intensities >75–80% $\dot{V}O_2$ max, GE is significantly reduced. When dehydration exceeds a 4% loss in body weight, and when hyperthermia is present, GE is significantly impaired and GI symptoms (nausea, vomiting, bloating, pain, etc.) emerge. In the most severe cases, the "barrier" function of the gut fails. This could produce GI bleeding, mucosal lesions, endotoxemia, the release of inflammatory cytokines, and circulatory impairment. Whether or not the ingestion of fluids and/or nutrients can help to sustain barrier function during stressful exercise is an intriguing question.

REFERENCES

1. American College of Sports Medicine. *The prevention of thermal injuries during distance running, American College of Sports Medicine, Position stands and opinion statements (1975–1985)*. Indianapolis: American College of Sports Medicine, 1985.
2. Armstrong, L.E., Hubbard, R.W., Jones, B.H., and Daniels, J.T. Preparing Alberto Salazar for the heat of the 1984 Olympic marathon. *Phys. Sportsmed.* 3(14): 73–81, 1986.
3. Arvanitakis, C., Chen, G.-H., Folscroft, J., and Greenberger, N.J. Effect of aspirin on intestinal absorption of glucose, sodium, and water in man. *Gut* 18: 187–190, 1977.
4. Barclay, G.R. and Turnberg, L.A. Effect of moderate exercise on salt and water transport in the human jejunum. *Gut* 29: 816–820, 1988.
5. Baska, R.S., Moses, F.M., Graeber, G., and Kearney, G. Gastrointestinal bleeding during an ultramarathon. *Dig. Dis. Sci.* 35(2): 276–279, 1990.
6. Bjarnason, I. Intestinal permeability. *Gut* (Suppl.) 1: S18–S22, 1994.
7. Bosenberg, A.T., Brock-Utne, J.G., Gaffin, L., Wells, M.T.B., and Blake, G.T.W. Strenuous exercise causes systemic endotoxemia. *J. Appl. Physiol.* 65(1): 106–108, 1988.
8. Brandsborg, O., Christensen, N.J., Galbo, H., Brandsborg, M., and Lovgreen, N.A. The effect of exercise, smoking and propranolol on serum gastrin in patients with duodenal ulcer and in vagotomized subjects. *Scand. J. Clin. Lab. Invest.* 38: 441–446, 1978.
9. Brener, W., Hendrix, R.R., and McHugh, P.R. Regulation of gastric emptying of glucose. *Gastroenterology* 85: 76–82, 1983.
10. Bristol, J.B., Williamson, R.C.N., and Chir, M. Nutrition, operations, and intestinal adaptation. *J. Parenteral Enteral Nutr.* 12(3): 299–309, 1988.
11. Brock-Utne, J.G., Gaffin, S.L., Wells, M.T., Gathiram, P., Sohar, E., James, M.F., Morrell, D.F., and Norman, R.J. Endotoxaemia in exhausted runners following a long-distance race. *S. Afr. Med. J.* 73: 533–536, 1988.
12. Brouns, F. and Beckers, E. Is the gut an athletic organ? Digestion, absorption and exercise. *Sports Med.* 15(4): 242–257, 1993.

13. Brouns, F., Saris, W.H.M., and Rehrer, N.J. Abdominal complaints and gastrointestinal function during long-lasting exercise. *Int. J. Sports Med.* 8: 175–189, 1987.
14. Campbell, J.M.H., Mitchell, G.O., and Powell, A.T.W. The influence of exercise on digestion. *Guy's Hosp. Rep.* 78: 279–293, 1924.
15. Carrio, I., Estorch, M., Serra-Grima, R., Ginjaume, M., Notivol, R., Calabuig, R., and Vilardell, F. Gastric emptying in marathon runners. *Gut* 30: 152–155, 1989.
16. Cervero, F. Sensory innervation of the viscera: Peripheral basis of visceral pain. *Physiol. Rev.* 74(1): 95–129, 1994.
17. Cheeseman, C.I. GLUT2 is the transporter for fructose across the rat intestinal basolateral membrane. *Gastroenterology* 205: 1050–1056, 1993.
18. Costill, D.L. Gastric emptying of fluids during exercise. In: *Perspectives in Exercise Science and Sports Medicine. Fluid Homeostasis During Exercise.* C.V. Gisolfi and D.R. Lamb, Eds. Indianapolis: Benchmark Press, 1990, 97–127.
19. Costill, D.L. and Saltin, B. Factors limiting gastric emptying during rest and exercise. *J. Appl. Physiol.* 37: 679–683, 1974.
20. Coyle, E.F., Coggan, A.R., Hemmert, M.K., and Ivy, J.L. Muscle glycogen utilization during prolonged strenuous exercise when fed carbohydrate. *J. Appl. Physiol.* 61(1): 165–172, 1986.
21. Coyle, E.F. and Montain, S.J. Carbohydrate and fluid ingestion during exercise: Are there trade-offs? *Med. Sci. Sports Exer.* 24(6): 671–678, 1992.
22. Cunningham, K.M., Daly, J., Horowitz, M., and Read, N.W. Gastrointestinal adaptation to diets of differing fat composition in human volunteers. *Gut* 32: 483–486, 1991.
23. Cunningham, K.M., Horowitz, M., and Read, N.W. The effect of short-term dietary supplementation with glucose on gastric emptying in humans. *Br. J. Nutr.* 65: 15–19, 1991.
24. Dantzker, D.R. The gastrointestinal tract. The canary of the body? *J. Am. Med. Assoc.* 270(10): 1247–1248, 1993.
25. Darlington, W. and Quastel, J. Absorption of sugars from isolated surviving intestine. *Arch. Biochem.* 43: 194–207, 1953.
26. Dempster, J.A., VanHoek, A.N., DeJong, M.D., and van Os, C.H. Glucose transporters do not serve as water channels in renal and intestinal epithelia. *Eur. J. Physiol.* 419: 249–255, 1991.
27. Duchman, S.M., Bleiler, T.L., Schedl, H.P., Summers, R.W., and Gisolfi, C.V. Effects of gastric function on intestinal composition of oral rehydration solutions. *Med. Sci. Sports Exer.* 22(2): S89, 1990.
28. Eichner, E.R. Gastrointestinal bleeding in athletes. *Physician Sportsmed.* 17(5): 128–140, 1989.
29. Elias, E., Gison, G.J., Greenwood, L.F., Hunt, J.N., and Tripp, J.H. The slowing of gastric emptying by monosaccharides and disaccharides in test meals. *J. Physiol.* 194: 317–326, 1968.
30. Evans, M.A. and Shronts, E.P. Intestinal fuels: Glutamine, short-chain fatty acids, and dietary fiber. *J. Am. Diet Assoc.* 92: 1239–1246, 1992.
31. Ferraris, R.P. and Diamond, J.M. Specific regulation of intestinal nutrient transporters by their dietary substrates. *Annu. Rev. Physiol.* 51: 125–141, 1989.
32. Ferraris, R.P., Yasharpour, S., Lloyd, K.C.K., Mirzayan, R., and Diamond, J.M. Luminal glucose concentrations in the gut under normal conditions. *Am. J. Physiol.* 259: G822–G837, 1990.
33. Fine, K.D., Ana, C.A.S., Porter, J.L., and Fordtran, J.S. Effect of D-glucose on intestinal permeability and its passive absorption in human small intestine in vivo. *Gastroenterology* 105: 1117–1125, 1993.
34. Fordtran, J.S. and Saltin, B. Gastric emptying and intestinal absorption during prolonged severe exercise. *J. Appl. Physiol.* 23(3): 331–335, 1967.
35. Gardner, M.L.G., Illingworth, K.M., Kelleher, J., and Wood, G. Intestinal absorption of the intact peptide carnosine in man, and comparison with intestinal permeability to lactulose. *J. Physiol.* 439: 411–422, 1991.

36. Gisolfi, C.V. and Duchman, S.M. Guidelines for optimal replacement beverages for different athletic events. *Med. Sci. Sports Exer.* 24(6): 679–687, 1992.
37. Gisolfi, C.V., Spranger, K.J., Summers, R.W., Schedl, H.P., and Bleiler, T.L. Effects of cycle exercise on intestinal absorption in humans. *J. Appl. Physiol.* 71(6): 2518–2527, 1991.
38. Gisolfi, C.V., Summers, R., and Schedl, H. Intestinal absorption of fluids during rest and exercise. In: *Perspectives in Exercise Science and Sports Medicine. Fluid Homeostasis During Exercise.* C.V. Gisolfi and D.R. Lamb, Eds. Indianapolis: Benchmark Press, 1990, 129–180.
39. Gisolfi, C.V., Summers, R.W., Schedl, H.P., and Bleiler, T.L. Intestinal water absorption from select carbohydrate solutions in humans. *J. Appl. Physiol.* 73(5): 2142–2150, 1992.
40. Gisolfi, C.V., Summers, R.W., Schedl, H.P., Bleiler, T.L., and Oppliger, R.A. Human intestinal water absorption: Direct vs indirect measurements. *Am. J. Physiol.* 258: G216–G222, 1990.
41. Green, D.W., Gomez, G., and Greeley, G.H. Gastrointestinal peptides. *Gastroenterol. Clin. North Am.* 18(4): 695–719, 1989.
42. Guslandi, M. Nitric oxide: An ubiquitous actor in the gastrointestinal tract. *Dig. Dis.* 2: 28–36, 1994.
43. Harris, A., Lindeman, A.K., and Martin, B.J. Rapid orocecal transit in chronically active persons with high energy intake. *J. Appl. Physiol.* 70(4): 1550–1553, 1991.
44. Hilsted, J., Galbo, H., Sonne, B., Schwartz, T., Fahrenkrug, J., Muckadell, O.B.S.D., Lauritesen, K.H., and Tronier, B. Gastroenteropancreatic hormonal changes during exercise. *Am. J. Physiol.* 239: G136–G140, 1980.
45. Hirschberg, A.L., Lindholm, C., Carlstrom, K., and Schoultz, B.V. Reduced serum cholecystokinin response to food intake in female athletes. *Metabolism* 43(2): 217–222, 1994.
46. Hunt, J.B., Elliott, E.J., Fairclough, P.D., Clark, M.L., and Farthing, M.J.G. Water and solute absorption from hypotonic glucose-electrolyte solutions in human jejunum. *Gut* 33: 479–483, 1992.
47. Hunt, J.B., Thillainayagam, A.V., Salim, A.F.M., Carnaby, S., Elliott, E.J., and Farthing, M.J.G. Water and solute absorption from a new hypotonic oral rehydration solution: Evaluation in human and animal perfusion models. *Gut* 33: 1652–1659, 1992.
48. Hunt, J.N. Mechanisms and disorders of gastric emptying. *Annu. Rev. Med.* 34: 219–229, 1983.
49. Hunt, J.N. and Stubbs, D.F. The volume and energy content of meals as a determinant of gastric emptying. *J. Physiol. London* 245: 209–215, 1975.
50. Karbach, U. Paracellular calcium transport across the small intestine. *J. Nutr.* 122: 672–677, 1992.
51. Kenney, M.J., Flatt, A., Summers, R.W., Brown, C.K., and Gisolfi, C.V. Changes in jejunal myoelectrical activity during exercise in fed untrained dogs. *Am. J. Physiol.* 254: G741–G747, 1988.
52. Khan, M.I., Read, N.W., and Grundy, D. Effect of varying the rate and pattern of gastric distension on its sensory perception and motor activity. *Am. J. Physiol.* 264: G824–G827, 1993.
53. Konturek, S.J. Opiates and the gastrointestinal tract. *Am. J. Gastroenterol.* 74: 285–291, 1980.
54. Konturek, S.J. and Konturek, J.W. Gastric adaptation: Basic and clinical aspects. *Digestion* 55: 131–138, 1994.
55. Lamb, D.R. and Brodowicz, G.R. Optimal use of fluids of varying formulations to minimize exercise-induced disturbances in homeostasis. *Sports Med.* 3: 247–274, 1986.
56. Langkamp-Henken, B., Glezer, J.A., and Kudsk, K.A. Immunologic structure and function of the gastrointestinal tract. *Nutr. Clin. Prac.* 7(3): 100–108, 1992.
57. Leiper, J.B. and Maughan, R.J. Absorption of water and electrolytes from hypotonic, isotonic and hypertonic solutions. *J. Physiol. London* 373: 90P, 1986.

58. Levens, N.R. Control of intestinal absorption by the renin-angiotensin system. *Am. J. Physiol.* 249: G3–G15, 1985.
59. Liddle, R.A., Rushakoff, R.J., Morita, E.T., Beccaria, L., Carter, J.D., and Goldfine, I.D. Physiological role of cholecystokinin in reducing postprandial hyperglycemia in humans. *J. Clin. Invest.* 81: 1675–1681, 1988.
60. Lifshitz, F. and Wapnir, R.A. Oral hydration solutions: experimental optimization of water and sodium absorption. *J. Pediatr.* 106: 383–389, 1985.
61. Lin, H.C., Elashoff, J.D., Gu, Y.-G., and Meyer, J.H. Nutrient feedback inhibition of gastric emptying plays a larger role than osmotically dependent duodenal resistance. *Am. J. Physiol.* 28: G672–G676, 1993.
62. Maggi, C.A. and Meli, A. The sensory-efferent function of capsaicin-sensitive sensory neurons. *Gen. Pharmacol.* 19(1): 1–43, 1988.
63. Maughan, R. Carbohydrate-electrolyte solutions during prolonged exercise. In: *Perspectives in Exercise Science and Sports Medicine*, Ergogenics: Enhancement of Performance in Exercise and Sport. D.R. Lamb and M.H. Williams, Eds. Indianapolis: Benchmark Press, 1991, 35–85.
64. Maughan, R.J., Leiper, J.B., and McGaw, B.A. Effects of exercise intensity on absorption of ingested fluids in man. *Exp. Physiol.* 75: 419–421, 1990.
65. Mei, N. Intestinal chemosensitivity. *Physiol. Rev.* 65: 211–237, 1985.
66. Mitchell, J.B. and Voss, K.W. The influence of volume on gastric emptying and fluid balance during prolonged exercise. *Med. Sci. Sports Exer.* 23(3): 314–319, 1991.
67. Moragas, G., Azpiroz, F., Pavia, J., and Malagelada, J.-R. Relations among intragastric pressure, postcibal perception, and gastric emptying. *Am. J. Physiol.* 264: G1112–G1117, 1993.
68. Moran, R.H. and McHugh, P.R. Distinctions among three sugars in their effects on gastric emptying and satiety. *Am. J. Physiol.* 241: 25–30, 1982.
69. Moseley, P.L. and Gisolfi, C.V. New frontiers in thermoregulation and exercise. *Sports Med.* 16: 163–167, 1993.
70. Moses, F.M. The effect of exercise on the gastrointestinal tract. *Sports Med.* 9(3): 159–172, 1990.
71. Murray, R. The effects of consuming carbohydrate-electrolyte beverages on gastric emptying and fluid absorption during and following exercise. *Sports Med.* 4: 322–351, 1987.
72. Murray, R., Eddy, D.E., Bartoli, W.P., and Paul, G.L. Gastric emptying of water and isocaloric carbohydrate solutions consumed at rest. *Med. Sci. Sports Exer.* 26(6): 725–732, 1994.
73. Neufer, P.D., Young, A.J., and Sawka, M.N. Gastric emptying during exercise: Effects of heat stress and hypohydration. *Eur. J. Appl. Physiol.* 58: 433–439, 1989.
74. Noakes, T.D., Rehrer, N.J., and Maughan, R.J. The importance of volume in regulating gastric emptying. *Med. Sci. Sports Exer.* 23(3): 307–313, 1991.
75. Notivol, R.I. Carrio, L., Cano, L., Estorch, M., and Vilardell, F. Gastric emptying of solid and liquid meals in healthy young subjects. *Scand. J. Gastroenterol.* 8: 1107–1113, 1984.
76. Oektedalen, O., Flaten, O., Opstad, P.K., and Myren, J. hPP and gastrin response to a liquid meal and oral glucose during prolonged severe excercise, caloric deficit, and sleep deprivation. *Scand. J. Gastroenterol.* 17: 619–624, 1982.
77. Oektedalen, O., Lunde, O.C., Opstad, P.K., Aabakken, L., and Kvernebo, K. Changes in the gastrointestinal mucosa after long-distance running. *Scand. J. Gastroenterol.* 27: 270–274, 1992.
78. Owen, M.D., Kregel, K.C., Wall, P.T., and Gisolfi, C.V. Effects of ingesting carbohydrate beverages during exercise in the heat. *Med. Sci. Sports Exer.* 18(5): 568–575, 1986.
79. Pappenheimer, J.R. and Reiss, K.Z. Contribution of solvent drag through intercellular junctions to absorption of nutrients by the small intestine of the rat. *Membrane Biol.* 100: 123–136, 1987.
80. Persson, B.E. and Spring, K.R. Gallbladder epithelial cell hydraulic water permeability and volume regulation. *J. Gen. Physiol.* 79: 481–505, 1982.

81. Qamar, M.I. and Read, A.E. Effects of exercise on mesenteric blood flow in man. *Gut* 28: 583–587, 1987.
82. Rehrer, N.J. The maintenance of fluid balance during exercise. *Int. J. Sports Med.* 15(3): 122–125, 1994.
83. Rehrer, N.J., Beckers, E., Brouns, F., TenHoor, F., and Saris, W.H.M. Exercise and training effects on gastric emptying of carbohydrate beverages. *Med. Sci. Sports Exer.* 21(5): 540–549, 1989.
84. Rehrer, N.J., Beckers, E.J., Brouns, F., TenHoor, F., and Saris, W.H.M. Effects of dehydration on gastric emptying and gastrointestinal distress while running. *Med. Sci. Sports Exer.* 22(6): 790–795, 1990.
85. Robert, A., Varannes, S.B.D., Bizais, Y., Roze, C., and Galmiche, J.-P. Simultaneous assessment of liquid emptying and proximal gastric tone in humans. *Gastroenterology* 105: 667–674, 1993.
86. Robinson, P.H., Clarke, M., and Barrett, J. Determinants of delayed gastric emptying in anorexia nervosa and bulimia nervosa. *Gut* 29: 458–464, 1988.
87. Rosensweig, N.S., Herman, R.H., and Stifel, F.B. Dietary regulation of small intestinal enzyme activity in man. *Am. J. Clin. Nutr.* 24: 65–69, 1971.
88. Rowell, L.B., Blackmon, J.R., and Bruce, R.A. Indocyanine green clearance and estimated hepatic blood flow during mild to maximal exercise in upright man. *J. Clin. Invest.* 43(8): 1677–1690, 1964.
89. Rozsa, Z., Mattila, J., and Jacobson, E.D. Substance P mediates a gastrointestinal thermoreflex in rats. *Gastroenterology* 95: 265–276, 1988.
90. Ryan, A., Lambert, G., Shi, X., Chang, R., Summers, R., and Gisolfi, C. Effect of hypohydration on gastric emptying and intestinal absorption during exercise. *Faseb J.*, 9(3), A292, 1995.
91. Ryan, A.J., Bleiler, T.L., Carter, J.E., and Gisolfi, C.V. Gastric emptying during prolonged cycling exercise in the heat. *Med. Sci. Sports Exer.* 21(1): 51–58, 1989.
92. Sabolic, I., Valenti, G., Verbavatz, J.-M., VanHock, A.N., Verikman, A.S., Ausiello, D.A., and Brown, D. Localization of the CHIP28 water channel in rat kidney. *Am. J. Physiol.* 263: C1225–C1233, 1992.
93. Schedl, H.P., Maughan, R.J., and Gisolfi, C.V. Intestinal absorption during rest and exercise: implications for formulating an oral rehydration solution (ORS). *Med. Sci. Sports Exer.* 26(3): 267–280, 1994.
94. Schiller, L.R., SantaAna, C.A., and Fordtran, J.S. Glucose stimulated Na absorption: Relative contribution of glucose-sodium cotransport and solvent drag during total intestinal perfusion. *Gastroenterology* 100: A702, 1991.
95. Scholer, J.F. and Code, C.F. Rate of absorption of water from stomach and small bowel of human beings. *Gastroenterology* 27(5): 565–577, 1954.
96. Shi, X., Summers, R.W., Schedl, H.P., Chang, R.T., Lambert, G.P., and Gisolfi, C.V. Effects of solution osmolality on absorption of select fluid replacement solutions in human duodenojejunum. *J. Appl. Physiol.* 77(3): 1178–1184, 1994.
97. Shi, X., Summers, R.W., Schedl, H.P., Flanagan, S.W., Chang, R.T., and Gisolfi, C.V. Effects of carbohydrate type and concentration and solution osmolality on water absorption. *Med. Sci. Sports*, 27(12), 1607–1615, 1995.
98. Sjovall, H. Sympathetic control of jejunal fluid and electrolyte transport: an experimental study in cats and rats. *Acta Physiol. Scand. Suppl.* 535: 1–63, 1984.
99. Sladen, G.E. and Dawson, A.M. Interrelationships between the absorptions of glucose, sodium and water by the normal human jejunum. *J. Clin. Sci.* 36: 119–132, 1969.
100. Soffer, E.E., Merchant, R.K., Duethman, G., Launspach, J., Gisolfi, C., and Adrian, T.E. Effect of graded exercise on esophageal motility and gastroesophageal reflux in trained athletes. *Dig. Dis. Sci.* 38(2): 220–224, 1993.
101. Soffer, E.E., Summers, R.W., and Gisolfi, C. The effect of exercise on intestinal motility and transit in trained athletes. *Am. J. Physiol.* 260(G698–G702): 1991.

102. Spiller, R.C., Trotman, I.F., Adrian, T.E., Bloom, S.R., Misiewicz, J.J., and Silk, D.B.A. Further characterisation of the "ileal brake" reflex in man — Effect of ileal infusion of partial digests of fat, protein, and starch on jejunal motility and release of neurotensin, enteroglucagon, and peptide YY. *Gut* 29: 1042–1051, 1988.
103. Sullivan, S.N., Chamption, M.C., Christofides, N.D., Adrian, T.E., and Bloom, S.R. Gastrointestinal regulatory peptide responses in long-distance runners. *Phys. Sportsmed.* 12(7): 77–82, 1984.
104. Takamata, A., Mack, G.W., Gillen, C.M., Jozsi, A.C., and Nadel, E.R. Acute recovery of osmotically inhibited sweating in humans by drinking. *FASEB* 8(4): A65, 1994.
105. Tapper, E.J. Local modulation of intestinal ion transport by enteric neurons. *Am. J. Physiol.* 244: G457–G468, 1983.
106. Thoren, P., Floras, J.S., Hoffmann, P., and Seals, D.R. Endorphins and exercise: Physiological mechanisms and clinical implications. *Med. Sci. Sports Exer.* 22: 417–428, 1990.
107. Wapnir, R.A. and Lifshitz, F. Osmolality and solute concentration — Their relationship with an oral hydration solution effectiveness: An experimental assessment. *Pediatr. Res.* 19: 894–898, 1985.
108. Wapnir, R.A., Litov, R.E., Zdanowicz, M.M., and Lifshitz, F. Improved water and sodium absorption from oral rehydration solutions based on rice syrup in a rat model of osmotic diarrhea. *J. Pediatr.* 118: S53–S61, 1991.
109. Williams, J.H., Mager, M., and Jacobson, E.D. Relationship of mesenteric blood flow to intestinal absorption of carbohydrates. *J. Lab. Clin. Med.* 63(5): 853–863, 1964.

Chapter 3

HORMONAL CONTROL OF BODY FLUID VOLUME

_____ Charles E. Wade

CONTENTS

I. Introduction..53

II. Water and Electrolyte Balance During Exercise 54
   A. Fluid Loss 54
   B. Electrolyte Loss..54
   C. Blood Volume Redistribution 55
   D. Thirst 55

III. Hormonal Responses to Exercise...........................55
   A. Catecholamines 56
   B. Arginine Vasopressin...................................57
   C. Atrial Natriuretic Peptide 63
   D. Renin–Angiotensin–Aldosterone Axis 64
   E. Modifying Factors......................................65

IV. Summary and Conclusions.................................67

References 69

I. INTRODUCTION

Hormones play a major role in the maintenance of fluid and electrolyte homeostasis during and following exercise. A variety of hormones modulate the distribution and conservation of fluids during exercise, and following exercise in the replacement of lost fluid and electrolytes. The loss of fluids and electrolytes during exercise is primarily via sweating and subsequently voluntary dehydration. The aim of this chapter is to describe the responses to exercise of the various hormones important in the maintenance of fluid and electrolyte homeostasis, and subsequently blood volume. Their regulation and actions will also be presented. Of interest are the hormones arginine vasopressin (AVP), atrial natriuretic peptide (ANP), the renin–angiotensin–aldosterone axis, and catecholamines. These hormones play major roles in the handling of fluid and electrolytes by the kidney, distribution of blood volume, and thirst.

II. WATER AND ELECTROLYTE BALANCE DURING EXERCISE

A. FLUID LOSS

During exercise there is a net loss of fluids and electrolytes that is tolerated until the bout of exercise is completed. The loss of fluid occurs via sweating necessitated by the increase in body heat associated with the performance of exercise. Even with access to fluids, moderate exercise at about 70% of maximum will result in a decrease in body weight of approximately 930 gm/h.[4,61,69] It is presumed that this loss in body weight is reflective of the loss in total body water. In a 70 kg human with a total body water of 48 l, this loss represents a 2% reduction. This loss is referred to as "voluntary dehydration" because it is tolerated even when supplemental fluids are provided.[28] The voluntary dehydration represents about 20–30% of the total loss of fluids. That is, only 70–80% of the fluids are replaced when access to fluids is provided. The inability to replace the fluid loss appears to be a conflict in the factors modulating thirst: plasma osmolality and blood volume.[15,42,49] That is, the rapid replacement with water dilutes plasma osmolality and expands blood volume. The primary drives for thirst, an increase in plasma osmolality and a decrease in blood volume, are then attenuated. Thus, full replacement is delayed as equilibration is achieved between the various body fluid compartments. The deficit in total body water is usually replaced within 24 h if access to fluids is available.[69]

B. ELECTROLYTE LOSS

There is a loss of electrolytes via the sweat as well. Although the concentration of electrolytes is low (hypotonic) in sweat compared to plasma, with sweat rates as high as 1500 ml/h the loss of solutes is significant. For example the concentration of sodium in sweat is 60 meq/l.[16,72] Thus, in an hour there would be a loss of 90 meq of sodium, or 3% of total body sodium. Most electrolytes present in sweat have a net loss in total body content with exercise. The net loss in the body levels is not reflected in the plasma, which shows an increase in concentrations of electrolytes as the loss of water exceeds that of solutes. Following exercise the plasma levels of sodium may increase from 140 to 145 meq/l, while osmolality is increased from 290 to over

300 mOsm/kg.[67] For this reason the net loss in total body solute during exercise is often not appreciated. Further, the replacement of solutes is not as rapid as water, and repeated daily exercise can exacerbate the condition.[69]

C. BLOOD VOLUME REDISTRIBUTION

With exercise there is a redistribution of the blood volume. This is necessitated by a variety of factors, such as metabolic demands and thermal loads in individual vascular beds.[16,17,50] During exercise there is usually a shift of blood flow away from the splanchnic region to active muscles and the heart.[39] This results in a three- to ten fold increase in blood flow to active muscles.[56] These changes in the distribution of cardiac output are predominantly due to alterations of local vascular resistance. Changes in resistance are due to local metabolic demands and the autonomic nervous system; however, hormones also play a role.[39,56] This redistribution of blood volume allows the maintenance of the "effective blood volume" compensating in part for the losses due to exercise.

D. THIRST

As mentioned above, fluid intake is a major component in the maintenance of fluid and electrolyte homeostasis during exercise.[41] When measured following exercise, there in an increase in thirst — the subjective sensation motivating the seeking and drinking of fluids.[61] There are a variety of factors that modulate thirst.[49] Some of these factors, such as plasma osmolality and blood volume, are regulated by hormones. Furthermore, hormones may have a direct effect on thirst. Another mechanism to maintain fluid balance is to decrease losses. This is done by decreasing the excretion by the kidneys of fluid and electrolytes, and to some extent altering the composition of sweat.[70,71,77] Hormones play major roles in these compensatory responses.

III. HORMONAL RESPONSES TO EXERCISE

Hormonal regulation of excretion by the kidneys and stimulation of intake both attenuate decreases in total body water and electrolytes during, and rectify losses after exercise. The actions of the hormones are assumed to be determined by the concentration of the hormones in blood. The concentration of a hormone is the product of the amount presently circulating, the quantity released, and the rate of metabolic clearance. During exercise, plasma concentrations of the hormones of interest are reported to be increased, and the reason for this may be the product of changes in both release and clearance. Further, a decrease in total body water during exercise reduces the volume of distribution for the hormones and would result in an increase in concentration if release were constant. During exercise, a number of changes may be contributing to the alteration in the plasma concentrations of hormones.

In recent years there have been numerous extensive reviews of the response of hormones to exercise.[20,24,58,62,65,68,70,71,77] For this reason, in the present chapter an overview is presented, and the focus is on new data as to the response, regulation, and actions of the hormones during exercise.

A. CATECHOLAMINES

Hormones of the sympathetic nervous system respond to exercise and play a major role in the redistribution of blood (fluid) during exercise.[5,23,59] Of prime interest is the effect of catecholamines on renal blood flow, which represents about 20% of the cardiac output at rest but is greatly reduced during exercise. Catecholamines also modulate metabolism, and the release of renin.[24,64,65]

The two hormones of interest are norepinephrine, released predominantly from the sympathetic nervous system, and epinephrine, derived from the adrenal medulla. Norepinephrine and epinephrine function in concert and are often referred to as the sympathoadrenal system. These hormones have resting plasma concentrations of 200–500 pg/ml for norepinephrine and 70–120 pg/ml for epinephrine.[23,24,59] In response to exercise, there is a progressive increase in both hormones (Figure 1).[23,24] Norepinephrine during maximal exercise may attain levels as high as 2000 pg/ml, a fourfold increase. Epinephrine reaches plasma concentration of up to 700 pg/ml following maximal exercise. These increases are not sustained and basal resting levels are attained within 30 min of completion of exercise.

Pharmacological blockade of the actions of sympathoadrenal hormones has elucidated a variety of actions. To demonstrate the role of catecholamines in the modulation of metabolism, blockade of beta receptors attenuates the response of plasma glucose, free fatty acids, and lactate to submaximal exercise.[65] Blockade also reduces heart rate at any given workload and may decrease blood pressure. These changes are associated with a reduced response of the renin–angiotensin system to exercise.[75] Sweat rate during exercise has been found to be unchanged or reduced with beta blockade.[1,36] Thus, blockade of the sympathoadrenal hormones results in a variety of changes in responses to exercise.

As mentioned earlier, a major role of catecholamines is the redistribution of blood flow during exercise.[2,50] It is often assumed that the shunting or diversion of blood from the kidneys is important in the cardiovascular adjustments to exercise.[4,31,77] However, the total amount of blood diverted is relatively small. The decrease is on the order of 300 ml/min, or less than 2% of the cardiac output during exercise. However, this change is a significant event for the kidneys, representing a 40–50% decrease in renal blood flow.[77] Recent work by Tidegren and colleagues[64] has demonstrated a relationship during exercise between the increase in catecholamines and renal blood flow reduction as well as the increase in renin release (Figure 2). When performing bicycle ergometer exercise in the supine position at workloads of 30, 60, and 80–90% of maximum, a progressive increase in arterial catecholamine concentrations and in norepinephrine overflow from the kidneys occurs. Norepinephrine overflow is believed to be indicative of the amount of norepinephrine released into the circulation from a circulatory bed, in this case the kidneys. The increase in catacholamine levels was correlated with an increase in renal vascular resistance and a reduction in renal venous blood flow (RVBF) (Figure 2).[64] The decrease in RVBF was 41%, from 639 ml/min at rest to 377 ml/min at the highest workload. This represents a significant reduction in the delivery of fluid to nephrons contributing to a reduction in glomerular filtration rate (GFR) and the conservation of fluid and electrolytes (Figure 3).

Catecholamines modulate the release of renin from the kidney. Renin is important in the regulation of angiotensin II (AII) and subsequently aldosterone (ALDO) release. During exercise, the blockade of catecholamine receptors reduces the response of renin to exercise.[3,30,76] The increase in catecholamines during exercise is correlated with the increase in renin (Figure 2).[64] The increase in catecholamines during exercise, via their actions contributing to a decrease in renal blood flow and increase in renin release (see below), contribute to the maintenance of fluid and electrolyte homeostasis.

B. ARGININE VASOPRESSIN

AVP is an octapeptide produced in the hypothalamus and stored in the posterior pituitary.[74] It is also referred to as antidiuretic hormone (ADH). Basal levels in the plasma range from 1 to 4 pg/ml. In response to maximal exercise, plasma concentrations increase four- to sixfold.[8,67,68,70] This increase may be sustained for 30 min following exercise. In response to submaximal exercise, the increase in AVP is variable. In most studies the increase in AVP during exercise is related to the intensity of the exercise (Figure 1).[60] There appears to be a threshold for the increase in AVP with increases noted at work intensities of 60–70% of maximum.[66,68] In a recent study Freund and co-workers[22] also report an increase in AVP to be related to the intensity of the exercise. Of note was their observation of a decrease in plasma AVP concentrations at a workload of 25% and subsequent increases at 60 and 100% of maximal exercise.

The increase in AVP during exercise appears to be due to the increase in plasma osmolality and a decrease in blood volume.[68] With exercise there is a reduction in blood volume of up to 7%.[7,8,29] In response to hemorrhage, the release of AVP is exponentially related to the decrease in blood volume.[52,74] However, the increase in blood pressure, as sensed by arterial baroreceptors, during exercise may provide a negative input as high-pressure baroreceptors are the prime sensors of the decrease in blood volume. This hypothesis is supported by the finding that in cardiac transplant patients the AVP response to maximal exercise is exaggerated.[46] Further, in the work of Freund et al.[22] the reduction in AVP at low work intensity was suggested to be due to an acute increase in blood volume at the onset of exercise. This may be related

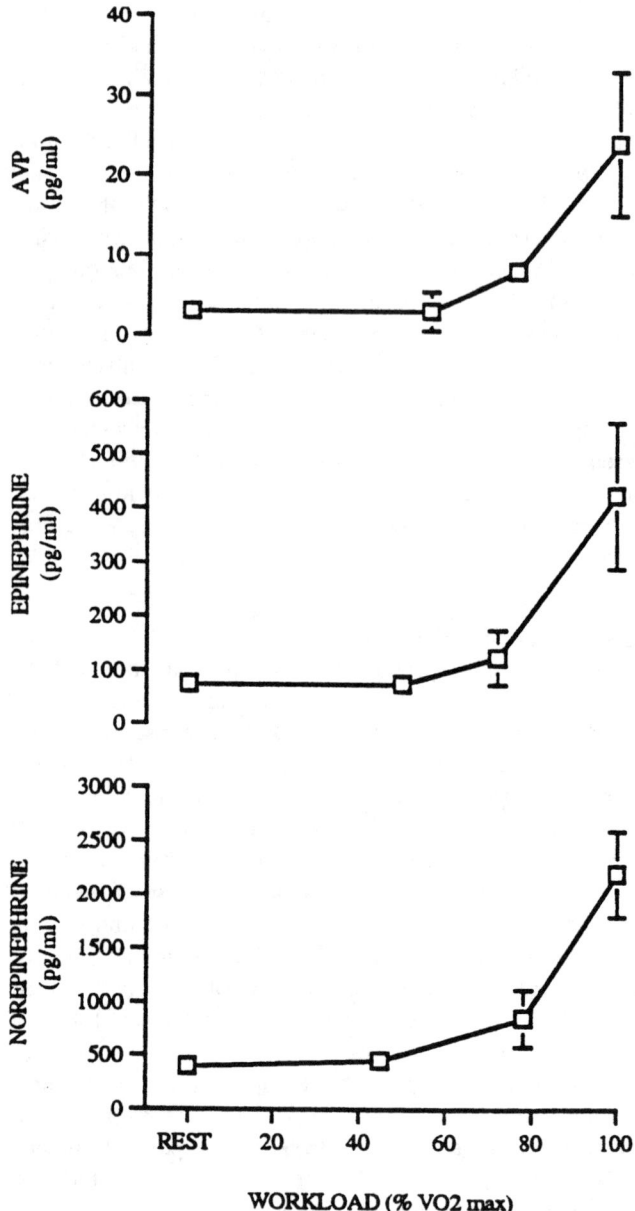

FIGURE 1 Responses of plasma vasopressin (AVP), norepinephrine, epinephrine, atrial natriuretic peptide (ANP), aldosterone (ALDO), and renin activity (PRA) to graded exercise of short duration on a bicycle ergometer. As work intensity is increased, there are significant

to low-pressure baroreceptors. In a study where the responses to bicycle ergometer exercise were assessed in air and during water immersion, plasma

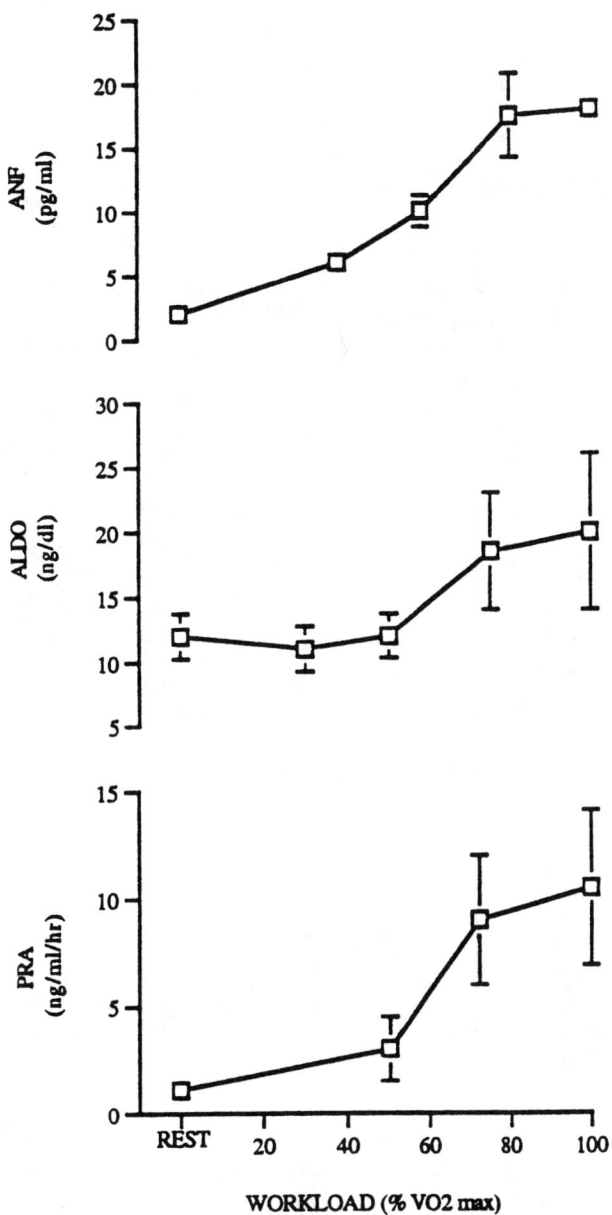

FIGURE 1 (continued) increases in all of the hormones. The increases occur above a threshold work intensity.[27,64] (Values are means ± SE. Redrawn from data in References 23, 24, and 60.)

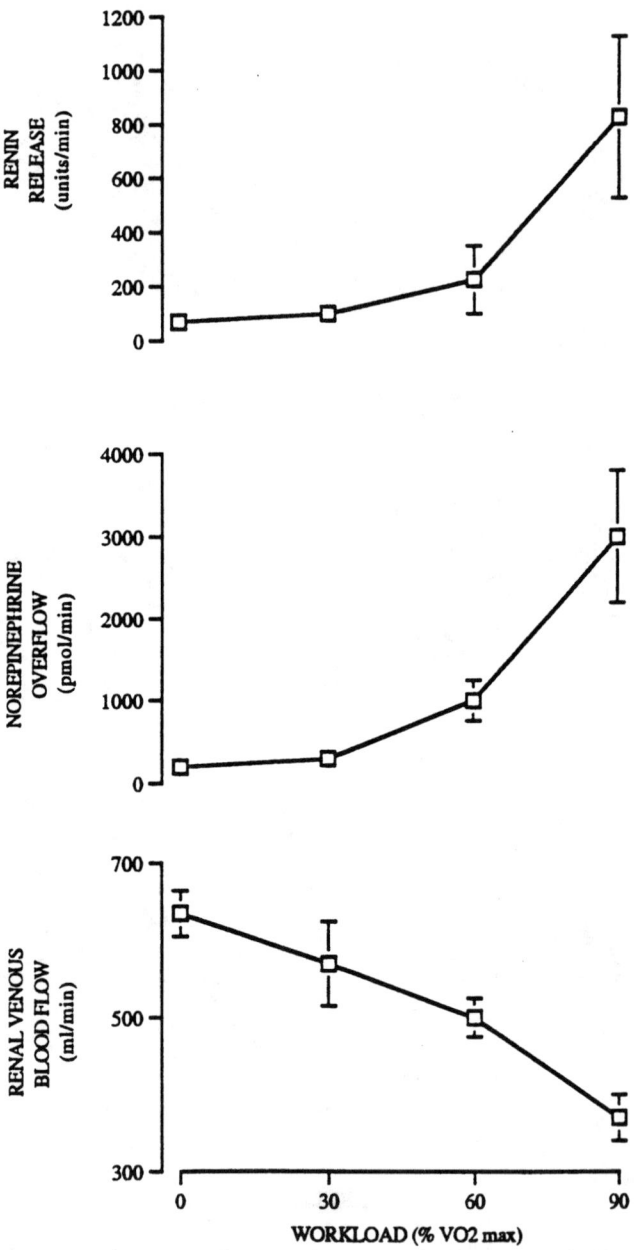

FIGURE 2 Effect of increasing work intensity on a supine bicycle ergometer on renal venous blood flow, norepinephrine overflow, and renin release. With the increase in work intensity, there is an increase in norepinephrine overflow, indicative of an increase in renal sympathetic nerve activity, which appears to contribute to the decrease in renal venous blood flow and the increase in release of renin (Values are means ± SE. Redrawn from data in Reference 64.)

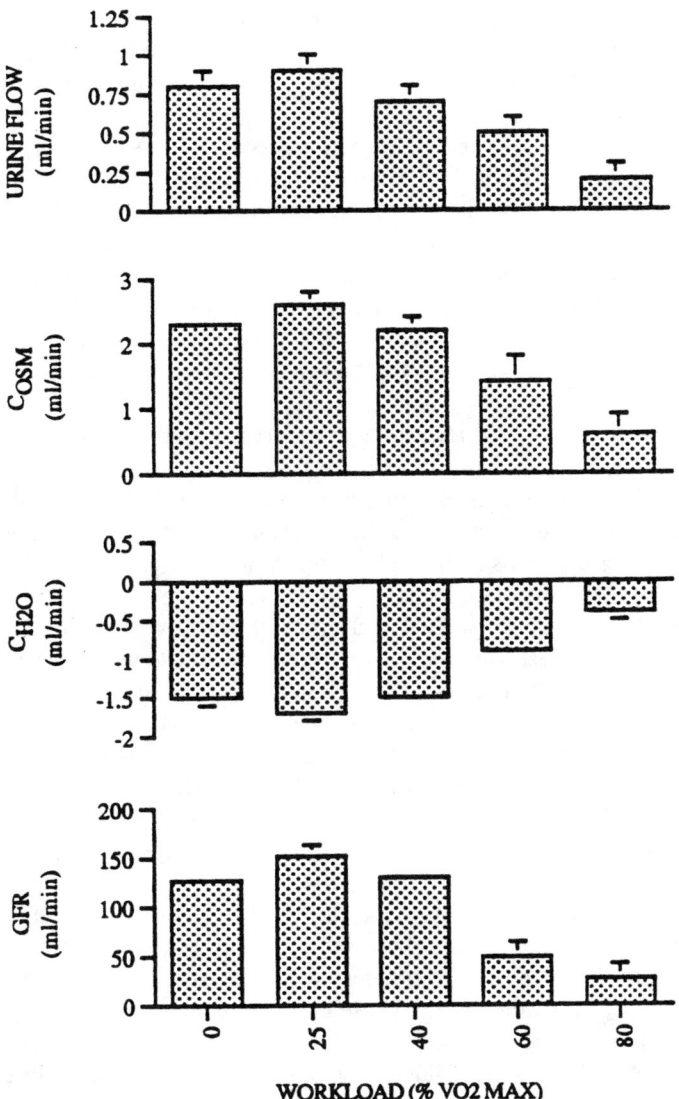

FIGURE 3 Change in urine flow, osmotic clearance (C_{osm}), free water clearance (C_{H2O}), and glomerular filtration rate (GFR) in response to increasing work intensities on a bicycle ergometer. With the increase in work intensity urine flow is decreased due to a reduction in GFR and C_{osm}. However, C_{H2O} is increased (less negative) contributing to an increase in urine flow. The net effect is a reduction in urine flow rates with increasing work intensity. (Values are means ± SE. Redrawn from the data of in Reference 22.)

AVP levels were reduced with immersion.[53] The decrease in the AVP response to exercise occurred with no differences in plasma osmolality noted between treatments and was presumed to be the result of expansion of the central blood volume altering stimulation of low-pressure baroreceptors and atrial stretch. In conclusion, the increase in AVP may in part be related to alterations in blood volume during exercise as sensed by high- and low-pressure baroreceptors.

AVP responds to increases in plasma osmolality in a linear manner once a threshold is exceeded.[74] With maximum treadmill exercise, there is an increase in plasma osmolality from resting levels of about 290 to over 300 mOsm/kg.[67] However, the AVP levels observed during exercise exceed those associated with the increases in plasma osmolality alone.[68] Although the increase in plasma osmolality accounts for the majority of the increase in AVP during exercise, other factors must be considered. These other factors include an increase in AII, elevation in body temperature, and psychological changes.[54,68]

The increase in AVP levels during exercise was believed to account partially for the decrease in urine output.[4,32] In resting subjects, urine output is closely related to the plasma concentration of AVP.[74] This decrease is due to a decrease in free water clearance (an increase in tubular water reabsorption). During exercise there is an increase in free water clearance (Figure 3).[22,47,67,77] The reason for the increase in urinary water loss in the presence of an increased AVP level during exercise is not clear. Following exercise may be another situation. The increase in AVP incurred during exercise may have an effect at this time. However, the increase in free water clearance is present for an hour after exercise, well after resting AVP levels are attained.

AVP also has been suggested to modulate extrarenal water loss. The increase in AVP has been related to alterations in the rate and composition of sweat when injected at the site of the gland.[14,26] However, this has not been confirmed during exercise because sweat rate has not been related to changes in plasma AVP levels.

Increases in AVP with exercise may play a role in the modulation of the arterial baroreflex, and thus the sensing of changes in blood volume. In exercising swine, blockade of AVP attenuated the increase in mean arterial pressure and increased cardiac output.[56] These changes demonstrate a role for AVP in the alterations in vascular resistance during exercise. Further, Stebbins[55] has demonstrated that AVP modulates the sympathetic response to brief muscle contractions. It was suggested that this change may be mediated via an effect of AVP on the arterial baroreflex. AVP appears to contribute to the cardiovascular responses to exercise.

Although AVP increases during exercise, it does not appear to influence fluid and electrolyte homeostasis directly. AVP may modulate the sensed reduction in blood volume during exercise and therefore have a role in the conservation of fluids following exercise.

C. ATRIAL NATRIURETIC PEPTIDE

ANP is released from the atria in response to distension associated with increases in atrial volume or filling pressure.[20] ANP is proposed to increase the excretion of sodium with an accompanying increase in water excretion. An increase in ANP during exercise should result in a loss of both fluid and electrolytes.

At rest, reported concentrations of ANP are variable due to difference in the techniques used for measurements. When assayed following extraction, values range from 10 to 40 pg/ml.[20,69] With maximal exercise, plasma concentrations of ANP may reach 100 pg/ml. During acute bouts of exercise, the plasma concentrations of ANP are related to the intensity of the exercise (Figure 1).[60] The increase with exercise appears to be transient. With submaximal exercise there is an initial increase, but with longer duration exercise ANP values return to resting levels or decrease.[20,71] Basal levels are also attained within 1 h after the completion of exercise.

The factor modulating the increase in ANP during exercise is believed to be an increase in atrial pressure.[20] At initiation of exercise there is an increase in atrial pressure.[44,50] However, as exercise continues and there is a redistribution of fluid (cardiovascular drift), atrial pressure is decreased.[50] This may explain the transient nature of the ANP response to exercise of long duration. Nose and co-workers[44] recently found the increase in ANP levels during exercise in the heat to be related to an increase in right atrial pressure at the onset of exercise (10 min) and to other factors after this period. Of note is the recent study of patients who had undergone cardiac transplant.[46] In response to maximal exercise there was a greater increase in ANP compared to control, suggesting the response is independent of cardiac innervation and is the result of mechanical distension of the atrium or other factors.

ANP has been shown to produce a diuresis due to an increase in the excretion of sodium, a natriuresis.[11,73] However, the plasma levels demonstrating this response are well beyond those attained with exercise. Further, with high-intensity exercise the renal responses, antidiuresis and conservation of sodium, are in contrast to the actions of ANP. With low-intensity exercise there is an increase in ANP, at which time there is a trend for an increase in urine flow rate and excretion of solutes, presumably sodium.[22,44] Increases in ANP during exercise may also modulate the release and actions of other hormones.[11,37,38] The release of AVP in response to a decrease in blood volume or an increase in plasma osmolality is reduced in the presence of elevated ANP levels.[10] Further, the infusion of ANP decreases plasma levels of PRA and ALDO. Of note is that all of these hormones have actions contrary to those of ANP. Though there is an increase in plasma concentrations during exercise, the actions of ANP in the maintenance of fluid and electrolyte homeostasis are not clear.

D. RENIN–ANGIOTENSIN–ALDOSTERONE AXIS

In the kidney, the enzyme renin is released from the juxtaglomerular apparatus and converts angiotensinogen to angiotensin I (AI).[48] In the lungs, AI is transformed to AII by angiotensin-converting enzyme. AII is a powerful vasopressor, modulates release of ALDO, and is dipsogenic. ALDO, from the adrenal cortex, has a profound effect on the conservation of sodium, and subsequently water, by the kidneys. This cascade is potentiated during exercise and is important in the maintenance of fluid and electrolyte homeostasis.[70,71]

Plasma renin measurements are usually presented as a function of its ability to convert angiotensinogen, and is referred to as plasma renin activity (PRA). At rest PRA ranges from 0.5 to 2.0 ng AI/ml/h. Following maximal exercise, values of 4.0–6.0 ng AI/ml/h are obtained.[70] With increases in exercise intensity, above a threshold of 60–70% of maximum, there are increases in PRA and renin levels (Figures 1 and 2).[27,60,64,66] Exercise duration affects the response of PRA. The performance of long-duration exercise may produce PRA levels that exceed those observed following acute maximal exercise.

The increase in AII with exercise is closely correlated with the increase in renin.[64] During exercise, the response of AII to intensity and duration is the same as those observed for PRA. Resting plasma levels of AII are on the order of 15–25 ng/l and reach values of 130–160 ng/l with maximal exercise.

With exercise, there is an increase in the steroid ALDO, which is in part modulated by AII.[48] At rest, plasma levels are highly variable being influenced by the history of sodium intake and the time of day. Resting plasma concentrations range from 3 to 30 ng/dl.[70] Following maximal exercise, values are 3 to 4 times higher than those at rest (Figure 1).[60] Exercise duration also affects the response of ALDO, with longer durations resulting in higher levels. Furthermore, this elevation may persist for hours after the completion of exercise.[61] With very heavy exercise, elevated plasma ALDO concentrations have been reported for days.[69]

The release of renin and ensuing increase in AII are regulated primarily by sympathetic nervous activity during exercise. As noted earlier, norepinephrine overflow is indicative of the sympathetic activity of the kidney. This is correlated with the increase in renin and plasma renin activity during increasing work intensities (Figure 2).[64] This is further supported by studies employing beta blockade which decreased the response to exercise.[3,30,76] The increase in sympathetic nerve activity during exercise has been addressed above in the discussion of catecholamines. The accompanying increase in AII may provide a negative feedback to renin release. Infusion of AII during exercise attenuated the increase in PRA.[13] AVP has also been demonstrated to have a negative effect on the release of renin,[48] but this has yet to be investigated during exercise. The primary modulator of the release of renin and AII during exercise therefore appears to be sympathetic nerve activity.

The increase in AII during exercise is the principal regulator of ALDO release.[40,70,71] Production of ALDO may also be increased. The increase in ALDO during exercise is closely correlated with the increase in the renin–angiotensin system, but other factors may be involved. These factors include an increase in ACTH, which occurs during exercise, and changes in plasma levels of sodium and potassium. The role of these factors in the regulation of ALDO during exercise is not clear.[35,70]

The renin–angiotensin–aldosterone axis plays a major role in the regulation of fluid and electrolyte balance during exercise. AII, besides stimulating the release of ALDO, may contribute by modulating fluid intake.[49,57] AII has been demonstrated to be a powerful dipsogen, especially in the presence of a reduction of extracellular water. Nose et al.[43] found that with exercise, the degree of rehydration was related to the decrease in plasma volume and to the increase in PRA. Inasmuch as the increase in PRA could be caused by the reduction in plasma volume, it is difficult to assess the role of the renin–angiotensin axis in thirst. However, when the subjects ingested saltwater, which resulted in a greater decrease in PRA compared to the rectification of plasma volume, satiety was achieved at a higher volume of rehydration. These data suggest a possible role for the renin–angiotensin system in fluid replacement.

AII may alter renal function during exercise by constriction of the efferent arterioles. During exercise, there is a decrease in renal blood flow due to constriction of the afferent arterioles by catecholamines from the sympathetic nervous system. The reduction in GFR should be proportional to this decrease, but it is not. The increase in the filtration fraction during exercise is indicative of this change.[4,77] This may be due in part to efferent vasoconstriction by AII maintaining filtration pressure and thus GRF. There are conflicting findings as to this idea. If true, AII would be contributing to an increased loss of fluid and electrolytes during exercise.

Elevation of ALDO concentration during exercise is related to an increase in renal sodium reabsorption, and with it water.[9,40,61,69] This effect persists for hours after the completion of exercise and the return of ALDO to resting levels.[61,69] In addition, Takamata and colleagues[61] found plasma levels of ALDO to increase 17 h after exercise in the heat and to be associated with a reduction in the excretion of sodium. This increase in ALDO corresponded to an increase in the palatability of salt solutions. During this period the increase in "sodium appetite" could contribute to replacement of fluid and electrolytes following exercise.[57,61] The increase in ALDO may also reduce losses via sweat as well.[6,33]

E. MODIFYING FACTORS

Various factors significantly affect hormonal responses to exercise and should be considered when comparing results between studies and in the design of studies to assess responses.

The *mode of exercise* greatly affects responses. For example, with maximal exercise on a treadmill PRA is increased by a factor of 6, and by only 3 when exercise is performed on a bicycle ergometer.[70]

Exercise duration influences the response of hormones to exercise. For example, long-duration submaximal exercise results in plasma catecholamine levels similar to those attained with short-duration maximal exercise.[23] With submaximal exercise, 70% of maximum, at 20 min AVP is not increased, but is elevated at 60 min to concentrations similar to those seen with maximal exercise.[67]

Environment may also affect hormonal responses. At an altitude of 4350 m, the response of PRA to maximal bicycle ergometer exercise was decreased from 5.1 ng AI/ml/h at sea level to 3.5 ng AI/ml/h.[3] ALDO responses are also attenuated, attaining concentrations of 0.39 nmol/l at altitude compared to 0.53 nmol/l at sea level.

The *hydration status* of the subject may influence hormonal responses.[41] Prior ingestion of water, 30 min before exercise, reduces the AVP response to maximal exercise by 65%.[67]

Age and gender of the subjects play a role in the responses of hormones to exercise. In older subjects (age 47) the ANP response to a 10-km run is exaggerated, 104 pg/ml, compared to young subjects (age 28), 43 pg/ml.[21] In women, hormonal responses may be influenced by menstrual status.[12] Resting plasma ALDO concentrations are elevated during the midluteal phase of the cycle and the response to exercise is exaggerated.

The *body position* in which the exercise is performed influences hormonal responses. In comparing upright and supine bicycle ergometry performed at 40–50% of maximum for 20 min, ALDO levels were increased by 90 and 49%, respectively.[75]

Diet and alteration of sleep patterns modify hormonal response to exercise. In subjects deprived of sleep for 3 days and given minimal food, the increase in ALDO concentration in response to exercise was doubled.[45]

The presence of *disease* may alter responses to exercise. In subjects with Type 1 diabetes, in the presence of hypoglycemia, the response of catecholamines to 60 min of exercise at 60–65% of maximum on a bicycle ergometer was attenuated by 50% compared to hypoglycemic control subjects.[51]

Exercise *training* does not affect final hormone concentrations in response to maximal exercise.[18,66] This is a result of the hormones' responses being related to relative workloads. Thus, at a given absolute workload the trained individual would have lower hormone levels. Other factors may be altered with training.[8,18,19] For example, trained subjects have an increased blood volume at rest, yet the AVP concentrations are not different from untrained values.[8] Further, following maximal exercise, trained subjects have a lower plasma osmolality compared to untrained subjects, yet the plasma AVP levels and changes in plasma volume are not different.[18] These findings suggest that training may increase the sensitivity of AVP to changes in osmolality and decrease the response to alterations in blood volume.

Of particular importance in the study of hormone responses to exercise is modulation by *fluid intake*. An oral pharyngeal reflex has been identified that results in the reduction of hormone concentrations prior to the absorption of fluid across the gut (Figure 4).[25,63] For example, a decrease in AVP occurs in a matter of minutes and is independent of changes in plasma osmolality or blood volume/pressure. Therefore, the intake of fluids before, during, or following exercise may alter the responses of the hormones to exercise via this reflex as well as by attenuation of the decrease in blood volume.[15,41,42,43] The ingestion of fluids (progressive rehydration) during exercise of long duration in the heat attenuates or negates the increase in hormones.[15] Fluid ingestion immediately following exercise returns AVP levels to control values.[6] Plasma ALDO attained basal levels, but was again increased 17 hours after exercise. The increase of plasma ALDO is similar to that seen after heavy bouts of daily exercise. Of note is that thirst, which is subjective, was also decreased upon the ingestion of fluids and increased 17 h after exercise, along with an increase in salt appetite. Thus, during and following exercise the intake of fluids may modulate hormone responses.

In summary, hormonal responses to exercise may be modified by a variety of factors, many of which are covered in greater detail in other chapters.

IV. SUMMARY AND CONCLUSIONS

In response to exercise, plasma hormone concentrations are increased. The elevation of hormones with short-duration exercise is related to the intensity of the exercise above 60% of maximum. Below work of this intensity some hormones, AVP for example, may be decreased or not changed, while ANP is increased. The duration of the exercise greatly influences the hormonal responses, with higher plasma concentrations observed for most hormones. In the case of ANP, values may decrease over time. There are also a number of factors, such as the type of exercise or hydration status of the subjects, which modify hormonal responses to exercise. The increase in plasma hormones appears to be related to the decrease in effective blood volume and the increase in plasma osmolality. These factors modulate the release of the hormones via baroreceptors and osmoreceptors. During exercise, the maintenance of fluid and electrolyte homeostasis appears to be predominantly by physical factors, with decreasing renal blood flow resulting in a reduction in GFR. This decrease in GFR results in a reduced delivery to the tubule and an increase in transit time facilitating reabsorption. The changes in renal blood flow are due to the increase in catecholamine and AII levels with exercise. These hormones both increase renal vascular resistance, but are acting in conflict with each other in modulating GFR. However, the net result is a decrease in urine flow rate. This is also partially due to the increase in the reabsorption of electrolytes. The increased reabsorption of electrolytes is facilitated by an increase in tubular transit time, as mentioned

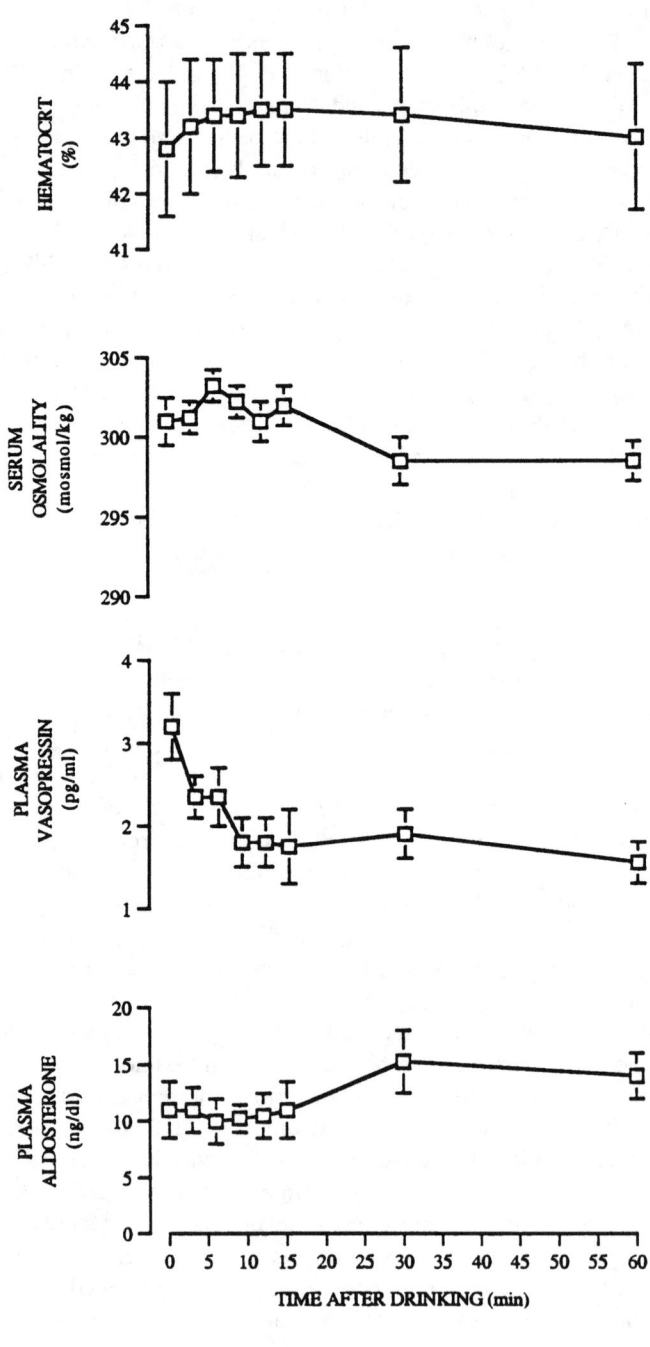

FIGURE 4

FIGURE 4 Plasma vasopressin, aldosterone, osmolality and hematocrit responses to water ingestion following 24 h of fluid restriction. Plasma vasopressin is decreased within minutes of water consumption. This decrease precedes a decrease in plasma osmolality, or an increase in blood volume as indicated by an absence a change in hematocrit. Plasma aldosterone is increased 30 min after fluid ingestion when osmolality is decreased and blood volume is expanded. These findings demonstrate the oral pharyngeal reflex and its possible influence on hormonal responses to exercise if fluids are ingested during exercise. (Values are means ± SE. Redrawn from the data in Reference 25.)

previously, and an increase in ALDO concentrations. With exercise there is an increase in free water clearance even though AVP is increased. The reason for the failure of an increase in AVP to result in a concentrated urine is not clear. The increase in AVP during exercise may have other roles such as modulation of vascular resistance and alteration of responsiveness of the arterial baroreflex. The elevation of ANP is also an anomaly. The increase in ANP and the reduction of AVP during exercise at low work intensities may account for the trend of an increase in urine flow rates; however, the continued elevation of ANP with higher work intensities does not appear to have a function in the maintenance of fluid and electrolyte homeostasis during exercise. Hormones may alter the loss of fluid and electrolytes in the sweat and modulate thirst thus stimulating fluid intake. The exact functions of hormones on these processes during exercise are not clear. In summary, while hormones, normally important at rest in the regulation of fluid and electrolyte balance, are elevated during exercise, their functions in the regulation of blood volume are modified and are still being defined.

REFERENCES

1. Allen, J. A., Jenkinson, D. J., and Roddie, I. C., The effect of beta-adrenoceptor blockade on human sweating, *Br. J. Pharmacol.*, 47:487, 1972.
2. Baer, P. G. and McGiff, J. C., Hormonal systems and renal hemodynamics, *Annu. Rev. Physiol.*, 42:589, 1980.
3. Bouissou, P., Richalet, J.-P., Galen, F. X., Lartigue, M., Larmignat, P., Devaux, F., Durban, C., and Keromes, A., Effect of β-adrenoceptor blockade on renin-aldosterone and a-ANF during exercise at altitude, *J. Appl. Physiol.*, 67:141, 1989.
4. Castenfors, J., Renal function during exercise, *Acta Physiol. Scand. Suppl.*, 70:1, 1967.
5. Clutter, W. E., Bier, D. M., Shad, S. D., and Cryer, P. E., Epinephrine plasma metabolic clearance rates and physiologic thresholds for metabolic and hemodynamic actions in man, *J. Clin. Invest.*, 66:94, 1980.
6. Collins, K. J., Action of exogenous aldosterone on the secretion and composition of drug-induced sweat, *Clin. Sci.*, 30:207, 1969.
7. Convertino, V. A., Keil, L. C., and Bernauer, E. M., Plasma volume, osmolality, vasopressin, and renin activity during graded exercise in man, *J. Appl. Physiol.*, 50:123, 1981.
8. Convertino, V. A., Keil, L. C., and Greenleaf, J. E., Plasma volume, renin and vasopressin responses to graded exercise after training, *J. Appl. Physiol.*, 54:508, 1983.
9. Costill, D. L., Branam, G., Fink, W., and Nelson, R., Exercise induced sodium conservation: Changes in plasma renin and aldosterone, *Med. Sci. Sports*, 8:209, 1976.
10. Crandall, M. E. and Gregg, C. M., *In vitro* evidence for an inhibitory effect of atrial natriuretic peptide on vasopressin release, *Neuroendocrinology*, 44:439, 1986.

11. Cuneo, R. C., Espiner, E. A., Nicholls, M. G., Yandle, T. G., Joyce, S. L., and Gilchrist, N. L., Renal, hemodynamic, and hormonal responses to atrial natriuretic peptide infusions in normal man, and effect of sodium intake, *J. Clin. Endocrinol.,* 63:946, 1986.
12. De Souza, M. J., Maresh, C. M., Maguire, M. S., Kraemer, W. J., Flora-Ginter, G., and Goetz, K. L., Menstrual status and plasma vasopressin, renin activity, and aldosterone exercise responses, *J. Appl. Physiol.,* 67:736, 1989.
13. Fagard, R., Lijnen, P., and Amery, A., Effects of angiotensin II on arterial pressure, renin and aldosterone during exercise, *Eur. J. Appl. Physiol.,* 54:254, 1985.
14. Fasciolo, J. C., Totel, G. L., and Johnson, R. E., Antidiuretic hormone and human eccrine sweating, *J. Appl. Physiol.,* 27:303, 1969.
15. Follenius, M., Candas, V., Bothorel, B., and Brandenberger, G., Effect of rehydration on atrial natriuretic peptide release during exercise in the heat, *J. Appl. Physiol.,* 66:2516, 1989.
16. Fortney, S. M., Wenger, C. B., Bove, J. U., and Nadel, E. R., Effect of blood volume on sweating rate and body fluids in exercising humans, *J. Appl. Physiol.,* 51:1594, 1981.
17. Fortney, S. M., Wenger, C. B., Bove, J. R., and Nadel, E. R., Effect of hyperosmolality on control of blood flow and sweating, *J. Appl. Physiol.,* 57:1688, 1984.
18. Freund, B. J., Claybaugh, J. R., Dice, M. S., and Hashiro, G. M., Hormonal and vascular fluid responses to maximal exercise in trained and untrained males, *J. Appl. Physiol.,* 63:669, 1987.
19. Freund, B. J., Claybaugh, J. R., Hashiro, G. M., and Dice, M. S., Hormonal and renal responses to water drinking in moderately trained and untrained humans, *Am. J. Physiol.,* 254:R417, 1988.
20. Freund, B. J., Wade, C. E., and Claybaugh, J. R., Effects of exercise on atrial natriuretic factor: Implications to fluid homeostasis, *Sports Med.,* 6:364, 1988.
21. Freund, B. J., Claybaugh, J. R., Hashiro, G. M., Buono, M., and Chrisney, S., Exaggerated ANF response to exercise in middle-aged vs. young runners, *J. Appl. Physiol.,* 69:1607, 1990.
22. Freund, B. J., Shizuru, E. M., Hashiro, G. M., and Claybaugh, J. R., Hormonal, electrolyte, and renal responses to exercise are intensity dependent, *J. Appl. Physiol.,* 70:900, 1991.
23. Galbo, H., Holst, J. J., and Christensen, N. J., Glucagon and plasma catecholamine responses to graded and prolonged exercise in man, *J. Appl. Physiol.,* 38:70, 1975.
24. Galbo, H., *Hormonal and Metabolic Adaptation to Exercise,* Thieme-Stratton, New York, 1983, 57.
25. Geelen, G., Keil, L. C., Kravik, S. E., Wade, C. E., Thrasher, T. N., Barnes, P. R., Pyka, G., Nesvig, C., and Greenleaf, J. E., Inhibition of plasma vasopressin after drinking in dehydrated humans, *J. Appl. Physiol.,* 247:R968, 1984.
26. Gibiniski, K., Kozbowski, S., Chwalbinksa-Moneta, J., Giec, L., Zmudzinski, J., and Markiewicz, A., ADH and thermal sweating, *Eur. J. Appl. Physiol.,* 42:1, 1979.
27. Gleim, G. W., Zabetakis, P. M., DePasquale, E. E., Michelis, M. F., and Nicholas, J. A., Plasma osmolality, volume, and renin activity at the "anaerobic threshold," *J. Appl. Physiol.,* 56:57, 1984.
28. Greenleaf, J. E. and Sargent, F., II, Voluntary dehydration in man, *J. Appl. Physiol.,* 20:719, 1965.
29. Harrison, M. H., Effects of thermal stress and exercise on blood volume in humans, *Physiol. Rev.,* 65:149, 1985.
30. Hespel, P., Lijnen, P., Vanhees, L., Fagard, R., and Amery, A., Beta-adrenoceptors and the regulation of blood pressure and plasma renin during exercise, *J. Appl. Physiol.,* 60:108, 1986.
31. Johnson, M. D. and Barger, A. C., Circulating catecholamines in control of renal electrolyte and water excretion, *Am. J. Physiol.,* 240:F192, 1981.
32. Kachadorian, W. A. and Johnson, R. E., Renal responses to various rates of exercise, *J. Appl. Physiol.,* 28:748, 1970.

33. Kirby, C. R. and Convertino, V. A., Plasma aldosterone and sweat sodium concentrations after exercise and heat acclimation, *J. Appl. Physiol.,* 61:967, 1986.
34. Kjær, M., Secher, N. H., Bach, F. W., Sheikh, S., and Galbo, H., Hormonal and metabolic responses to exercise in humans: Effect of sensory nervous blockade, *Am. J. Physiol.,* 257:E95, 1989.
35. Luger, A., Deuster, P. A., Debolt, J. E., Loriaux, D. L., and Chrousos, G. P., Acute exercise stimulates the renin-angiotensin-aldosterone axis: Adaptive changes in runners, *Horm. Res.,* 30:5, 1988.
36. Mack, G. W., Shannon, L. M., and Nadel, E. R., Influence of beta-adrenergic blockage on the control of sweating in humans, *J. Appl. Physiol.,* 61:1701, 1986.
37. Mannix, E. T., Palange, P., Aronoff, G. R., Manfredi, F., and Farber, M. O., Atrial natriuretic peptide and the renin-aldosterone axis during exercise in man, *Med. Sci. Sports Exer.,* 22:785, 1990.
38. Masotto, C. and Negro-Vilar, A., Inhibition of spontaneous or angiotensin II-stimulated water intake by atrial natriuretic factor, *Brain Res. Bull.,* 15:523, 1985.
39. Mitchell, J. H., Neural control of the circulation during exercise, *Med. Sci. Sports Exer.,* 22:141, 1990.
40. Morris, D. J., The metabolism and mechanism of action of aldosterone, *Endocr. Rev.,* 2:234, 1981.
41. Nadel, E. R., Mack, G. W., and Nose, H., Influence of fluid replacement beverages on body fluid homeostasis during exercise and recovery, in *Perspectives in Exercise Science and Sports Medicine, Vol. 3: Fluid Homeostasis During Exercise,* Lamb, D. R. and Gisolfi, C. V., Eds., Benchmark Press, Carmel, IN, 1990, chap. 5.
42. Nose, H., Mack, G. W., Shi, V., and Nadel, E. R., Role of osmolality and plasma volume during rehydration in humans, *J. Appl. Physiol.,* 65:325, 1988.
43. Nose, H., Mack G. W., Shi, X., and Nadel, E. R., Involvement of sodium retention hormones during rehydration in humans, *J. Appl. Physiol.,* 65:332, 1988.
44. Nose, H., Takamata, A., Mack, G. W., Kawabata, T., Oda, Y., Hashimoto, S., Hirose, M., Chihara, E., and Morimoto, T., Right atrial pressure and ANP release during prolonged exercise in a hot environment, *J. Appl. Physiol.,* 76:1882, 1994.
45. Opstad, P. K., Oktedalen, O., Aakvaag, A., Fonnum, F., and Lund, P. K., Plasma renin activity and aldosterone during prolonged physical strain, *Eur. J. Appl. Physiol.,* 54:1, 1985.
46. Perrault, H., Melin, B., Jimenez, C., Dureau, G., Dureau, P., Allevard, A. M., Cottet-Emard, J. M., Gauquelin, G., and Charib, C., Fluid-regulating and sympathoadrenal hormonal responses to peak exercise following cardiac transplantation, *J. Appl. Physiol.,* 76:230, 1994.
47. Poortmans, J. R., Exercise and renal function, *Sports Med.,* 1:125, 1984.
48. Reid, I. A. and Ganong, W. F., Control of aldosterone secretion, in *Hypertension: Pathophysiology and Treatment,* Genest, J., Koiw, E., and Kuchel, O., Eds., McGraw-Hill, New York, 1977, 265.
49. Rolls, B. J. and Rolls, E. T., *Thirst - Problems in the Behavioral Sciences,* Gray, J., Ed., Cambridge University Press, Cambridge, 1982.
50. Rowell, L. B., Human cardiovascular adjustments to exercise and thermal stress, *Physiol. Rev.,* 54:75, 1974.
51. Schneider, S. H., Vitug, A., Ananthakrishnan, R., and Khachadurian, A. K., Impaired adrenergic response to prolonged exercise in type 1 diabetes, *Metabolism,* 40:1219, 1991.
52. Share, L. and Claybaugh, J., Regulation of body fluids, *Annu. Rev. Physiol.,* 34:235, 1972.
53. Sheldahl, L. M., Tristani, F. E., Connelly, T. P., Levandoski, S. G., Skelton, M. M., and Cowley, A. W., Jr., Fluid-regulating hormones during exercise when central blood volume is increased by water immersion, *Am. J. Physiol.,* 262:R779, 1992.
54. Stebbins, C. L., Symons, J. D., McKirnan, M. D., and Hwang, F. F. Y., Factors associated with vasopressin release in exercising swine, *Am. J. Physiol.,* 266:R118, 1994.

55. Stebbins, C. L., Reflex cardiovascular response to exercise is modulated by circulating vasopressin, *Am. J. Physiol.*, 263:R1104, 1992.
56. Stebbins, C. L. and Symons, J. D., Vasopressin contributes to the cardiovascular response to dynamic exercise, *Am. J. Physiol.*, 264:H1701, 1993.
57. Stricker, E. M. and Verbalis, J. G., Hormones and behavior: The biology of thirst and sodium appetite, *Am. Scientist*, 76:261, 1988.
58. Sutton, J. R. and Farrett, P., Endocrine responses to prolonged exercise. Perspectives in exercise, *Sci. Sports Med.*, 1:153, 1988.
59. Svedenhag, J., The sympatho-adrenal system in physical conditioning, *Acta Physiol. Scand. Suppl.*, 125:3, 1985.
60. Tanaka, G., Shindo, M., Gutkowska, J., Kinoshita, A., Urata, H., Ikeda, M., and Arakawa, K., Effect of acute exercise on plasma immunoreactive - atrial natriuretic factor, *Life Sci.*, 39:1685, 1986.
61. Takamata, A., Mack, G. W., Gillen, C. M., and Nadel, E, R., Sodium appetite, thirst, and body fluid regulation in humans during rehydration without sodium replacement, *Am. J. Physiol.*, 266:R1493, 1994.
62. Terblanche, S. E., Recent advances in hormonal response to exercise, *Comp. Biochem. Physiol.*, 93B:727, 1989.
63. Thrasher, T. N., Nistal-Herrera, J. F., Keil, L. C., and Ramsay, D. J., Satiety and inhibition of vasopressin secretion after drinking in dehydrated dogs, *Am. J. Physiol.*, 240: E394, 1981.
64. Tidgren, B., Hjemdahl, P., Theodorsson, E., and Nussberger, J., Renal neurohormonal and vascular responses to dynamic exercise in humans, *J. Appl. Physiol.*, 70:2279, 1991.
65. Viru, A., *Hormones in Muscular Activity*, CRC Press, Boca Raton, FL, 1985.
66. Viru, A., Plasma hormones and physical exercise: A review, *Int. J. Sports Med.*, 13:201, 1992.
67. Wade, C. E. and Claybaugh, J., Plasma renin activity, vasopressin concentration, and urinary excretory responses to exercise in men, *J. Appl. Physiol.*, 49: 930, 1980.
68. Wade C. E., Response, regulation, and actions of vasopressin during exercise: A review, *Med. Sci. Sports Exer.*, 16:506, 1984.
69. Wade, C. E., Hill, L. C., Hunt, M. M., and Dressendorfer, R. H., Plasma aldosterone and renal function in runners during a 20-day road race, *Eur. J. Appl. Physiol.*, 54:456, 1985.
70. Wade, C. E., Freund, B. J., and Claybaugh, J. R., Fluid and electrolyte homeostasis during and following exercise: Hormonal and non-hormonal factors, in *Hormonal Regulation of Fluids and Electrolytes: Environmental Effects*, Claybaugh, J. R. and Wade, C. E., Eds., Plenus, New York, 1989, 1.
71. Wade, C. E. and Freund, B. J., Hormonal control of blood volume during and following exercise, *Perspectives in Exercise Science and Sports Medicine, Vol. 3: Fluid Homeostasis During Exercise*, Lamb, D. R., and Gisolfi, C. V., Eds., Benchmark Press, Carmel, IN, 1990, chap. 6.
72. Weidmann, P., Hasler, L., Gnadinger, M. P., Lang, R. E., Uehlinger, D. E., Shaw, S., Rascher, W., and Reubi, F. C., Blood levels and renal effects of atrial natriuretic peptide in normal man, *J. Clin. Invest.*, 77:734, 1986.
73. Weitzman, R. and Kleeman, C. R., Water metabolism and neurohypophyseal hormones, *Clinical Disorders of Fluid and Electrolyte Metabolism*, Maxwell, M. H. and Kleeman, C. R., Eds., McGraw-Hill, New York, 1980, 531.
74. Wilkerson, J. E., Horvath, S. M., Gutin, B., Molnar, S., and Diaz, F. J., Plasma electrolyte content and concentration during treadmill exercise in humans, *J. Appl. Physiol.*, 53:1529, 1982.
75. Wolf, J. P., Nguyen, N. U., Dumoulin, G., and Berthelay, S., Plasma renin and aldosterone changes during twenty minutes' moderate exercise, *Eur. J. Appl. Physiol.*, 54:602, 1986.

76. Zambraski, E. J., Tucker, M. S., Lakas, C. S., Grassl, S. M., and Scanes, C. G., Mechanisms of renin release in exercising dog, *Am. J. Physiol.,* 246:E71, 1984.
77. Zambraski, E. J., Renal regulation of fluid homeostasis during exercise, *Perspectives in Exercise Science and Sports Medicine, Vol. 3: Fluid Hemeostasis During Exercise,* Gisolfi, C. V. and Lamb, D. R., Eds., Benchmark Press, Carmel, IN, 1990, chap. 7.

Chapter **4**

THE KIDNEY AND BODY FLUID BALANCE DURING EXERCISE

Edward J. Zambraski

CONTENTS

I. Introduction 76

II. Review of Renal Physiology 76
   A. Glomerular Filtration 77
   B. Tubular Reabsorption of Electrolytes 78
   C. Reabsorption of Water 78

III. Changes in Renal Function with Acute Exercise 79
   A. Hemodynamics 79
      1. Renal Blood Flow 79
      2. Glomerular Filtration Rate 80
   B. Urine Flow Rate 80
   C. Sodium Excretion 81
   D. Renal Function in a Dehydrated State 81

IV. Factors Controlling Renal Function During Exercise 83
   A. Endocrine Control 83
   B. Sympathetic Control 86
   C. Summary 87

V. Quantitative Importance of the Renal Response to Exercise .. 87
   A. Renal Blood Flow Redistribution 87
   B. Conservation of Sodium and Water 88
   C. Control of Total Body Sodium 88
   D. Other Important Roles of the Kidney with Exercise 89

VI. Problems with Renal Function During Exercise 90
   A. Exercise Proteinuria 90
   B. Water Intoxication..90
   C. Acute Renal Failure 91

VII. Summary...93

Reference 93

I. INTRODUCTION

The focus of this chapter will be to describe the role of the kidney as a homeostatic organ, with respect to fluid and electrolyte balance during exercise. The approach to be used will focus on the quantitative importance of the kidneys in this regard and on the mechanisms responsible for the changes seen in renal function. While other reviews have detailed the renal response to acute exercise,[2,20,21,34] the issue of the relative importance of the kidneys in terms of fluid and sodium conservation during exercise is something that has not been directly addressed.

As will be discussed, there are significant misconceptions about the kidneys and exercise that can be found in the majority of exercise physiology textbooks; fallacies are thus being perpetuated in our teaching. The purpose of this review will be to focus on and attempt to clarify some of the fundamental issues.

II. REVIEW OF RENAL PHYSIOLOGY

To understand what the kidneys do with respect to fluid/electrolyte homeostasis during exercise, and the constraints that may exist, a review of renal physiology is required.

The ability of the kidney to act as a homeostatic organ to control body fluid and electrolyte levels is derived from: (1) the ability of the kidney to filter or translocate large amounts of plasma (approximately 170 l/day) and solute such as electrolytes, glucose, and urea into the renal tubule, (2) to reabsorb approximately 99% of the filtered water and solute back into the systemic circulation with the nonreabsorbed residual amount being excreted as urine, and (3) selectively transporting specific molecules, such as potassium and hydrogen ions, into the renal tubule for their elimination in the urine. These processes are referred to as glomerular filtration, tubular reabsorption, and tubular secretion, respectively. The outcome of these three processes will be that in a normal individual at rest approximately 1 ml of urine will be produced each minute; urine containing approximately 140 meq/l sodium, and 40 meq/l potassium ions. In situations such as exercise, when fluid/electrolyte deficits are incurred, the renal conservation fluid and electrolytes is achieved by decreasing the amount excreted. As will be discussed, it should be obvious that the maximum amount of fluid and electrolyte conservation by the kidney is totally limited by the amount excreted in the basal state.

A. GLOMERULAR FILTRATION

Glomerular filtration, or the movement of ultrafiltrate of plasma through the glomerular capillary membrane into the renal tubule, is determined primarily by the glomerular capillary hydrostatic pressure and the surface area/permeability characteristics of the glomerular membrane. Glomerular capillary pressure will be determined by the systemic or renal perfusion pressure and the relative amount of preglomerular vs. postglomerular vascular resistance. Constriction of the preglomerular afferent arteriole would decrease glomerular capillary pressure, and thus glomerular filtration rate (GFR), whereas constriction of the postglomerular efferent arteriole would increase glomerular pressure and GFR. The vascular smooth muscle, particularly of the afferent arteriole, is densely innervated with sympathetic adrenergic nerves and alpha adrenergic receptors. Increases in peripheral sympathetic nerve activity and/or circulating catecholamines will increase preglomerular resistance and decrease GFR.

In addition to the hydrostatic pressure, the permeability characteristics of the glomerular membrane will also determine GFR. Acting through either a change in surface area or an inherent change in permeability, compounds such as catecholamines, vasopressin, and angiotensin II will decrease glomerular membrane permeability, whereas compounds such as PGE_2, PGI_2, or possibly nitric oxide tend to increase glomerular permeability.

The combined resultant effect of all of the factors is such that GFR in a normal person at rest is approximately 120 ml/min. The kidneys receive approximately 20% of the 5 l of cardiac output at rest, consequently total renal blood flow (RBF) is approximately 1.0 l/min. Inasmuch as only plasma and not blood cells is filtered, if one corrects RBF for hematocrit, renal plasma flow is approximately 650 ml/min. This means that of all of the plasma received by the kidneys, only about 20% is filtered (e.g., 120/650).

As will be discussed, both GFR and RBF will decrease with exercise. It must be emphasized that the most efficacious way the kidney has to conserve both water and electrolytes, via a reduction in the amount excreted, is to decrease the amount being filtered. If GFR is decreased, with less water and sodium getting into the renal tubule, the effect on excretion will be relatively abrupt and dramatic.

B. TUBULAR REABSORPTION OF ELECTROLYTES

Of the electrolytes that gain access to the renal tubule, there is active reabsorption of sodium, chloride, and potassium. Factors that promote tubular reabsorption of sodium and chloride include: renal sympathetic nerve activity, aldosterone, angiotensin II, and circulating catecholamines; whereas, atrial natriuretic peptide (ANP), dopamine, prostaglandin, and nitric oxide decrease sodium reabsorption. Potassium may be reabsorbed and/or secreted. A mineralocorticoid, such as aldosterone, will increase sodium reabsorption and stimulate potassium secretion.

Although many of these endocrine control factors change with acute exercise, there are several important points to emphasize. The first is that the time course for the onset of an endocrine effect is relatively slow (i.e., minutes/hours), with a much more prolonged residual effect (i.e., hours/days). Secondly, the endocrine effect on tubular sodium reabsorption is influencing a relatively small percentage of potentially excreted electrolyte. For example, if the actions of aldosterone are pharmacologically inhibited, the resultant change in sodium excretion will be in the range of 1–3%. During a 1- to 2-h period of acute exercise, changes of this magnitude will be small and, for the most part, of limited consequence. The importance of the endocrine-mediated increase in sodium reabsorption will be the cumulative effect on total excretion over the 12- to 24-h period following exercise. The last point is that endocrine mediated changes in tubular reabsorption often involve complex interactions of more than one hormone. For example, ANP will significantly increase sodium excretion if administered to a normal subject. However, if ANP is given to a person with elevated renal sympathetic activity, increased angiotensin II and/or aldosterone, it is without effect. Such interactions make it more difficult to predict or quantify the effect of a specific hormone on tubular reabsorption in a setting such as exercise, where numerous factors may be changing simultaneously.

C. REABSORPTION OF WATER

Some 170 l of water is filtered every 24 h, or 120 ml each minute; tubular reabsorption is responsible for returning 99% of this amount back to the circulation. About 85% of this water reabsorption is accounted for via isoosmotic reabsorption, two thirds of which occurs early in the nephron before the loop of Henle. Isoosmotic reabsorption involves the reabsorption of water due to the osmotic gradient caused by the reabsorption of solute. As molecules such as glucose, sodium, chloride, small amino acids, etc., are reabsorbed into the renal interstitium and peritubular capillaries, water will follow. Consequently, any factor that increases the tubular reabsorption of solute will also increase the reabsorption of water.

The osmolarity of the plasma filtered into the renal tubule at the glomerulus is approximately 290 mOsm/l. By definition, isoosmotic reabsorption means that the osmolarity of the tubular fluid will be unchanged, even though approximately 150 l of water is being reabsorbed by this mechanism. If this were the only mechanism by which the kidneys reabsorbed water, it would mean that the final osmolarity of the urine produced must be isoosmotic with plasma. Obviously, this is not the case because in a normally hydrated individual the final urine osmolarity ranges from 600 to 800 mOsm/l (i.e., about twice as concentrated as plasma). The ability of the kidneys to make a urine that is more concentrated than plasma will assist in the conservation of water. This is achieved as a consequence of the action of vasopressin or antidiuretic hormone (ADH) at the collecting duct. With increased ADH, the permeability of the collecting duct is increased. This causes the abstraction of water from the tubule due to the extremely high tonicity of the medullary interstitium, which normally ranges around 1200 mOsm/l. Consequently, with maximally elevated levels of ADH the final urine could be four times as concentrated as plasma. This ability to make urine more concentrated than plasma accounts for about 15% of all of the water filtered.

It should be noted that there are two major limitations concerning the ability of ADH to maximally concentrate urine. The first is the tonicity of the medullary interstitium. If this is decreased, the maximum urine osmolarity will also be lowered. The second factor, which is perhaps more relevant to the exercise setting, is "free-water" delivery to the collecting duct. If tubular reabsorption of electrolytes, and consequently water, is elevated along the proximal segments of the renal tubule, the amount of pure water reaching the collecting duct will be minimal. If this is the case, the ability of ADH to maximally concentrate urine will be compromised.

III. CHANGES IN RENAL FUNCTION WITH ACUTE EXERCISE

As with many metabolic and cardiovascular parameters, the response to acute exercise is intensity dependent. The renal response to exercise is no exception.[6] Whether the focus is on exercise-induced changes in renal hemodynamics, excretory function, or endocrine release, the level of exercise intensity must be defined.

A. HEMODYNAMICS
1. Renal Blood Flow

The hemodynamic responses to acute exercise have been quantified in humans using clearance techniques (e.g., para-aminohippurate, PAH) that indirectly assess renal plasma flow (RPF). Because RPF and RBF will change in parallel, to avoid confusion the discussion will focus on RBF.

Various studies evaluating the RBF responses to exercise have been reviewed previously.[2,20,34] Studies in humans evaluating the effects of light exercise show minimal change in RBF. As the exercise workloads approach

50% of one's work capacity, the decreases in RBF become proportional to the exercise intensity. In general, with maximal or heavy workloads the decrease in RBF can range from 40 to 60%. On an absolute scale this would mean a 400–600 ml/min reduction of RBF. Because arterial or renal perfusion pressure is increased with acute exercise, decrements in RBF are due to an elevation in renal vascular resistance.

Studies in animals have examined the RBF response to exercise using either Doppler or electromagnetic flowprobes. The responses in miniature swine[17,24] and monkeys[8] are similar to what is seen in humans, in contrast to the dog, where RBF is unchanged.[29] Studies in instrumented animals suggest that the decrease in RBF occurs quickly at the onset of exercise. This may be seen even at the start of light exercise, with an eventual increase in RBF once a steady-state workload is achieved. The pattern of this response suggests a neurally mediated renal vasoconstriction.

2. Glomerular Filtration Rate

GFR responses to acute exercise are also exercise-intensity dependent, but they may differ somewhat from what is seen for RBF.[6] With exercise loads up to 40–50% of one's $\dot{V}O_2$ max, even if the exercise is for a prolonged period, GFR is either slightly increased or unchanged. With heavy or maximal exercise, GFR is decreased in the range of 30–50% of the resting value. In general, comparable levels of moderate to heavy exercise workloads, as compared to RBF the decrements in GFR tend to be less severe.[20] This may be due to a selective vasoconstriction of the efferent arteriole mediated by angiotensin II — an effect that would elevate or would maintain glomerular capillary hydrostatic pressure. A change in GFR could also be due to alterations in the glomerular capillary permeability. The problem is that from an experimental or technical standpoint, this is essentially impossible to assess. It has been well documented, and summarized in a recent review, that glomerular permeability is increased to proteins during acute exercise.[21] However, this effect would have no bearing on the filtration of water or electrolytes.

B. URINE FLOW RATE

During light exercise, urine flow rate may be unchanged or slightly increased.[34] With moderate to heavy exercise, urine flow rate is decreased. Depending on the hydration status of the subject, normal urine production at rest may range from 0.8 to 1.5 ml/min. Controlled laboratory studies and studies of athletes under competitive conditions have reported decreases in urine production ranging from 20–60%.[2,20] In addition to a decrease in urine volume, many exercise studies have reported that exercise also causes an increase in the concentration or osmolarity of the urine. However, several studies have also shown that there may be a decrease in urine osmolarity or an increase in free water clearance with heavy exercise.[6,31] It is difficult to consistently duplicate this response in a laboratory setting. Although the possibilities of medullary "wash-out" and/or a prostaglandin inhibition of ADH have been suggested to explain why the kidneys would be excreting a more dilute urine during exercise, the exact mechanism has not been identified.[31]

With regard to changes in the urine flow rates during exercise, it is important to understand exactly how much water is being conserved. With a typical resting urine flow rate of 0.8 to 1.5 ml/min, a decrease of even 60% will only amount to 0.5–0.9 ml/min, or less than 60 ml/h of actual renal water conservation.

C. SODIUM EXCRETION

Changes in sodium excretion with acute exercise tend to parallel what was discussed for both GFR and urine volume. With light to moderate exercise, sodium excretion, along with chloride, may be unchanged or even increased. With moderate (50% $\dot{V}O_2$ max) and heavier workloads, significant declines in sodium excretion occur. The decreases in sodium excretion usually exceed the decreases in the amount being filtered, which suggests increased tubular sodium reabsorption.[20] In field studies of various distance and marathon runners and cross-country skiers, the decrements in sodium excretion during competition are approximately 40–60% of resting levels.[2,34]

D. RENAL FUNCTION IN A DEHYDRATED STATE

In a nonexercise situation, the effects of hypohydration on dehydration result in significant changes in renal function. In general, the renal excretory responses to dehydration are similar to those described for acute exercise, namely, decreased urine volume, increased urine osmolarity, and a decrease in sodium excretion. Although one can easily induce quantifiable levels of dehydration in subjects in the laboratory in order to characterize changes in renal function, a classic example of this in the real world is seen in wrestlers: individuals who are using dehydration as a means of making weight.[33] Figure 1 shows the changes in the urinary profile of a group of collegiate wrestlers over a 3-day period prior to the Saturday "weigh-in" for a wrestling meet. It can be seen that the urinary profile observed on Thursday was relatively "normal." After that, however, the changes in the urinary profile were quite dramatic and by Saturday the increases in urine osmolarity and decreased urine sodium were characteristic of renal response to a severely dehydrated state. Of note are the significantly large increases in urine potassium. As discussed earlier, with increased aldosterone there is an increase in sodium reabsorption along with increased potassium secretion. The possibility that some of this potassium is also derived from renal tubule cells damaged by dehydration has also been suggested.[33]

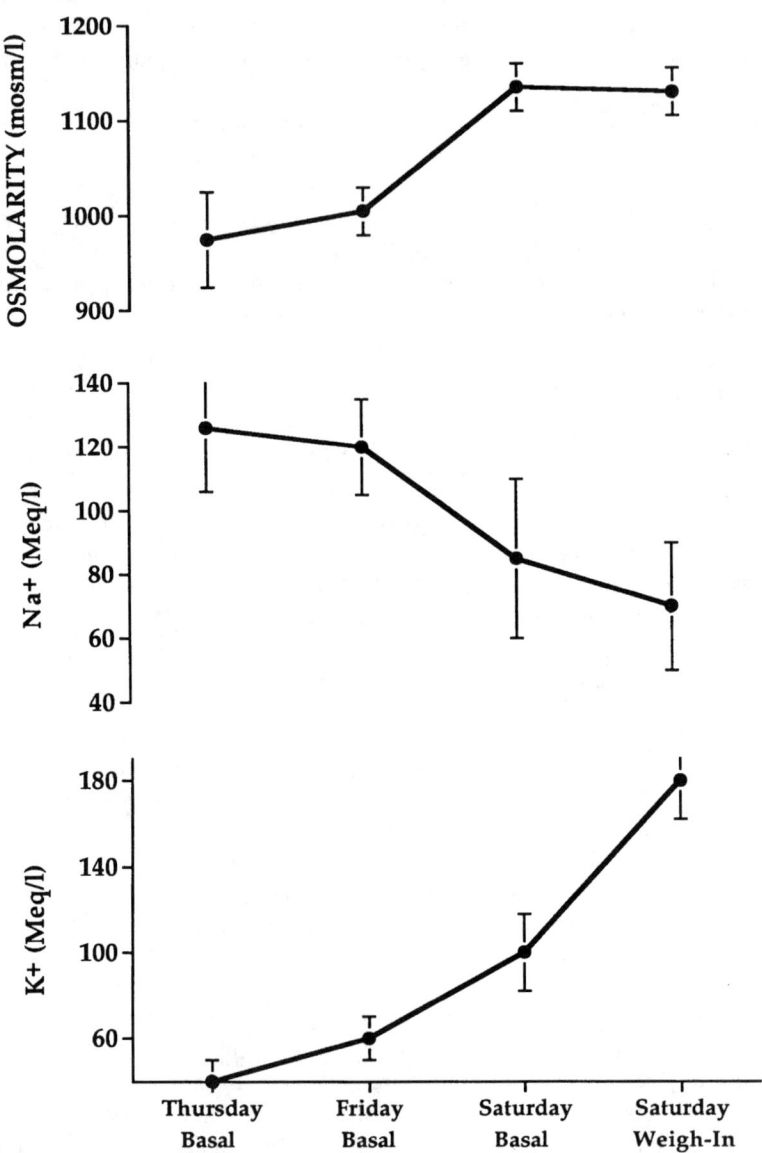

FIGURE 1 Changes in the urinary profile of wrestlers over a 3-day period prior to a "weigh-in." The changes seen reflect progressive dehydration. (Adapted from Zambraski, E.J., et al., *Med. Sci. Sport* 8:105–108, 1976. With permission.)

Many athletes, such as wrestlers, may begin exercise while in a dehydrated state. In other athletes who are performing over a prolonged period of time, the dehydrated state may develop as they continue to exercise. The renal hemodynamic response to a given level of moderate–heavy exercise (i.e., decreased GFR, RBF) may be exaggerated in dehydrated individuals.[22] The changes in excretory function or the urinary profile of a dehydrated subject, as illustrated in Figure 1, will probably not be significantly altered by the additional stress of exercise, simply because tubular reabsorption will already be near maximal levels.

IV. FACTORS CONTROLLING RENAL FUNCTION DURING EXERCISE

A. ENDOCRINE CONTROL

With dehydration, sodium deprivation, and acute exercise there will be various inputs responsible for an increase in sympathetic nerve activity and various endocrines that potentially can alter renal function. Figure 2 illustrates how these factors would be predicted to function in an interactive fashion to promote the renal conservation of sodium and water.[34]

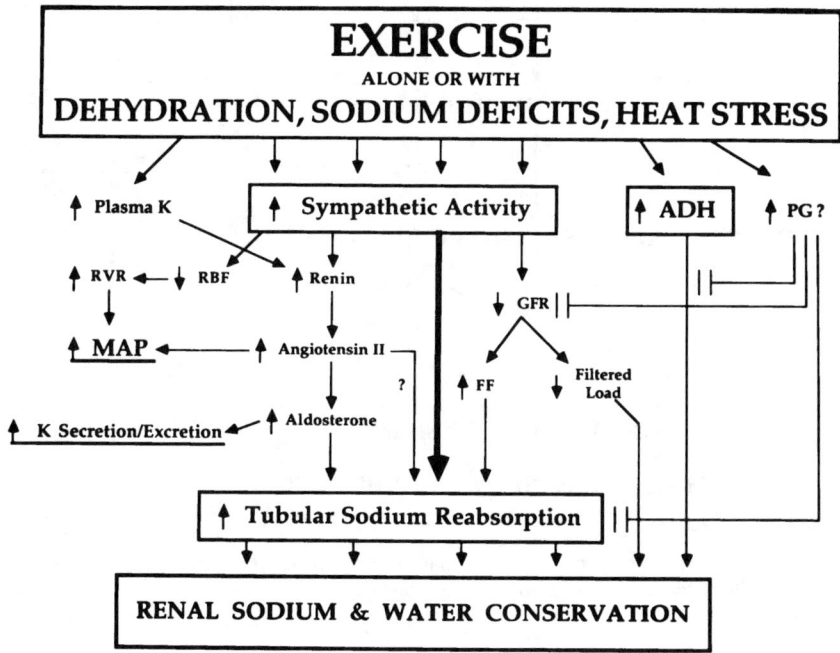

FIGURE 2 Factors controlling renal function during acute exercise that result in the renal conservation of sodium and water. (From Zambraski, E.J., in *Fluid Homeostasis During Exercise,* Gisolfi, C.V. and Lamb, D.R., Eds., Benchmark Press, Indianapolis, 1990. With permission.)

The basis for such a schema comes largely from studies employing interventions such as dehydration, sodium deprivation, or heat stress. For these perturbations, studied under relatively long-term, steady-state conditions, one can easily delineate an important role for ADH, renin–angiotensin, and/or aldosterone. In such situations there are measured increases in these endocrines, and if you block a specific factor pharmacologically, a change in renal function is demonstrable. This is not the case with acute exercise. In fact, there is very little direct evidence to substantiate the role of endocrines in terms of controlling renal function during acute exercise. The problem is that many conclusions about endocrine control of renal function during exercise are being based on "associative" changes between a hormone level and an alteration in renal function. As illustrated in Figure 3, these associative changes are being used to make inferences about causality. What has been historically lacking in the area of exercise and kidney function are intervention studies that, as shown in Figure 3, block a specific endocrine and actually demonstrate a modified response.

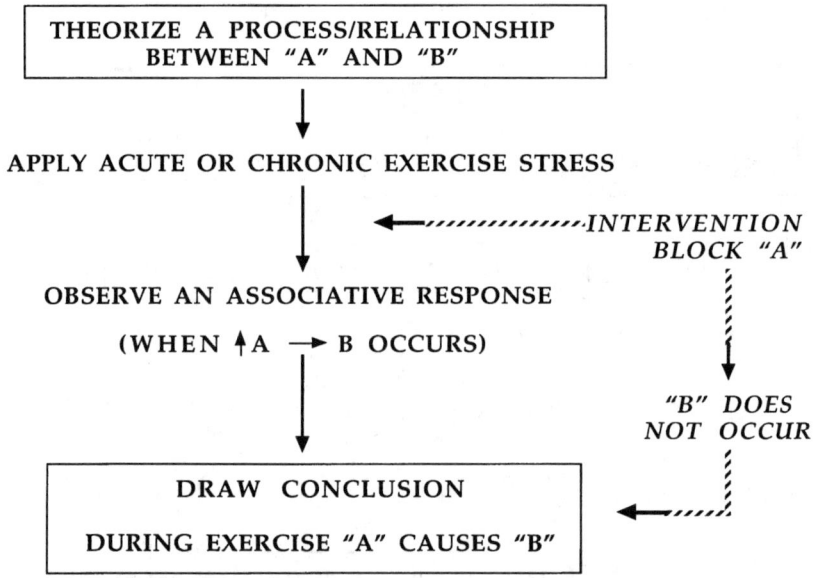

FIGURE 3 Basing conclusions on "associative" responses. Until interventions are employed to block the suspected mediator and alter the response, "causality" should not be presumed.

For example, even though there is a statistically significant inverse correlation between plasma aldosterone and sodium excretion at various levels of exercise,[34] there are no data to indicate that aldosterone is actually changing renal function during exercise. No published studies have shown that if one blocks aldosterone with a compound such as spironolactone, the renal response to exercise is significantly altered. Similarly, inasmuch as we know that with acute exercise the renin–angiotensin-aldosterone axis is activated, one presumes that it has an important effect during exercise. However, there are no data to support such a conclusion. In fact, the data suggest a lack of involvement. A study by Wade et al.[32] blocked the renin–angiotensin system by administering an angiotensin I–angiotensin II-converting enzyme inhibitor, captopril. During maximal exercise there was no effect on GFR or sodium excretion, and despite the lack of angiotensin II, the increase in aldosterone with exercise was unchanged. Studies from the author's lab demonstrated that the renal hemodynamic and excretory responses to acute exercise in minature swine are not modified if the animals are experimentally renin depleted.[17] Lastly, studies in humans using converting enzyme inhibitors suggest that the sodium conservation seen with exercise is not dependent on renin–angiotensin.[13]

Mechanistic studies examining the role of vasopressin or ADH during acute exercise are lacking. This issue has been reviewed by Wade.[31] In general, although vasopressin increases with exercise, it is unclear as to whether it has a definitive effect on the excretion of water. As indicated earlier, several exercise studies have reported a paradoxical increase in free water clearance, despite increased ADH. Drugs that block vasopressin receptors are available. Studies using this pharmacological approach in exercising miniature swine have been published recently by Stebbins and Symons.[27] Although these studies have implicated vasopressin as being important for systemic cardiovascular changes, these ongoing studies have not as yet evaluated renal function.

Another example in which an erroneous conclusion could be made based on an associative change of a compound during exercise and alterations in renal pertains to prostaglandins. Prostaglandins have the capacity to influence various aspects of renal function. They may alter RBF, GFR, sodium reabsorption, or medullary blood flow/toxicity; mediate the release of renin; and antagonize the hydroosmotic effects of vasopressin.[4] Studies in humans and animals have also shown that exercise increases the renal synthesis and release of prostaglandins. However, numerous studies using compounds that inhibit renal prostaglandin synthesis — such as indomethacin, sulindac, or aspirin — have failed to show that any definitive aspect of renal function is controlled by prostaglandins during exercise in normal health subjects.[13,17]

With the discovery of ANP, and the ability to measure this compound in the plasma, numerous studies soon followed demonstrating that ANP is increased with acute and prolonged exercise.[10,19] The fundamental effect of ANP is an increase in water/sodium excretion due primarily to an increase in GFR, with an additional effect being an inhibition of tubular sodium reabsorption. It has been suggested and is reasonable to postulate that with light exercise, increases in ANP may be responsible for the increases or minimal changes in GFR, urine volume, and/or sodium excretion discussed earlier.[6] Even though tremendously large increases in ANP are seen with heavy workloads (80–100% $\dot{V}O_2$ max), at these exercise intensities ANP probably is not directly influencing renal function. Numerous studies have shown that neither endogenous nor exogenously administered ANP has any renal vasodilatory or natriuretic effects if renal sympathetic nerve activity, renin–angiotensin, or aldosterone is elevated. Inasmuch as all of these factors increase with moderate–heavy exercise, at these workloads the ANP effect on renal function is probably being overridden. With light exercise, even though the changes in ANP are consistent with some of the alterations in renal hemodynamics and excretory function, direct evidence confirming its involvement is required. A nonpeptide ANP receptor antagonist is now available.[9] Exercise studies using such a compound will be required to delineate the degree that ANP influences renal function at various exercise workloads.

B. SYMPATHETIC CONTROL

For its size, the kidney is one of the most densely innervated organs in the body. The great majority of the nerves going to the kidney are sympathetic and adrenergic. The renal nerves innervate all of the vascular and tubular elements of the nephron. Functionally, the renal nerves have the capacity to decrease RBF and GFR, cause the release of renin, and increase renal tubular sodium reabsorption. Although most of the evidence so far is indirect, it is reasonable to postulate that most, if not all, of the changes in renal function seen with acute exercise are mediated by increased renal sympathetic nerve activity.

It has been well documented that with acute exercise, peripheral sympathetic nerve activity increases. Using chronically instrumented animals, studies have been able to directly measure increases in renal sympathetic nerve activity during exercise.[16] In human subjects, because renal neurograms cannot be obtained, renal sympathetic nerve activity is estimated by the renal release of norepinephrine.[5] This approach has been used to verify that during acute exercise renal nerve activity is elevated.[5,28] Sympathetic neural outflow is not homogenous, and studies in animals during exercise and humans at rest suggest that the kidneys receive a disproportionate amount of sympathetic activity.[5] With acute exercise in humans, changes in peripheral sympathetic outflow, as estimated by increased circulating norepinephrine, are a linear function of the relative workload; a situation similar to that of changes in RBF, GFR, and sodium excretion.[34] In addition, as mentioned earlier, the time course for changes in renal function with acute exercise, being relatively rapid in nature, suggests a neural control mechanism.

Studies to directly implicate neural control of renal function during exercise are difficult to carry out, and they are complicated by certain issues. If one surgically denervates the kidney(s) in an experimental animal, the denervated kidney will develop a hypersensitivity to circulating catecholamines. Such an effect could confound the results when looking at the renal response to exercise in a surgically denervated animal. To utilize adrenergic receptor blockade is also difficult because of systemic effects. If an animal is administered an alpha-1 adrenoreceptor blocker systemically in order to determine whether the renal vasoconstriction during exercise is sympathetically mediated, the results may be uninterpretable because of the profound hypotension that will occur. Even if such drugs are infused intrarenally, the problem of systemic spillover still may exist. If one can apply a specific sympatholytic agent during exercise and not induce confounding systemic changes, very definitive data can be obtained. For example, studies employing beta-1 adrenoreceptor blockade were able to conclusively demonstrate that renin release by the kidneys during exercise is totally mediated by increases in renal sympathetic nerve activity.[35]

C. SUMMARY

Although various hormones or compounds such as renin–angiotensin, aldosterone, ANP, and prostaglandins increase with exercise, very little evidence exists to confirm that they are responsible for mediating the changes in renal function during exercise. The major control factors that alter kidney function with acute exercise are probably elevated renal sympathetic nerve activity, and possibly circulating catecholamines and vasopressin or ADH. It is likely that augmented renal sympathetic nerve activity is responsible for the decrease in RBF and GFR with moderate–heavy exercise, as well as an increase in the renal tubular reabsorption of sodium. These effects would decrease the amount of filtered sodium and water, increase the reabsorption of sodium, and facilitate the isoosmotic reabsorption of water in order to conserve water and sodium. Vasopressin's primary effect would be to facilitate the formation of a concentrated urine.

V. QUANTITATIVE IMPORTANCE OF THE RENAL RESPONSE TO EXERCISE

A. RENAL BLOOD FLOW REDISTRIBUTION

As indicated earlier, with moderate to heavy exercise there is an increase in renal vascular resistance, such that despite the increase in systemic or renal perfusion pressure, RBF decreases. Although the concept of a "redistribution" of RBF to metabolically active skeletal muscle during exercise is correct, the overall quantitative importance of this is poorly understood. As discussed earlier, and as pointed out by Rowell,[23] the actual absolute amount of RBF being redistributed is very small, ranging from 300 to 600 ml/min at most. The misconception about the importance of this event is largely due to the fact that textbooks and diagrams explain the redistribution of RBF in terms of a percentage of cardiac output. When this is done, a presentation of RBF being 20% of cardiac output at rest and only 4–5% of cardiac output with maximal exercise, leads one to conclude that large amounts of RBF are being redistributed. The point that is not made is that cardiac output is changing from 5 to 25–30 l/min with heavy exercise. Even though RBF as a percentage of cardiac output is decreased substantially (i.e., from 20 to 4%), the 4% is of a much larger quantity. Consequently, the change in absolute RBF is actually very small (300–600 ml), especially in comparison to a cardiac output of 25–30 l.

However, the renal vasoconstriction seen during acute exercise is important for another reason. With exercise there is a decrease in total peripheral vascular resistance. This is primarily due to neural and metabolic vasodilation of muscle tissue. The decrease in total peripheral resistance is offset by an increase in cardiac output such that systemic mean blood pressure is slightly elevated or maintained. Because the kidneys receive such a large amount of blood flow, and therefore potentially contribute a large fraction to total peripheral resistance, if renal vasoconstriction did not occur with exercise, the fall in peripheral vascular resistance would be so great that it could not be matched by increased cardiac output. This would result in a marked fall in systemic blood pressure, which would compromise blood flow to all peripheral tissues.

B. CONSERVATION OF SODIUM AND WATER

The predominant thought is that with acute exercise the kidneys are important in conserving water and sodium to offset the sweat losses. As indicated earlier, because the kidneys are excreting so little urine and sodium in the basal-resting state, even with dramatic decreases in urine production and/or sodium excretion relative to the amount of water/sodium lost in the sweat, the amount conserved by the kidneys will be negligible. A study by Meyer et al.[12] calculated sweat and electrolyte losses in subjects of varied age and gender. Using their data from young adults, and the changes in urine flow rates and urine sodium concentrations that would be expected at the workloads utilized, it can be calculated that the renal conservation of water would be about 4% of that lost and only about 8% for the sodium. These fractions would be even smaller if one used the sweat rate data from highly trained athletes; sweat rates that would be severalfold greater than those reported by Meyer et al.[12] for untrained subjects.

While the contribution of the kidneys to conserved fluid/electrolytes during exercise is negligible, the renal response during the recovery phase is of paramount importance.[34] The kidneys will adjust the amount and chemical composition of the urine until such time that fluid and electrolyte losses are corrected. These changes are probably hormonally mediated. Depending upon the severity of the dehydration and sodium depletion, and changes in fluid intake as driven by the thirst mechanism, the renal restoration of body water/electrolytes may take anywhere from several hours to several days.

C. CONTROL OF TOTAL BODY SODIUM

As described by Guyton,[7] the kidneys have infinite gain and the ultimate responsibility for controlling total body sodium. Because sodium is the major extracellular electrolyte, by doing so the kidneys will be determining total body water. If an individual experiences an increase in the volume of a given fluid compartment, such as blood volume, without a concomitant decrease in fluid from the intracellular space or other extracellular zones, this means that total body water and sodium must have increased. For this to happen, a change in renal function must have occurred.

The issue of steady-state vs. transient changes in total body sodium balance with exercise has been discussed elsewhere.[34] However, if a person is in steady-state and plasma volume is altered, such changes will only occur if there is a change in the renal handling of sodium. There are numerous situations where there may be steady-state changes in blood or plasma volume. Examples would include the effects of acute exercise, exercise training, altitude, microgravity, water immersion, and certain disease states such as hypertension and cirrhosis. A point not recognized is that for these changes to become established, the perturbation involved must be altering renal function.

D. OTHER IMPORTANT ROLES OF THE KIDNEY WITH EXERCISE

Aside from the issues of the redistribution of RBF and fluid/electrolyte conservation and/or restoration, there are several other important functions of the kidneys during exercise.

It is well known that the kidney releases renin, which will result in the formation of angiotensin II. Angiotensin II is important during exercise in terms of the thirst response, a contribution to systemic vascular resistance, and possibly a determinant of sympathetic outflow. In addition to renin, the kidneys also release large amounts of norepinephrine, neuropeptide Y, dopamine, and probably urodilatin into the systemic circulation during exercise.[28] These compounds can have a wide array of metabolic and cardiovascular effects.

There is a debate as to what tissue type or organ may be responsible for the increase of circulating norepinephrine with acute exercise. Some of the early animal and human studies suggest that norepinephrine spillover from muscle tissue is the primary site of origin.[18] More recent work in humans by Esler and colleagues suggests that at rest the kidneys may be responsible for as much as 25–30% of total norepinephrine release[5]; an amount that would clearly increase with exercise because, as discussed earlier, renal sympathetic nerve activity increases with exercise.

Although the issue of the kidneys being the major source of norepinephrine during exercise is not resolved, one point should be made. It has been well documented that exercise-trained individuals have lower plasma norepinephrine concentrations to any given level of absolute work, or at rest if their starting values are elevated (e.g., hypertensives). It is also known that the sympathetic outflow to a stressor such as exercise is not uniform; it differs widely to various tissues/organs. Putting these things together, it has been shown that in humans with exercise training there is a decrease in renal sympathetic nerve activity; a decrease that is responsible for the majority of the reduction in total circulating norepinephrine.[11] In contrast, studies using microneurographic techniques in humans to measure muscle sympathetic activity show no changes with training.[25] Putting these facts together suggests that the kidneys, and not muscle, may be contributing the majority of norepinephrine; if it were muscle tissue, changes in circulating norepinephrine with training would not be expected.

VI. PROBLEMS WITH RENAL FUNCTION DURING EXERCISE

There are at least three problems or complexities that may occur with renal function during exercise — namely, proteinuria, water intoxication, and acute renal failure.

A. EXERCISE PROTEINURIA

As indicated earlier, the glomerular capillary performs an important barrier function between the systemic circulation and the renal tubule. Because of their size and electrical charge characteristics, normally proteins are not filtered; hence, the amount of protein in the urine is usually negligible. With exercise, however, glomerular barrier function and possibly the tubular reabsorption of protein may be altered such that exercise proteinuria occurs. Because there are no performance consequences of exercise proteinuria and the fact that an excellent review on this topic was recently published by Poortmans,[210] only a few comments will be offered.

Exercise proteinuria is a transient and benign condition, in contrast to the proteinuria that exists in persons with established renal disease. The traditional historical belief that exercise proteinuria was due to renal vasoconstriction (i.e., decreased GFR, and RBF), is not supported by various mechanistic studies. Exercise proteinuria probably results from an interaction of hemodynamic and endocrine changes that occur with exercise, in addition to actual changes in the glomerular capillary wall. More importantly, the changes in glomerular membrane protein permeability appear to be similar to what is seen in various capillaries during exercise — changes that will affect the movement of molecules and water across different extracellular compartments. Consequently, exercise-induced proteinuria could serve as an appropriate model system for changes in systemic function.[21]

B. WATER INTOXICATION

There have been several reports of "water intoxication" in athletes.[1,15] For individuals in a long-term endurance event, such as a marathon, in some cases the amount of fluid being ingested may exceed that lost via sweating and urine production. This situation can adversely affect fluid volumes and plasma electrolyte levels. There is also controversy as to whether water intoxication due to excessive fluid ingestion or sodium loss via sweating is the determining factor in causing exercise-induced hyponatremia.[1,14] Aside from this debate is the question of why the kidney does not excrete large amounts of free water when a person is ingesting copious amounts of water during exercise, in order to prevent water intoxication.

As indicated in an earlier paper, the failure of the kidney to excrete the excess of fluid being consumed is probably not due to an abnormality in renal function, but rather to changes in the control factors that exist.[34] It was shown most convincingly by Poortmans[20] that in overly hydrated subjects who continue to drink 200 ml of water every 20 min, with resultant urine flow rates of 10–12 ml/min, if heavy exercise is superimposed then urine flow rates are decreased to 2–3 ml/min, even if the person continues drinking water. As explained earlier, this is probably due to the fact that heavy exercise is decreasing GFR. If water is not filtered, it cannot be excreted. Also, with heavy exercise the various factors enhancing tubular sodium reabsorption will be causing the isoosmotic reabsorption of water to increase. Combining this with a reduction in GFR will mean that the amount of free water being delivered to the collecting duct will be reduced. If this occurs, even with appropriately suppressed levels of ADH, total urine production will be limited.

C. ACUTE RENAL FAILURE

Acute renal failure is defined as an abrupt decrease in renal function associated with a significant decline in GFR. Factors that decrease renal perfusion, such as volume depletion, hypotension, elevated renal sympathetic activity, increased catecholamines, and/or angiotensin II could contribute to acute renal failure.[34] In addition, rhabdomyolysis may also induce renal injury and acute renal failure. Despite the fact that many of the factors and neural and endocrine changes listed above increase with heavy exercise, the incidence of exercise-induced acute renal failure is extremely low. If one separates out acute renal failure due to rhabdomyolysis or other medical complications, exercise-induced renal failure is rare. This is an extremely fortunate and surprising fact.

With an exercise-induced activation of the various neural and endocrine controls that have been described, it would be predicted that acute renal failure should occur to a much greater extent than is seen. In a laboratory setting, if one experimentally applied the increases in renal sympathetic nerve activity that are believed to occur with exercise to an experimental animal at rest, as well as infused angiotensin II, ADH, and aldosterone to achieve the plasma levels seen with exercise, renal function would be severely compromised. With acute exercise, and the activation of various renal vasoconstriction and anti-natriuretic control factors, there is probably some other factor(s), yet to be identified, that is serving to counterbalance and thereby preserve or protect renal function. Such a system has been defined for various physiological and pathophysiological states involving prostaglandins.[4] However, prostaglandins, probably do not modulate increases in sympathetic nerve activity and angiotensin II during exercise. Exercise studies that have employed renal prostaglandin inhibition using nonsteroidal antiinflammatory drugs (NSAIDs) and/or aspirin do not show that renal function is significantly or deleteriously altered.[13,16] In addition, because a very large number of runners are using NSAIDs or aspirin to treat musculoskeletal injuries, if prostaglandins were important in this regard exercise-induced renal failure would be much more prevalent.

There are at least two known compounds that may be important in this regard — ANP and endothelial-derived relaxing factor (EDRF), which is believed to be nitric oxide (NO).

As discussed earlier, ANP is increased with acute exercise and it is a renal vasodilator. Although one does not see increases in GFR and a natriuresis at the heavy exercise workloads when ANP is markedly elevated, it may be that ANP is important in modulating renal vasoconstrictor tone (i.e., in the absence of ANP the decreases in GFR and RBF would be more severe). Studies will now be able to address this possibility with the availability of ANP receptor antagonists.[9]

The renal vasculature has a large capacity to synthesize NO, a potent renal vasodilator that also has natriuretic capacities. NO is synthesized from l-arginine. A way to evaluate a role for NO is to inhibit NO synthesis by administering an analogue of arginine such as l-arginine methyl ester (l-NAME). Studies suggest that NO modulates renal sympathetic nerve activity and other factors responsible for renal vasoconstriction tone. If l-NAME is given to a resting animal, mean blood pressure will increase, as will renal vascular resistance. A recent study evaluated the role of NO in exercising dogs.[26] It was demonstrated that during exercise, renal vascular resistances tended to be higher when NO was inhibited. As indicated earlier, it should be noted that in the exercising dog, renal sympathetic nerve activity does not increase to the extent that RBF declines, as is seen in humans.[29] Consequently, evaluating the effect of NO inhibition in an exercising dog may underestimate the full involvement of NO in controlling renal function. Recently, a study was conducted in which exercise was "mimicked" in anesthetized dogs.[30] This involved increasing renal sympathetic nerve activity to the kidney by altering baroreceptor input. This maneuver decreased GFR and RBF. When experiments were repeated with NO blocked, the decreases in RBF and GFR were significantly greater. These data suggest that EDRF/NO may be very important as a modulator of sympathetic and renal vasoconstriction with exercise — an effect that could be preventing acute renal failure with exercise.

VII. SUMMARY

This chapter reviews basic renal physiology as it pertains to changes in kidney function during acute exercise. The various changes that occur in renal function are described, the major factors being a decrease in RBF and water/electrolyte conservation. Several misconceptions about kidney function and exercise are discussed, including the quantitative importance of the fluid/electrolyte conservation and the degree to which associative changes in various hormones, such as aldosterone or renin–angiotensin, actually alter kidney function during exercise. An important role of the neural control of kidney function during exercise is emphasized. Lastly, some abnormal and/or potentially detrimental changes in kidney function with exercise are described. These include exercise-induced proteinuria, water intoxication, and acute renal failure. Mechanisms responsible for these changes, and factors that may prevent acute renal failure with strenuous exercise, are discussed.

REFERENCES

1. Armstrong, L.E., Curtis, W.C., Hubbard, R.W., Francesconi, R.P., Moore, R., and Askew, E.W., Symptomatic hyponatremia during prolonged exercise in the heat. *Med. Sci. Sports Exer.* 25:543–549, 1993.
2. Castenfors, J., Renal function during prolonged exercise. *Ann. N.Y. Acad. Sci.* 301:151–159, 1977.
3. DiBona, G.F., The functions of the renal nerves. *Rev. Physiol. Biochem. Pharmacol.* 94:76–181, 1982.
4. Dunn, M.J. and Zambraski, E.J., Renal effect of drugs that inhibit prostaglandin synthesis. *Kidney Int.* 18:609–622, 1980.
5. Esler, M., Clinical application of noradrenaline spillover methodology: delineation of regional human sympathetic nervous responses. *Pharmacol. Toxicol.* 73:243–253, 1993.
6. Freund, B.J., Shizuru, E.M., Hashiro, G.M., and Claybaugh, J.R., Hormonal, electrolyte, and renal responses to exercise are intensity dependent. *J. Appl. Physiol.* 70:900–906, 1991.
7. Guyton, A.C., The surprising kidney-fluid mechanism for fluid control — Its infinite gain. *Hypertension* 16:725–730, 1990.
8. Hohimer, A.R. and Smith, O.A., Decreased renal blood flow in the baboon during mild dynamic leg exercise. *Am. J. Physiol.* 236:H141–H150, 1970.
9. Imura, R., Sano, T., Goto, J., Yamada, K. and Matsuda, Y., Inhibition by HS 142-1, a novel nonpeptide atrial natriuretic peptide antagonist of microbial origin, of atrial natriuretic peptide — Induced relaxation of isolated rabbit aorta through the blockade of guanylyl cyclase-linked receptors. *J. Pharmacol. Exp. Therap.* 42:982–990, 1992.
10. Lijnen, P., Hespel, P. M'Buyamba-Kabangu, J.R., Goris, M., Lysens, R., VandenEynde, E., Fagard, R., and Amery, A., Plasma atrial natriuretic peptide and cyclic nucleotide levels before and after a marathon. *J. Appl. Physiol.* 63:1180–1184, 1987.
11. Meredith, I.T., Friberg, P., Jennings, G.L., Dewar, E.M., Fazio, V.A., Lambert, G.W., and Esler, M.D., Exercise training lowers resting renal but not cardiac sympathetic activity in humans. *Hypertension* 18:575–582, 1991.
12. Meyer, F., Bar-or, O., MacDougall, D., and Heigenhauser, G.J.F., Sweat and electrolyte loss during exercise in the heat: Effects of gender and maturation. *Med. Sci. Sports Exer.* 24:776–781, 1992.

13. Mittleman, K.D. and Zambraski, E.J., Exercise-induced proteinuria is attenuated by indomethacin. *Med. Sci. Sports Exer.* 24:1069–1074, 1992.
14. Noakes, T.D., Hyponatremia during endurance running: A physiological and clinical interpretation. *Med. Sci. Sports Exerc.* 24:403–405, 1992.
15. Noakes, T.D., Goodwin, N., Rayner, B.L., Branken, T., and Taylor, R.K.N., Water intoxication: A possible complication during endurance exercise. *Med. Sci. Sports Exer.* 17:370–375, 1985.
16. O'Hagan, K.P., Bell, L.B., Mittelstadt, S.W., and Clifford, P.S., Effect of dynamic exercise on renal sympathetic nerve activity in conscious rabbits. *J. Appl. Physiol.* 74:2099–2104, 1993.
17. O'Hagan, K.P., Hora, D., and Zambraski, E.J., Indomethacin attenuates exercise-induced proteinuria in hypertensive swine. *Am. J. Physiol.* 236:R954–R961, 1992.
18. Peronnet, F., Beliveau, L., Boudreau, G., Trudeau, F., Brisson, G., and Nadeau, R., Regional catecholamine removal and release at rest and exercise in dogs. *Am. J. Physiol.* 254:R663–R672, 1988.
19. Perrault, H., Cantin, M., Thibault, G., Brisson, G.R., Brisson, G., and Beland, M., Plasma atrial natriuretic peptide during brief upright and supine exercise in humans. *J. Appl. Physiol.* 66:2159–2167, 1989.
20. Poortmans, J., Exercise and renal function. *Sports Med.* 1:125–153, 1984.
21. Poortmans, J.R. and Vanderstraeten, J., Kidney function during exercise in healthy and diseased humans. *Sports Med.* 18:419–437, 1994.
22. Radigan, L.R. and Robinson, S., Effects of environmental stress and exercise on renal blood flow and filtration rate. *J. Appl. Physiol.* 2:185–191, 1949.
23. Rowell, L.B., Human cardiovascular adjustments to exercise and thermal stress. *Physiol. Rev.* 54:75–159, 1974.
24. Sanders, M., Rasmussen, S., Cooper, D., and Bloor, C., Renal and intrarenal blood flow distribution in swine during severe exercise. *J. Appl. Physiol.* 40:932–935, 1976.
25. Seals, D.R., Sympathetic neural adjustments to stress in physically trained and untrained humans. *Hypertension* 17:36–43, 1991.
26. Shen, W., Lunborg, M., Wang, J., Stewart, J.M., Xu, X., Ochoa, M., and Hintze, T.H., Role of EDRF in the regulation of regional blood flow and vascular resistance at rest and during exercise in conscious dogs. *J. Appl. Physiol.* 77:165–172, 1994.
27. Stebbins, C.L. and Symons, J.D., Vasopressin contributes to the cardiovascular response to dynamic exercise. *Am. J. Physiol.* 264:H1701–1707, 1993.
28. Tidgren, B., Hjemdahl, P., Theodorsson, E., and Nussberger, J., Renal neurohormonal and vascular responses to dynamic exercise in humans. *J. Appl. Physiol.* 70:2279–2286, 1991.
29. Vatner, S.F., Higgins, C.B., and Franklin, D., Regional circulatory adjustments to moderate and severe chronic anemia in conscious dogs at rest and during exercise. *Circ. Res.* 30:731–740, 1972.
30. Vogl, H. and Zambraski, E.J., Nitric oxide mediates the renal hemodynamic responses to increased sympathetic nerve activity during mimicked exercise. *Med. Sci. Sports Exer.* 26:S150, 1994.
31. Wade, C.E., Response, regulation, and actions of vasopressin during exercise: A review. *Med. Sci. Sports Exer.* 16:506–511, 1984.
32. Wade, C.E., Ramee, S.R., Hunt, M.M., and White, C., Hormonal and renal responses to converting enzyme inhibition during maximal exercise. *J. Appl. Physiol.* 63:1796–1800, 1987.
33. Zambraski, E.J., Foster, D.T., Gross, P.M., and Tipton, C.M., Iowa wrestling study: Weight loss and urinary profiles of collegiate wrestlers. *Med. Sci. Sports* 8:105–108, 1976.
34. Zambraski, E.J., Renal regulation of fluid homeostasis during exercise. In: *Fluid Homeostasis During Exercise*, Gisolfi, C.V. and Lamb, D.R., Eds. Benchmark Press, Indianapolis, 1990, Chap. 7.

35. Zambraski, E.J., Tucker, M.S., Lakas, C.S., Grassl, S.M., and Scanes, C.G., Mechanism of renin release in exercising dog. *Am. J. Physiol.* 246:E71–E78, 1984.

Chapter 5

FLUID AND ELECTROLYTE BALANCE OF THE LUNG DURING EXERCISE

Eric K. Birks
Richard M. Effros

CONTENTS

I. Introduction..98

II. Cardiopulmonary Adjustments During Exercise.................98

III. Evidence for Pulmonary Edema During Exercise...............98

IV. Structure of the Lungs....................................100

V. Filtration Across the Pulmonary Capillaries..................101

VI. Role of Lymphatics, Cuffs, and Pleura......................103

VII. Passive Transport of Fluid Across the Pulmonary Epithelium.....104

VIII. Active Transport Across the Pulmonary Epithelium............106

IX. Water Transport in the Lungs..............................107

X. Stress Failure in Pulmonary Capillaries......................108

XI. Conclusions..110

References...110

I. INTRODUCTION

Maintenance of optimal gas exchange in the lungs is of utmost importance during exercise. As blood flow increases in response to exercise demands, pulmonary arterial pressures also increase, and there is distension and/or recruitment of vessels throughout the lungs. These changes in the pulmonary circulation serve to increase the amount of blood that is oxygenated during transit through the pulmonary vasculature, but they may also predispose the lungs to interstitial or even airspace edema, thereby impairing gas exchange. Evidence that some edema can occur in well-trained athletes during extreme exercise will be discussed in this chapter, and consideration will be given to the mechanisms that normally keep the pulmonary interstitium and alveoli free of edema. In addition, the possibility that extreme increases in vascular pressure may be responsible for damage to the pulmonary vascular barrier will also be addressed.

II. CARDIOPULMONARY ADJUSTMENTS DURING EXERCISE

With increases of oxygen consumption from 0.3 l/min at rest to 4 l/min with vigorous exercise, cardiac output increases from approximately 7 l/min to 25 l/min in average, exercising humans (see Table 1). This is associated with linear increases in pulmonary arterial and left atrial pressures (as estimated by wedge pressures) (Figure 1). Although direct measurements of capillary pressures have not been possible during exercise, animal studies indicate that pressures taken as an average of arterial and left atrial pressures represent reasonable approximations of capillary pressures.[7,43,78,106] It seems likely that pulmonary capillary pressures might reach levels greater than 35 mmHg in this population.[99,100] Much higher intravascular pressures are encountered in trained athletes during maximal exercise[77] and, as discussed below, these pressures may be sufficient to damage the blood–gas barrier and predispose to pulmonary edema.

III. EVIDENCE FOR PULMONARY EDEMA DURING EXERCISE

High levels of exercise in trained athletes can result in increased A-a O_2 gradients, and in some individuals, arterial hypoxia and desaturation are observed. These abnormalities have been attributed to abnormal diffusion or $\dot{V}/\dot{Q}_2$ ratios in the lungs.[23,58,98] Acceleration of red cell transit through the capillaries can decrease the opportunity for full saturation of hemoglobin, particularly if the blood returning to the lungs is very unsaturated.[77] It is also quite

TABLE 1 Pulmonary Hemodynamics at Rest and During Exercise

Rest				Exercise				
$\dot{V}O_2$ (l/min)	P_{PA} (mmHg)	P_{WEDGE} (mmHg)	$\dot{Q}_T$ (l/min)	$\dot{V}O_2$ (l/min)	P_{PA} (mmHg)	P_{WEDGE} (mmHg)	$\dot{Q}_T$ (l/min)	Ref.
0.3	13.8	5.3	6.4	1.2	25.5	10.6	13.2	103
0.4	13.2	3.4	6.9	3.7	37.2	21.1	23.9	94
0.3	14	8	7.6	4	35	24	25.4	77
NA	15	7	6.7	NA	33	21	27.2	43
0.36	15	6.9	6.6	3.1	29	16	26.7	79
0.3	NA	NA	6	3.6	NA	NA	25	93

Note: NA = data not given in cited reference.

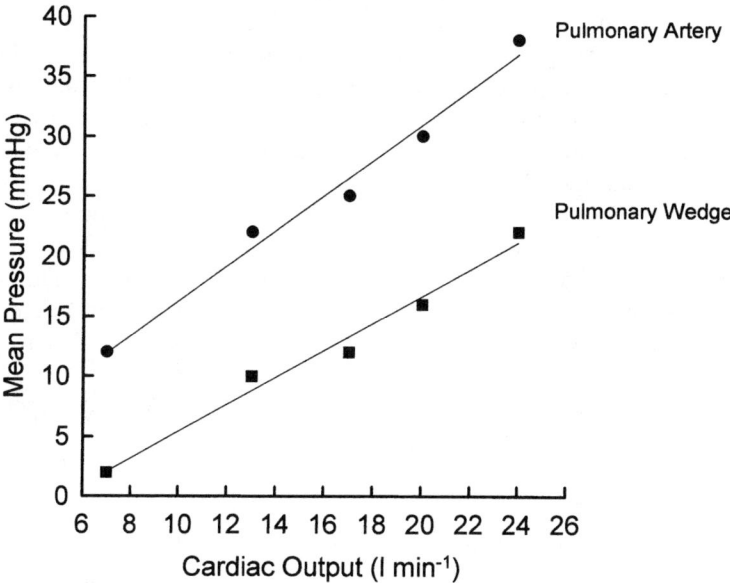

FIGURE 1 Rise in pulmonary arterial pressure (●) and wedge pressure (■) as cardiac output increases with exercise. (Redrawn from Reference 94.)

possible that some areas of the lungs do not receive adequate ventilation for local blood flow to maintain full saturation. However, a number of investigators have found that hypoxia may persist for as long as 20 min after exercise has been terminated.[46,57,58] Younes and Burks,[105] and more recently Caillaud et al.[14] found that this hypoxia may be associated with a rapid shallow pattern of breathing, which in turn has been associated with stimulation of J-receptors in the pulmonary interstitium by edema formation.[72] Schaffartzik et al.[82] observed that in subjects who retained low $\dot{V}/\dot{Q}_2$ ratios after exercise, vital capacities tended to be low, cardiac indices were higher, and arterial pH was lower than in those who had more abnormal $\dot{V}/\dot{Q}_2$ ratios. They suggested that interstitial edema might be responsible for altered gas exchange.

Double indicator dilution measurements have also been conducted in man during exercise and these appeared to indicate an increase in the amount of water in the lungs.[41,61] These studies must be interpreted carefully because increases in the detected water in the lungs may reflect better tissue perfusion rather than a real increase in lung water.[28] Transthoracic measurements of water have also suggested that lung water may be increased following exercise.[13] However, chest X-rays taken at full inspiration within 2 min after maximal exercise did not show changes expected with early interstitial edema.[38] More precise detection of edema formation might be possible with modern high-resolution computerized tomography or magnetic resonance imaging.

Evidence has been reported by two groups that strenuous exercise can increase the permeability of the pulmonary epithelium to hydrophilic solutes.[55,65] These investigators utilized a radioaerosol approach that is based upon the clearance of aerosolized ^{99m}Tc-DTPA from the lungs.[80] The cause of this apparent increase in epithelial permeability remains unclear, but increased stress applied to the alveolar membranes during exercise or elevations of intravascular and interstitial pressures (see Section V) might be responsible.

Although these observations suggest that there may be some lung injury and/or edema formation during vigorous exercise, frank pulmonary edema is decidedly unusual in normal subjects at sea level.[64,93] However, pulmonary edema is frequently associated with exercise in patients with increased pulmonary vascular pressures, such as in chronic congestive heart failure. Furthermore, it is observed under a variety of circumstances that are associated with elevations in pulmonary artery pressure, such as high altitude exposure[56] or acute central nervous system injuries.[59]

IV. STRUCTURE OF THE LUNGS

With the evolution of the mammalian lung, the barrier separating the blood from the airspaces has become progressively more attenuated.[95] Although this arrangement favors efficient gas exchange, it may also facilitate movement of water and solute into the interstitium and airspaces.

The barriers separating the pulmonary vasculature from the airspaces in the lungs comprise two cellular membranes: the endothelium and the epithelium, which are separated by an interstitium of variable width. The endothelium is continuous and the vessels are arranged in a complex network that has been described in terms of two sheets. More than 95% of the alveolar epithelial surface is covered by the type I cells. These cells are very attenuated and extend out in plates to several adjoining alveoli. Similar numbers of type II cells are also present on the alveolar surface, but these cells are more cuboidal in shape and account for less than 5% of the surface area of the alveoli. The type II cells tend to be located in the corners of the alveoli and are responsible for the secretion of surfactant within the lungs. They represent the precursors of the type I cells. Following injury, there is loss of type I cells and replacement by type II cells, which then mature to form new type I cells.[1,34,90,104]

The early studies of Schneeberger and Karnovsky[85] showed that the pulmonary epithelium is significantly less permeable to macromolecules (horseradish peroxidase) than the endothelium. When intravascular pressures are increased, this indicator makes its way through the spaces between endothelial cells and can be found in the interstitium, but passage through the intercellular spaces between the epithelial cells is blocked by the intercellular junctions. Utilizing freeze-fracture technology, Schneeberger and Karnovsky[84] showed that whereas the endothelial cells are joined by one or two rows of sealing beads, multiple rows of sealing strands connect the epithelial cells.

Cottrell et al.[20] demonstrated that the pulmonary capillaries are asymmetrical, with a thin portion facing the airspaces and a thicker region facing the interstitium of the lungs. They speculated that whereas gas exchange occurs primarily through the portion of the capillaries that is associated with the airspaces, solute and water movement is primarily restricted to the interstitial surfaces of the capillaries. Once fluid escapes the capillaries and enters the interstitium, it must find its way to the lymphatics, which do not descend in the airways below the level of the respiratory bronchioles. It has been proposed that edema fluid is carried along preferential pathways in the interstitium surrounding the alveoli to the lymphatics.[97]

A thin layer of fluid, frequently referred to as the epithelial lining fluid, normally covers the epithelial surface. The depth of this layer tends to be greater at the corners of the alveoli. The epithelial lining fluid is itself covered by a layer of laminar surfactant.

V. FILTRATION ACROSS THE PULMONARY CAPILLARIES

As in most other circulatory beds, fluid transport across the endothelium is governed by Starling forces. The flow of fluid across the endothelium is related to the difference between hydrostatic pressures and osmotic pressures across this barrier:

$$J_v = L_p S(\Delta p - \sigma_d \Delta \pi) \tag{1}$$

where L_p is the permeability of the capillary barrier and S is the surface area of the capillary bed, Δp designates the hydrostatic pressure difference between the capillary lumen and the interstitium, $\Delta \pi$ indicates the corresponding protein oncotic pressure difference and σ_d is the solute reflection coefficient of the endothelium, which is related to the leakiness of the endothelium to the proteins. This equation is simplified because it assumes that there is a single solute (a protein) that is playing a role in fluid transport. It is assumed that small solutes such as the normal electrolytes in the plasma and tissues freely pass through the endothelium, as originally posited by Starling.[87,88] Thus, J_v refers to the movement of protein-free fluid containing electrolytes.

The equation is useful because it indicates a variety of factors that could contribute to edema formation during exercise: (1) an increase in the permeability (L_p) of the endothelium to the movement of fluids, (2) an increase in the area of exchange (S), (3) an increase in the hydrostatic pressure difference (Δp) that drives fluid transport into the interstitium, and (4) a decrease in the plasma protein concentration, which has been observed during vigorous exercise.[35,47] It is not known if exercise has any effect upon σ_d, in other words, leakage of the protein across the endothelial barrier. Ultrafiltration of fluid into the interstitium during exercise would have two effects that act to reduce further transudation from the vasculature: (1) interstitial pressure would increase and (2) protein concentrations would decrease as fluid containing low concentrations of protein enters the interstitium.

The potential influence of exercise on fluid accumulation within the lungs is most readily detectable in patients who have congestive heart failure or mitral stenosis, in whom left atrial pressures increase with work and can result in the prompt development of pulmonary edema.

It has been suggested that very large increases in transmural pressures can increase capillary permeability to both fluid and proteins.[98-101] Formation of exudative edemas within the lungs following head trauma, high altitude exposure, and both cocaine and opiate overdosage has been attributed to vascular damage associated with marked elevations in capillary pressures.[17,54] These events would presumably increase Δp and decrease σ_d.

The early studies of Guyton and Lindsey[44] indicated what appeared to be a "safety factor" in the lungs that permitted lungs to withstand increases in hydrostatic pressure gradient up to 20 cm H_2O without developing edema. In these studies of dog lungs, edema developed at much lower pressures when protein was removed from the plasma. They hypothesized that the lungs are protected from edema formation by the low hydrostatic pressures (Δp) that prevail in the pulmonary capillaries as compared to systemic capillaries. They also hypothesized that large differences in plasma and tissue protein concentrations ($\Delta \pi$) would keep the interstitium free of edema fluid. It was therefore something of a surprise when it was subsequently discovered that lymphatic protein concentrations are only slightly less than those in the plasma.[33] This makes it more difficult to explain how $\Delta \pi$ could play an important role in keeping the lungs dry. It should be added that although hypoalbuminemia promotes peripheral edema in patients with nephrotic syndrome and liver disease, pulmonary edema is relatively uncommon in these conditions.

Some additional insight into the mechanisms that are responsible for keeping the lungs relatively "dry" is provided by considering the forces that are responsible for setting interstitial protein concentrations. The rate J_s at which a solute, in this case a protein, leaves the capillaries and enters the interstitium can be approximated by the equation:

$$J_s = P_d S \Delta c + (1 - \sigma_f) \overline{C} J_v \qquad (2)$$

where P_d is the permeability of the membrane to the solute, Δc is the concentration difference between the capillary and interstitium, σ_f is the solvent drag reflection coefficient, C is an average concentration in the capillary wall and J_v is the convectional flow through the capillary wall (see Equation 1). This is an approximate equation which was derived by Kedem and Katchalsky that applies to near-equilibrium conditions. More accurate equations have been derived by Patlak et al.[74] and Bressler et al.[10]

It is evident that protein concentrations in the interstitium will depend upon the balance between diffusion (the first term on the right side of Equation 2) and ultrafiltration (the second term on the right side of Equation 2). As ultrafiltration increases, protein concentrations will tend to fall. In contrast, increases in protein leakage, caused either by an increase in P_d or S, or a decrease in σ_f, will promote increases in interstitial protein concentration. Thus, the relatively high concentrations of protein found in the pulmonary interstitium could reflect either a relatively rapid rate of protein diffusion into the interstitium or a very slow rate of ultrafiltration. The observed resistance of the lungs to edema formation suggests that it is the slow rate of ultrafiltration and low values of Δp that are responsible for much of the immunity of the lungs to edema formation. However, as ultrafiltration increases, decreases in the oncotic pressure of the interstitium and increases in tissue pressure also inhibit further fluid accumulation within the lungs.

VI. ROLE OF LYMPHATICS, CUFFS, AND PLEURA

Once fluid and protein have reached the interstitium, subsequent clearance is presumably dependent upon lymphatic clearance. The actual magnitude of pulmonary lymph flow is difficult to measure with any accuracy. As emphasized by Drake and Gabel,[25] the fraction of the lung drained by the lymphatics that are under study can only be estimated, some of the lymph may be derived from nonpulmonary structures and cannulation of the ducts alters the amount of lymph carried within them. Despite these problems, they have estimated that lymph flow is normally between 3 and 4 ml/h/100 g lung weight in anesthetized sheep and can increase by tenfold or more when the lungs become edematous.

Some uncertainty persists regarding the manner in which the lymphatics convey fluid out of the lungs. Postnodal lymphatics have smooth muscle and are capable of pumping fluid with regular contractions.[11,53] This process is aided by the presence of one-way valves along the lymphatics that prevent backflow of fluid. Pumping is increased in the presence of edema, which may stimulate lymphatic contraction in a manner analogous to the effect that distension of the heart serves to increase cardiac output.

In addition to active contraction of lymphatics, there is good reason to believe that much of the flow of lymph is due to the passive effects of ventilation, which intermittently compresses these vessels.[3] Because vascular pulsations are transmitted all along the pulmonary circulation, the kinetic energy of this pulsation may also help to promote lymphatic flows. It is therefore possible that exercise can enhance lymph flow out of the lungs by increasing both ventilatory excursions and the force and rate of cardiac contractions. Animal studies indicate that increases in lymph flow during exercise exceed those observed when left atrial pressures are increased to levels comparable to those that occur during exercise. This suggests that hyperpnea contributes to increased lymph clearance.[66,67]

Despite the relative efficiency with which lymphatics can remove fluid from the interstitium, this mechanism can be overwhelmed. When this occurs, the fluid tends to accumulate in the loose interstitium that surrounds the larger airways and vessels in the form of "cuffs."[92] To what extent these cuffs can also conduct fluid to the mediastinum, where fluid can be drained by systemic lymphatics, remains uncertain. Regardless of whether much fluid can actually be removed in this fashion, the loose interstitium acts as a reservoir and may delay emergence of fluid into the airspaces of the lungs. However, edema of the airways as well as vascular congestion can interfere with the flow of gases in the bronchi, resulting in a clinical presentation of cardiac asthma.

Some attention has been given recently to the possible role of the pleura in transporting fluid from the surface of the lungs.[51] This route is particularly likely to be of importance in smaller animals, where the ratio between the pleural surface area to the volume of the lung is more favorable, but increases in fluid flow from the visceral surfaces of the lung have been observed when sheep lungs have been made edematous by volume overloading. Whether this provides a possible route for edema fluid during exercise remains uncertain. There appear to have been no radiologic studies to determine the frequency with which pleural effusions occur following exercise. Like the loose adventitia of the bronchi and larger vessels of the lung, the pleural space could act as a reservoir for excess fluid, though compression of the lung by larger effusions would obviously impair ventilation.[53] It could be speculated that the rate at which fluid is removed from the pleura is increased by vigorous ventilatory movements, which might increase fluid flow in the parietal lymphatics draining the pleural spaces.

VII. PASSIVE TRANSPORT OF FLUID ACROSS THE PULMONARY EPITHELIUM

Whereas Starling forces play an important role in governing the flow of fluids across the endothelium, they presumably have relatively little effect on fluid transport across the pulmonary epithelium, which is much less permeable to solutes of all sizes than the endothelium. Implicit in the Starling "law" is the assumption that although the endothelium is relatively impermeable to proteins, small solutes and electrolytes readily cross the capillary walls.[87,88] It is this difference in permeability to small and large solutes that is responsible for the importance of protein concentrations in avoiding edema formation. As noted above, evidence had been obtained that the pulmonary epithelium is much less permeable to macromolecules than the endothelium. The pulmonary epithelium, much like most other epithelial beds, is also much less permeable to small solutes than the endothelium.[81,89] The effects of small solutes on passive fluid movement across the epithelium can be conceptualized by generalizing the Starling equation:

$$J_v = PS\left(\Delta p \pm \sum_{i=1}^{n} \sigma_{d,i} \Delta \pi_i\right) \qquad (3)$$

where the contribution of each of the n solutes in the extracellular fluid is considered. If the reflection coefficients of common solutes such as Na^+ and Cl^- are close to 1.0, then the relative importance of concentration differences of proteins becomes much less important. Whereas protein concentrations in the plasma and interstitium are generally in the range of 1 mM, there are a total of about 280 mM of other, smaller solutes in these fluids. Indeed, it can be assumed that the rate at which fluid crosses the epithelium in response to increases in interstitial pressure would be restrained by the development of osmotic pressure differences related to the development of small differences in the concentrations of electrolytes across the epithelium. For example, the flow of a very small amount of water across the epithelium would lower interstitial Na^+ concentrations by 1 mM, a change in concentration that would be difficult to measure. If the reflection coefficients of Na^+ and its associated anions are close to 1.0, then a force equal to 40 cm H_2O would develop that would resist further transudation of fluid into the airspaces. The relative unimportance of proteins in governing fluid flow across the pulmonary epithelium was demonstrated by showing that over a range of protein concentration differences between the vasculature and airspace fluid that varied from +10 to −10 grams of albumin, no differences in the rates at which fluids were absorbed from the airspaces could be found.[31]

Provided that the integrity of the epithelium is not compromised, then the rate of filtration of fluid across the epithelium would be effectively governed by the permeability of this barrier. However, there is evidence that increases in interstitial pressure can have dramatic effects on the permeability of other epithelial membranes that can be either transient or may persist.[91] For example, although the mucosa of the gall bladder can remain relatively impermeable to the flow of fluid and solutes when luminal pressure is increased in this organ, even slight increases in the pressure on the adventitial surface of no more than 5 cm H_2O can increase filtration coefficients manyfold. This asymmetrical response of epithelial membranes can be attributed to alterations that occur in the interepithelial junctions. Because the tight junctions of these cells are located near the apical surfaces, increases in luminal pressures have little effect on the structure of the intercellular junctions unless they actually rupture the tight junctions. In contrast, increases in the interstitial pressure result in widening of these junctions and are more apt to result in disruption of the sealing strands that help to keep adjoining cells in contact.

Increases in interstitial pressure that might occur during exercise are presumably moderated by the ability of the loose portions of the interstitium to accommodate storage of fluid. However, local increases in pressure may lead to failure of the pulmonary epithelium and fluid entry into the airspaces. The common appearance of regional collections of edema fluid in the lung during acute congestive heart failure could reflect local failure of the alveolar-capillary wall with flooding of nearby airspaces. Of importance is the observation that the fluid that enters the airspaces is generally transudative — that is, it contains low concentrations of protein but concentrations of electrolytes are very similar to those found in the plasma. This would not be expected for an epithelial membrane, which is nearly as impermeable to small solutes as it is to proteins. However, it must be remembered that protein has been sieved by the endothelium from the fluid that enters the interstitium and reaches the epithelium. It is also possible that increases in interstitial pressure may make the interepithelial junctions more permeable to small solutes while maintaining their relative impermeability to protein molecules.

To the extent that exercise might increase tension on the intercellular junctions of the epithelium, one might expect an increase in their permeability. Marked increases in alveolar pressures during the ventilation of patients with adult respiratory distress syndrome have been blamed for further lung injury and edema formation.[27]

VIII. ACTIVE TRANSPORT ACROSS THE PULMONARY EPITHELIUM

Evidence that the pulmonary epithelium can actively absorb fluid from the airspaces was first found by Olver and Strang in fetal animals near the time of birth.[70] Prior to this time, the lungs actually secrete airway fluid. A variety of factors appear to be responsible for the reversal of flow near the time of birth. Secretion of epinephrine represents an important component of this process, but other hormones have also been implicated. Evidence that adult, air-filled lungs also reabsorb Na^+ from the airspaces was derived by a number of investigators in intact lungs, and it was subsequently shown that monolayers of type II pneumocytes are capable of transporting Na^+ from the apical to the basolateral surfaces.[4,5,30,40,63] It is not known whether the type I cells also participate in fluid transport. Not surprisingly, a complex variety of transporters have been associated with type II cells. As in most other cells, the energy needed for transport is provided primarily by the Na^+-K^+-ATPase transporter on the basolateral surfaces of type II cells (see Figure 2).[62] Beta-adrenergic agents act to increase transport across these cells by elevating intracellular cAMP concentrations and the resulting kinase-specific systems. It has also been shown that β-adrenergic agonists can increase alveolar fluid clearance *in vivo*.[6] Thus, it might be anticipated that increases in circulating catecholamines that are observed during exercise increase transport of fluid out of the airspaces.

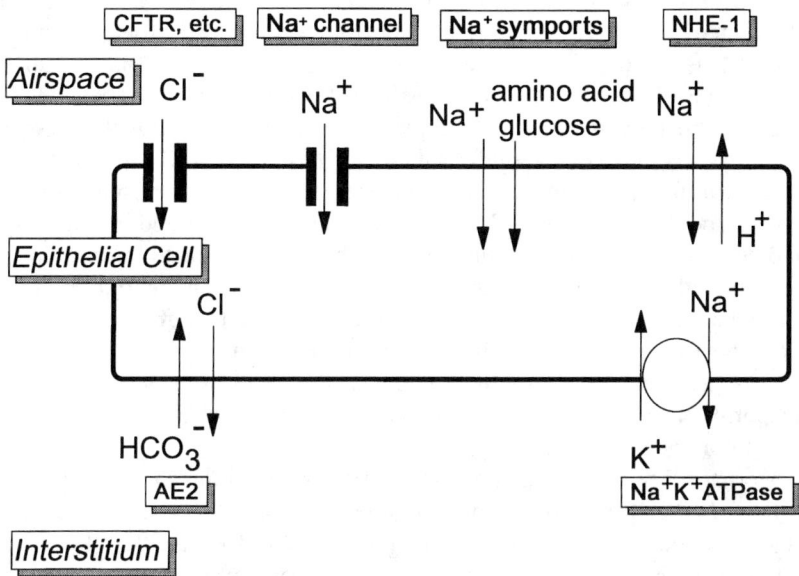

FIGURE 2 Some of the transport mechanisms that may be involved in minimizing fluid accumulation in the airways are shown in this schematic diagram of an alveolar epithelial cell. To what extent these transport functions are met by the type I and type II cells remains unclear. It will be noted that most of the energy expenditure in transporting solutes from the airspaces to the interstitium is related to operation of Na^+/K^+-ATPase on the basolateral surfaces of the cells. This pump acts to lower intracellular Na^+ concentrations, thereby increasing movement of Na^+ into the cells through a variety of pathways in the apical surface of the alveolar cells. Chloride movement accompanies that of Na^+ and is mediated by several transport mechanisms in the apical and basolateral surfaces of the cells.

IX. WATER TRANSPORT IN THE LUNGS

As far back as the mid-1950s, Solomon and his coinvestigators had shown that the permeability (P_f) of red cells to osmotic flows of water considerably exceeded the permeability (P_d) of these cells to tracer exchange.[71] They attributed this difference to the existence of "pores" in the red cell membranes that could accommodate bulk flow of fluid. After many failed attempts to identify the structures responsible for this process, Agre et al.[2] found the first of a family of "aquaporins" that are principally involved with the movement of water across cellular membranes. This aquaporin was a glycoprotein of which the polypeptide was of 28,000 daltons molecular weight, and the protein was referred to as the channel-forming integral membrane protein (or CHIP28). A tetramer of these molecules is present in the red cell membranes and water molecules are believed to traverse the center of each of these units in a single file.

In early studies of water transport in the lung, we had found that injections of hypertonic solutions of small solutes into the pulmonary artery result in the extraction of essentially solute-free water from the lungs.[28] Subsequent studies showed that when fluid-filled lungs are perfused with hypertonic solutions, the fluid lost from the airspaces was also very hypotonic.[29] These studies suggested the movement of water molecules had occurred through cell membranes that excluded extracellular solutes such as Na^+ and Cl^-. It is likely that transport through aquaporins was responsible for this phenomenon. Both the m-RNA and protein of the CHIP28 aquaporin have been found in a variety of endothelial membranes, including those of the lungs.[36,69] In addition, evidence was obtained that CHIP28 might also be present in the epithelium. However, more recent studies in our laboratory indicated that although water transport across the alveolar epithelium is probably conducted through a water channel, it is probably not the CHIP28 protein that is involved. A variety of other aquaporins have now been described that may participate in water flows across the pulmonary epithelium.[48,76]

Perhaps because there are less CHIP28 aquaporins in the pulmonary epithelium, the epithelium of the lung appears to be less permeable to water than the endothelium. This arrangement could help decrease fluid losses that occur during the hyperventilation that occurs during exercise. The abundance of these aquaporins in the endothelium suggests that contrary to conventional thought, much of the water that crosses capillary membranes in the lung traverses specialized channels that do not permit movement of Na^+ and other electrolytes. Presumably these electrolytes must traverse other channels to keep osmotic differences from accumulating, but it is not clear to what extent this would occur through the intercellular junctions or transport mechanisms in the cell membranes. Another advantage of the apparently asymmetrical permeability of the epithelium to water is the tendency for this arrangement to keep the osmolality of the cells in the alveolar membranes closer to those of the plasma, thereby decreasing the likelihood that these cells will become rapidly dehydrated with potentially catastrophic changes in cell volumes.[32,49]

X. STRESS FAILURE IN PULMONARY CAPILLARIES

It has been proposed recently that increased capillary transmural pressure may lead to separation of capillary endothelial cells, and, should the pressure become sufficiently elevated, stress failure of pulmonary capillaries may ensue.[9,19,98-101] Capillary stress failure may play a role in the development of several pulmonary disease states associated with increased pulmonary vascular pressures. These include neurogenic pulmonary edema, high altitude pulmonary edema, adult respiratory distress syndrome, and exercise-induced pulmonary hemorrhage seen in thoroughbred racehorses.[105] Moderate increases in vascular pressures can result in fluid transudation in accordance with the Starling relationship.[37,67] At higher pressures, disruption of capillary endothelial cells may occur with the formation of exudative edema. If vascular pressures become sufficiently elevated, complete failure of the blood–gas barrier may occur, resulting in frank pulmonary hemorrhage as observed frequently in racehorses.[100]

Using an *in situ* perfused rabbit lung model, pulmonary capillary transmural pressures of 40 mmHg and higher have been shown to cause significant disruption of the blood–gas barrier, leading to edema and the appearance of red cells in the interstitium and alveoli. In dog and horse lung models, similar changes were observed when pressures were raised to 68 and 100 mmHg, respectively.[9] These species differences may be related to differences in resting basement membrane thickness and capillary radius of curvature.[9] Although similar experimental data are unobtainable from humans, measurements of increased pulmonary vascular pressures during moderate exercise suggest that these same forces may be responsible for increased transvascular fluid movement in human lungs during extreme exercise. Fluid accumulation around vessels and/or airways can lead to changes in lung compliance as well as providing an impediment to gas exchange.[93] Both of these effects can lead to ventilation–perfusion inhomogeneities that may be contributing factors to the development of hypoxemia with extreme exercise. For the elite athlete, these may well provide a basis for limiting maximal exercise.[23,24,77,93,94]

Complete stress failure probably only occurs during bouts of extreme exercise, when pulmonary vascular pressures become sufficiently elevated to disrupt the integrity of the blood–gas barrier. The fact that practically 100% of thoroughbred racehorses in race training exhibit exercise-induced pulmonary hemorrhage[73,102] is evidence of the "design" dilemma of having a blood–gas barrier sufficiently thin to maximize gas exchange, yet strong enough to withstand elevated pulmonary vascular pressures that result from the increased cardiac output required to support the aerobic demands of racing. Genetic selection has led to what appears to be thickening of the alveolar–capillary barrier in thoroughbred horses, which is presumably at least partially responsible for protecting the lungs of racehorses from the extremely high pulmonary vascular pressures encountered during intense exercise.[8,9,52,100] Despite this thickening of the barrier, it is still apparently unable to cope with the high pressures that occur during extreme exercise.[9,99,100]

Many thoroughbred racehorses (and possibly greyhound dogs) show signs of complete capillary stress failure during intense exercise, as evidenced by bleeding into the lungs. That this phenomenon is not observed in man may reflect the fact that exercise in the average person is limited by factors other than those that demand high left atrial pressures, and thus, elevated pulmonary capillary pressures. It is possible that with advances in both exercise training techniques and detection methods, more evidence of stress failure of pulmonary capillaries in human athletes will be noted.

XI. CONCLUSIONS

Evolution of the gas exchange regions of the mammalian lung has been closely associated with increasing attenuation of the membranes that separate the blood traversing the lungs and the air with which it exchanges. This situation is fraught with the risk that fluid will enter the airspaces, thereby frustrating efficient exchange. The fact that edema and even capillary hemorrhage is observed in some species during vigorous exercise seems to be related in part to the level to which capillary pressures increase in animals. The infrequency with which edema occurs in man may be related in part to the fact that capillary pressures do not reach levels that would promote edema formation. Excessive amounts of fluid escape from the capillaries when capillary pressures reach sufficiently high levels in congestive heart failure and after exposure to high altitude, opiates, or central nervous system injuries. Although lymphatic and perhaps pleural transport can keep pace with some edema formation, these mechanisms may become overwhelmed. Fluid may then be stored in the pulmonary interstitium and pleural cavities. So long as the integrity of the epithelium is maintained, the airspaces remain open and the only inconvenience that is likely is some airway congestion, edema, and asthmatic symptoms. However, the pulmonary epithelium is probably unable to withstand more than minimal increases in interstitial pressure without rupturing, followed by the airway filling with fluid and even blood. Species bred to run, such as racehorses and greyhounds, require increased left atrial pressures to guaranty adequate cardiac output. Whether training advances for human athletes will eventually predispose to clinically important pulmonary edema remains to be seen. Presumably, some of the potentially beneficial aspects of exercise, such as increased lymph flow related to hyperpnea and increased reabsorption of alveolar fluid stimulated by high levels of catecholamines, will minimize edema formation within the lungs. However, persistence of some indirect physiological signs of edema accumulation within the lungs should serve as a warning that as exercise becomes more extreme, pulmonary edema may well become a significant problem.

REFERENCES

1. Adamson, I. Y. R. and Bowden, D. H., The type II cell as a progenitor of alveolar epithelial regeneration, *Lab. Invest.*, 30: 35–42, 1974.

2. Agre, P., Preston, G. M., Smith, B. L., Jung, J. S., Raina, S., Monon, C., Guggino, W. B., and Nielsen, S., Aquaporin CHIP: The archetypal molecular water channel, *Am. J. Physiol.*, 265: F463–F476, 1993.
3. Aukland, K. and Reed, R. K., Interstitial-lymphatic mechanisms in the control of extracellular fluid volume. *Physiol. Rev.*, 73:1–78, 1993.
4. Basset, G., Crone, C., and Saumon, G., Fluid absorption by rat lung *in situ*: Pathways for sodium entry in the luminal membrane of alveolar epithelium, *J. Physiol. London*, 384:325–345,1987.
5. Basset, G., Crone, C., and Saumon, G., Significance of active ion transport in transalveolar water absorption: A study on isolated rat lung, *J. Physiol. London*, 384:311–324,1987.
6. Berthiaume, Y., Staub, N. C., and Matthay, M. A., β-Adrenergic agonists increase lung liquid clearance in anesthetized sheep, *J. Clin. Invest.*, 79:335–343, 1987.
7. Bhattacharya, J., Nanjo, S., and Staub, N. C., Micropuncture measurement of lung microvascular pressure during 5-HT infusion, *J. Appl. Physiol.*, 52:634–637, 1982.
8. Birks, E. K., Giri, S. N., Li, C., and Jones, J. H., Effects of exercise on plasma concentrations of prostaglandins and thromboxane B_2, in *Equine Exercise Physiology 3*, Persson, S. G. B., Lindholm, A., and Jeffcott, L. B., Eds., ICEEP Publications, Davis, CA, 1991, 374–379.
9. Birks, E. K., Mathieu-Costello, O., Fu, Z., Tyler, W. S., and West, J. B., Comparative aspects of the strength of pulmonary capillaries in rabbit, dog, and horse, *Respir. Physiol.*, 97:235–246, 1994.
10. Bresler, E. H., Mason, E. A., and Wendt, R. P., Appraisal of equations for neutral solute flux across porous sieving membranes, *Biophys. Chem.*, 4:229–236, 1976.
11. Broaddus, V. C., Wiener-Kronish, J. P., and Staub, N. C., Clearance of lung edema in the pleural space of volume-loaded anesthetized sheep, *J. Appl. Physiol.* 68:2623–2630, 1990.
12. Brower, R. and Permutt, S., Exercise and the pulmonary circulation in exercise, in *Lung Biology in Health and Disease, Vol. 52*, Wipp, B. J. and Wasserman, K., Eds., Marcel Dekker, New York, 1991, pp. 201–221.
13. Buono, M. J., Wilmore, J. H., and Roby, F. B., Jr., Evidence of increased thoracic extravascular fluid following intense exercise in man (Abstract), *Physiologist*, 25:201, 1982.
14. Caillaud, C. F., Anselme, J., Mercier, and Préfaut, C., Pulmonary gas exchange and breathing pattern during and after exercise in highly trained athletes, *Eur. J. Appl. Physiol.*, 67:431–437, 1993.
15. Colice, G., Neurogenic pulmonary edema, *Clin. Chest Med.*, 6:473–489, 1985.
16. Collee, G. G., Lynch, K. E., Hill, R. D., and Zapol, W. M., Bedside measurement of pulmonary capillary pressure in patients with acute respiratory failure, *Anesthesiology*, 66:614–620, 1987.
17. Cooper, Jr., J. A. D., White, D. A., and Matthay, R. A., State of the art: drug induced pulmonary disease, *Am. Rev. Respir. Dis.*, 133:321–340, 488–505, 1986.
18. Cope, D. K., Allison, R. C., Parmentier, J. L., Miller, J. N., and Taylor, A. E., Measurement of effective pulmonary capillary pressure using the pressure profile after pulmonary artery occlusion, *Crit. Care Med.*, 14:16–22, 1986.
19. Costello, M. L., Mathieu-Costello, O., and West, J. B., Stress failure of alveolar epithelial cells studied by scanning electron microscopy, *Am. Rev. Respir. Dis.*, 145:1446–1455, 1992.
20. Cottrell, T. S., Levine, O. R., Senior, R. M., Wiener, J., Spiro, D., and Fishman, A. P., Electron microscopic alterations at the alveolar level in pulmonary edema, *Circ. Res.*, 21: 783–797, 1967.
21. Dawson, C. A., Role of pulmonary vasomotion in physiology of the lung, *Physiol. Rev.*, 64:544–616, 1984.
22. Dawson, C. A., Linehan, J. H., and Rickaby, D. A., Pulmonary microcirculatory haemodynamics, *Ann. N.Y. Acad. Sci.*, 384:90–106, 1982.
23. Dempsey, J. A., Some exercise-induced imperfections in pulmonary gas exchange, *Can. J. Sport Sci.*, 12:66–71, 1987.

24. Dempsey, J. A., Is the lung built for exercise? *Med. Sci. Sports Exer.*, 18:143–155, 1986.
25. Drake, R. E. and Gabel, J. C., Pulmonary edema fluid clearance pathways, *N.I.P.S.*, 10:107–111, 1995.
26. Drake, R. E. and Laine, G. A., Pulmonary microvascular permeability to fluid and macromolecules, *J. Appl. Physiol.*, 64:487–501, 1988.
27. Dreyfuss, D., Soler, P., Basset, G., and Saumon, G., High inflation pressure pulmonary edema: Respective effects of high airway pressure, high tidal volume and positive end-expiratory pressure, *Am. Rev. Respir. Dis.*, 137:1159–1164, 1988.
28. Effros, R.M., Lung water measurements with the mean transit time approach, *J. Appl. Physiol.*, 59:673–683, 1985.
29. Effros, R. M., Mason, G. R., Sietsema, K., Hukkanen, J., and Silverman, P., Pulmonary epithelial sieving of small solutes in rat lungs, *J. Appl. Physiol.*, 65:640–648, 1988.
30. Effros, R. M., Mason, G. R., Hukkanen, J., and Silverman, P., New evidence for active sodium transport in fluid-filled rat lungs, *J. Appl. Physiol.*, 66:909–919, 1989.
31. Effros, R. M., Hacker, A., Silverman, P., and Hukkanen, J., Protein concentrations have little effect on reabsorption of fluid from isolated rat lungs, *J. Appl. Physiol.*, 70:416–422, 1991.
32. Effros, R.M., Darin, C., and Krenz, G. S., Evidence for asymmetrical distribution of CHIP28 aquaporins in alveolar-capillary barrier, *FASEB J.*, 9:A279, 1995.
33. Erdman, A. J., Vaughan, T. R., Brigham, K. L., Woolverton, W. C., and Staub, N.C., Effect of increased vascular pressure on lung fluid balance in unanesthetized sheep, *Circ. Res.*, 37:271–284, 1975.
34. Evans, M. F. J., Cabral, L. F., Stephens, R. J., and Freeman, G., Transformation of alveolar type II cells to type I cells following exposure to nitrogen dioxide, *Exp. Mol. Path.*, 22:142–150, 1975.
35. Fellmann, N., Hormonal and plasma volume alterations following endurance exercise, *Sports Medicine*, 13:37–49, 1992.
36. Folkesson, H., Matthay, M. A., Hasegawa, H., Kheradmand, F., and Verkman, A. S., Transcellular water transport in lung alveolar epithelium through mercurial-sensitive water channels, *Proc. Natl. Acad. Sci. U.S.A.*, 91:4970–4974, 1994.
37. Gaar, K. A., Taylor, A. E., Owens, L. J., and Guyton, A. C., Pulmonary capillary pressure and filtration coefficient in the isolated perfused lung, *Am. J. Physiol.*, 213:910–914, 1967.
38. Gallagher, G. G., Huda, W., Rigby, M., Greenberg, D., and Younes, M., Lack of radiographic evidence of interstitial pulmonary edema after maximal exercise in normal subjects, *Am. Rev. Respir. Dis.*, 137:474–476, 1988.
39. Goodman, B. E. and Crandall, E. D., Dome formation in primary cultured monolayers of alveolar epithelial cells, *Am. J. Physiol.*, 243:C96–100, 1982.
40. Goodman, B. E., Kim, K. J., and Crandall, E. D., Evidence for active sodium transport across alveolar epithelium of isolated rat lung, *J. Appl. Physiol.*, 62:2460–2466, 1987.
41. Goresky, C. A., Warnica, J. W., Burgess, J. H., Cronin, R. F. P., and Nadeau, B. E., Changes during exercise in man, *Fed. Proc.*, 31:307–311, 1972.
42. Grimbert, F. A., Effective pulmonary capillary pressure, *Eur. Respir. J.*, 1:297–301, 1988.
43. Groves, B. M., Reeves, J. T., Sutton, J. R., Wagner, P. D., Cymerman, A., Malconian, M. K., Rock, P. B., Young, P. M., and Houston, C. S., Operation Everest II: Elevated high-altitude pulmonary resistance unresponsive to oxygen, *J. Appl. Physiol.*, 63:521–530, 1987.
44. Guyton, A. C. and Lindsey, A. W., Effect of elevated left atrial pressure and decreased plasma protein concentration on the development of pulmonary edema, *Circ. Res.*, 7:649–657, 1959.
45. Hackett, P. H., Bertman J., Rodriguez, G., and Tenney, J., Pulmonary edema fluid protein in high-altitude pulmonary edema, *J. Am. Med. Assoc.*, 256:36, 1986.

46. Hammond, M. D., Gale, G. E., Kapitan, K. S., Ries, A., and Wagner, P. D., Pulmonary gas exchange in humans during exercise at sea level, *J. Appl. Physiol.*, 60:1590–1598, 1986.
47. Harrison, M. H., Effects of thermal stress and exercise on blood volume in humans, *Physiol. Rev.*, 65:149–209, 1985.
48. Hasegawa, H., Ma, T., Skach, W., Matthay, M. A., and Verkman, A. S., Molecular cloning of a mercurial-insensitive water channel expressed in selected water-transporting tissues, *J. Biol. Chem.*, 269:5497–5500, 1994.
49. Hasegawa, H., Lian, S. C., Finkbeiner, W. E., and Verkman, A. S., Extrarenal tissue distribution of CHIP28 water channels by in situ hybridization and antibody staining, *Am. J. Physiol.*, 266:C893–903, 1994.
50. Holloway, H., Perry, M., Downey, Parker, J., and Taylor, A., Estimation of effective pulmonary capillary pressure in intact lungs, *J. Appl. Physiol.: Respir. Environ. Exer. Physiol.*, 54:846–851, 1983.
51. Johnston, M. G., Involvement of lymphatic collecting ducts in the physiology and pathophysiology of lymph flow, in *Experimental Biology of the Lymphatic Circulation*, M. G. Johnson, Ed., Elsevier Amsterdam: 1985, 81–120.
52. Jones, J. H., Smith, B. L., Birks, E. K., Pascoe, J. R., and Hughes, T. R., Left atrial and pulmonary arterial pressures in exercising horses (Abstract), *FASEB J.*, 6:A2020, 1992.
53. Lai-Fook, S. J. and Rodarte, J. R., Pleural pressure distribution and its relationship to lung volume and interstitial pressure, *J. Appl. Physiol.*, 70:967–978, 1991.
54. Lang, S. A. and Maron M. B., Hemodynamic basis for cocaine-induced pulmonary edema in dogs, *J. Appl. Physiol.*, 71:1166–1170, 1991.
55. Lorino, A. M., Meignan, M., Bouissou, P., and Atlan, G., Effects of sustained exercise on pulmonary clearance of aerosolized 99mTc-DTPA, *J. Appl. Physiol.*, 67: 2055–2059, 1989.
56. Malik, A. B., Pulmonary vascular response to increase in intracranial pressure: Role of sympathetic mechanisms, *J. Appl. Physiol.*, 42:335–343, 1977.
57. Manier, G., Moinard, J., Techoueyres, P., Varene, P., and Guenard, H., Pulmonary diffusion limitation after prolonged strenuous exercise, *Respir. Physiol.*, 83:143–154, 1991.
58. Manier, G., Moinard, J., and Stoicheff, H., Pulmonary diffusing capacity after maximal exercise, *J. Appl. Physiol.*, 75:2580–2585, 1993.
59. Maron, M. B., Analysis of airway fluid protein concentration in neurogenic pulmonary edema, *J. Appl. Physiol.*, 62:470–476, 1987.
60. Maron, M. B., Holcomb, P. H., Dawson, C. A., Rickaby, D. A., Clough, A. V., and Linehan, J. H., Edema development and recovery in neurogenic pulmonary edema, *J. Appl. Physiol.*, 77:1155–1163, 1994.
61. Marshall, B. E., Teichner, R. L., Kallos, T., Sugerman, H. J., Wyche, M. Q., and Tantum K. R., Effects of posture in exercise on the pulmonary extravascular water volume in man, *J. Appl. Physiol.*, 31:375–379, 1971.
62. Mason, R. J., Williams, M. C, Widdicombe, J. H., Sanders, M. J., Misfeldt, D. S., and Berry, L. C., Jr., Transepithelial transport by pulmonary alveolar type II cells in primary culture, *Proc. Natl. Acad. Sci. U.S.A.*, 79:6033–6037, 1982.
63. Matthay, M. A., Lundult, C. C., and Staub, N. C., Differential liquid and protein clearance from the alveoli of anesthetized sheep, *J. Appl. Physiol.*, 53:96–104, 1982.
64. McKechnie, J. K., Leary, W. P., Noakes, T. D., Kallmeyer, J. C., MacSearraigh, E. T. M., and Olivier, L. R., Acute pulmonary oedema in two athletes during a 90-km running race, *S. Afr. Med. J.*, 56:261–265, 1979.
65. Meignan, M., Rosso, J., Leveau, J., Katz, A., Cinotti, L., Medallion, G., and Gable, P., Exercise increases the lung clearance of inhaled technetium 99mDTPA, *J. Nucl. Med.*, 27: 274–280, 1986.
66. Newman, J. H., Butka, B. J., Parker, R. E., and Roselli, R. J., Effect of progressive exercise on lung fluid balance in sheep, *J. Appl. Physiol.*, 64:2125–2131, 1988.

67. Newman, J. H., Cochran, C. P., Roselli, R. J., Parker, R. E., and King L. S., Pressure and flow changes in the pulmonary circulation in exercising sheep: Evidence for elevated microvascular pressure, *Am. Rev. Respir. Dis.*, 147:921–926, 1993.
68. Nicolaysen, G., Waaler, B. A., and Aarseth P., On the existence of stretchable pores in the exchange vessels of the isolated rabbit lung preparation, *Lymphology*, 12:201–207, 1979.
69. Nielsen, S., Smith, B. L., Christensen, E. I., and Agre, P., Distribution of the aquaporin CHIP in secretory and resorptive epithelia and capillary endothelia, *Proc. Natl. Acad. Sci. U.S.A.*, 90:7275–7279, 1993.
70. Olver, R. E. and Strang, L. D., Ion fluxes across the pulmonary epithelium and the secretion of lung liquid in the foetal lamb, *J. Physiol. London*, 241:327–357, 1974.
71. Paganelli, C. V., and Solomon, A. K., The rate of exchange of tritiated water across the human red cell membrane, *J. Gen. Physiol.*, 41:259–277, 1957.
72. Paintal, A. S., Vagal sensory receptors and their reflex effects, *Physiol. Rev.*, 53:159–227, 1973.
73. Pascoe, J. R., Ferraro, G. L., Cannon, J. H., Arthur, R. M., and Wheat, J. D., Exercise-induced pulmonary hemorrhage in racing thoroughbreds: A preliminary study, *Am. J. Vet. Res.*, 42:703–707, 1981.
74. Patlack, C. S., Goldstein, D. A., and Hoffman, J. F., The flow of solute and solvent across a two membrane system, *J. Theor. Biol.*, 5:425–442, 1963.
75. Preston, G. M., Smith, B. L., Zeidel, M. L., Moulds, J. J., and Agre, P., Mutations in aquaporin-1 in phenotypically normal humans without functional CHIP water channels, *Science*, 265:1585–1587, 1994.
76. Raina, S, Preston, G. M., Guggino, W. B., and Agre, P., Molecular cloning and characterization of an aquaporin cDNA from salivary, lacrimal, and respiratory tissues. *J. Biol. Chem.*, 270:1908–1912, 1995.
77. Reeves, J. T., Dempsey, J. A., and Grover, R. F., Pulmonary circulation during exercise, in *Lung Biology in Health and Disease, Vol. 38*, Weir, E. K. and Reeves, J. T., Eds., Marcel Dekker, New York, 1988, 107–133.
78. Reeves, J. T., Groves, B. M., Cymerman, A., Sutton, J. R., Wagner, P. D., Turkevich, D., and Houston, C. S., Operation Everest II: Cardiac filling pressures during cycle exercise at sea level, *Respir. Physiol.*, 80:147–154, 1990.
79. Reeves, J. T., Groves, B. M., Sutton, J. R., Wagner, P. D., Cymerman, A., Malconian, M. K., Rock, P. B., Young, P. M., and Houston, C. S., Operation Everest II: Preservation of cardiac function at extreme altitude, *J. Appl. Physiol.*, 63:531–539, 1987.
80. Rinderknecht, J., Shapiro, L., Krauthammer, M., Taplin, G., Wasserman, K., Uszler, J. M., and Effros, R. M., Accelerated clearance of small solutes from the lungs in interstitial lung disease, *Am. Rev. Respir. Dis.*, 121:105–117, 1980.
81. Saumon, G. and Basset, G., Electrolyte and fluid transport across the mature alveolar epithelium, *J. Appl. Physiol.*, 74:1–15, 1993
82. Schaffartzik, W., Poole, D. C., Derion, T., Tsukimoto, K., Hogan, M. C., Arco, J. P, Bebout, D. E and Wagner, P.D., V̇/Q̇ distribution during heavy exercise and recovery in humans: Implications for pulmonary edema, *J. Appl. Physiol.*, 72:1657–1667, 1992.
83. Schaffartzik, W., Arcos, J., Tsukimoto, K., Mathieu-Costello, O., and Wagner, P. D., Pulmonary interstitial edema in the pig after heavy exercise, *J. Appl. Physiol.*, 75:2535–2540, 1993.
84. Schneeberger, E. E. and Karnovsky, M. J., Substructure of intercellular junctions in freeze–fractured alveolar-capillary membrane of mouse lung. *Circ. Res.* 38:404–411, 1976.
85. Schneeberger, E. E. and Karnovsky, M. J., The ultrastructural basis of alveolar–capillary membrane permeability to peroxidase used as a tracer. *J. Cell Biol.*, 37:781–793, 1968.
86. Sidel, V. W. and Solomon, A. K., Entrance of water into human red cells under an osmotic pressure gradient, *J. Gen. Physiol.*, 41:243–257, 1957.
87. Starling, E. H., On the absorption of fluids from the connective tissue, *J. Physiol. London*, 19:312–326, 1895–1896.

88. Starling, E. H., Physiological factors involved in the causation of dropsy, *Lancet*, 1:1267-1270, 1896.
89. Taylor, A. E. and Gaar, K. A., Estimation of equivalent pore radii of pulmonary capillary and alveolar membranes, *Am. J. Physiol.*, 218:1133–1140, 1970.
90. Valimaki, M., and Ninikoski, J., Development and reversibility of pulmonary oxygen poisoning in the rat, *Aerosp. Med.* 44: 533–538, 1973.
91. van Os, C.H., Wiedner, G., and Wright, E. M., Volume flow across gallbladder epithelium induced by small hydrostatic and osmotic gradients. *J. Membr. Biol.*, 49: 1–20, 1979.
92. Vreim, C. E., Snashall, P. D., Demling, R. H., and Staub, N.C., Lung lymph and free interstitial fluid protein composition in sheep with edema, *Am. J. Physiol.*, 230: 1650–1653, 1976.
93. Wagner, P. D., Ventilation-perfusion matching during exercise, *Chest*, 101:192S–198S, 1992.
94. Wagner, P. D., Gale, G. E., Moon, R. E., Torre-Bueno, J. R., Stolp, B. W., and Saltzman, H. A., Pulmonary gas exchange in humans exercising at sea level and simulated altitude, *J. Appl. Physiol.*, 61:260–270, 1986.
95. Weibel, E. R., Functional morphology of lung parenchyma, in *Handbook of Physiology*, Macklem, P. T. and Mead, J., Eds., American Physiological Society, Bethesda, MD, 1986 89–111.
96. Weibel, E. R., Oxygen demand and the size of respiratory structures in mammals, In: *Evolution of Respiratory Processes. A Comparative Approach*, Wood, S. C. and Lenfant, C., Eds., Marcel Dekker, New York, 1979, pp. 289–346.
97. Weibel, E.R. and Bachofen, H., Structural design of the alveolar septum and fluid exchange, in *Pulmonary Edema*, Fishman, A.P. and Renkin, E. M., Eds., American Physiological Society, Bethesda, MD, 1979, 1–20.
98. West, J. B. and Mathieu-Costello, O., Stress failure of pulmonary capillaries in the intensive care setting, *Schweiz. Med. Wochenschr.*, 122:751–757, 1992.
99. West, J. B. and Mathieu-Costello, O., Stress failure of pulmonary capillaries as a limiting factor for maximal exercise, *Eur. J. Appl. Physiol.*, 70:99-108, 1995.
100. West, J. B., Mathieu-Costello, O., Jones, J. H., Birks, E. K., Logemann, R. B., Pascoe, J. R., and Tyler, W. S., Stress failure of pulmonary capillaries in racehorses with exercise-induced pulmonary hemorrhage, *J. Appl. Physiol.*, 75:1097-1109, 1993.
101. West, J. B., Tsukimoto, K., Mathieu-Costello, O., and Prediletto, R., Stress failure in pulmonary capillaries, *J. Appl. Physiol.*, 70:1731-1742, 1991.
102. Whitwell, K. E. and Greet, T. R. C., Collection and evaluation of tracheobronchial washes in the horse, *Equine Vet. J.*, 16:499-508, 1984.
103. Widimsky, J., Berglund, E., and Malmberg, R., Effect of repeated exercise on the lesser circulation, *J. Appl. Physiol.*, 18:983–986, 1963.
104. Witsch, I. H., Proliferation of type II cells: a review of common responses in toxic lung injury, *Toxicology*, 5:267–277, 1976.
105. Younes, M. and Burks. J., Breathing pattern during and after exercise of different intensities. *J. Appl. Physiol.* 59:898–908, 1985.
106. Younes, M., Bshouty, Z., and Ali, J., Longitudinal distribution of pulmonary vascular resistance with very high pulmonary blood flow, *J. Appl. Physiol.*, 62:344–358, 1987.

Chapter **6**

INTEGRATED CONTROL OF BODY FLUID BALANCE DURING EXERCISE

Patricia C. Szlyk-Modrow
Ralph P. Francesconi
Roger W. Hubbard

CONTENTS

I. Historical Perspective and Overview 118
   A. Voluntary Dehydration 118
   B. Insensible Water Loss 118
   C. Renal Water Loss 118
   D. Vasopressin Release 119
   E. Osmoregulation......................................119
   F. Blood Volume 120

II. Behavior and Physiology 120
   A. Drinking and Palatibility..............................120
   B. Thirst, Missing Osmols, and Rehydration 121
   C. Osmoreceptors and Sodium Receptors...................122
   D. Aging..122

III. Hormonal Integration 123
   A. Atrial Natriuretic Peptide 123
   B. AVP, Plasma Renin Activity, and Aldosterone..............124

IV. Hepatic, Renal and CNS Receptors 127
   A. Hepatic and Portal Osmoreceptors......................127
   B. CNS and Peripheral Interactions 127
   C. Intestinal Osmoreceptors and Effects....................129

V. Conclusion 129

Acknowledgments 130

References 130

I. HISTORICAL PERSPECTIVE AND OVERVIEW

A. VOLUNTARY DEHYDRATION

Euhydration is maintained as a dynamic balance between body water loss (sweating and urination) and fluid replacement as the perception of thirst strengthens into a drive.[76] Without a conscious effort to drink in the absence of thirst, some hypohydration usually occurs before water is consumed, especially during exercise. This delay in drinking has been referred to by Rothstein et al.[110] as "voluntary dehydration" and occurs because "thirst is an inadequate stimulus to drinking".[76] Moreover, Pitts et al.[104] emphasized that, during work in the heat, humans rarely voluntarily drink as much water as they lose and usually replace only two thirds of net water loss.

B. INSENSIBLE WATER LOSS

Evaporative water loss by a nonsweating individual comprises respiratory water loss and insensible perspiration, and is called insensible water loss.[76] Under normal conditions respiratory water loss is about 200 ml per day but may reach 350 ml per day for men working in a dry climate and approach 1500 ml per day for men working at altitude in cold, dry air.[76] Insensible perspiration may be as low as 500 ml per day in a moist climate, and even with a minimum urine volume (<300 ml/day), obligate losses of 1000 ml/day must be replenished.

C. RENAL WATER LOSS

Urine usually comprises a maximum of 1.4 osmoles/l of catabolites (mostly urea) and surplus electrolytes when a subject is consuming a mixed diet. Maximal water loss by the kidneys during hyperhydration is directly correlated with the glomerular filtration rate and the solute load.[70] Without arginine vasopressin (AVP) action, nearly all of the urine that reaches the distal tubules is excreted,[131] and this represents the maximal rate of renal water loss. In Kleeman's subjects,[70] this rate was equivalent to 23.7 ml/min or 1422 ml/h which is similar to the maximal rate of gastric emptying, 15 to 20 ml/min or

---

* The views, opinions, and findings in this report are those of the authors, and should not be construed as an official Department of the Army position, policy, or decision, unless so designated by other official documentation. Citations of commercial organizations and trade names in this report do not constitute an official Department of the Army endorsement or approval of the products or services of these organizations.

900 to 1200 ml/h.[29] Thus, the greater rate of water loss in a healthy individual may occur through eccrine sweating, which can exceed 3 l/h for short periods, while prolonged sweating can be sustained at over 1 l/h for 12–18 h.

D. VASOPRESSIN RELEASE

Vokes[129] contends that "one of the best examples of a perfectly functioning homeostatic system is water balance." Because the homeostatic control of body temperature benefits from both behavioral and physiological adjustments, it is not surprising that the thirst mechanism employs similar strategies in dealing with environmental challenge. Increases in osmolality stimulate osmoreceptors (supraoptic region of the hypothalamus) resulting in AVP release that stimulates renal water reabsorption.[127] Thirst was regarded by Elkinton and co-workers[34,35] as central in origin and closely correlated with antidiuresis, hypertonicity, and intracellular water deficit. The threshold for AVP release and renal water conservation occurs at lower osmolalities than the thirst threshold; polydipsic patients manifest aberrations in AVP release in response to hypertonicity.[90] Thus, thirst behavior does not become prominent until the osmotic dehydration exceeds the renal capacity to deal with it physiologically.

E. OSMOREGULATION

Although the solute composition of the extracellular compartment is markedly different from the intracellular space, the total osmolality (solute concentration, not content) is very similar[25] because most cell membranes are permeable to water. The major intracellular osmotic solutes are potassium, magnesium, organic phosphates, and protein. The major solutes in extracellular fluid are sodium (Na) and its anions, chloride and bicarbonate. They are impermeant and are kept on the proper side of the membrane by molecular size, electrical charge, or active pumps. Net movement of water is determined by the osmolalities of the intra- and extracellular compartments.[100]

The osmoregulatory system displays large interindividual differences in both sensitivity and threshold. Generally, the range of body fluid osmolality in health is 280–295 mOsm/kg of water, and at 280 mOsm/kg water, AVP release is inhibited and urine osmolality is minimal (<100 mOsm/kg of water). Although there is wide variation in the individual thirst threshold, Vokes[129] estimates the average at 295 mOsm/kg, with significant decrements in thirst sensitivity occurring with age.[83] Thus, at the thirst threshold the increased AVP concentration elicits maximum urinary concentration (UOsm>800–1000 mOsm/kg of water).

The most important stimulus for thirst and AVP release is hypohydration characterized by reduced intracellular fluid volume, hyperosmolality of the body fluids, or elevated "extracellular" Na.[105] Andersson[3] has described those conditions that result in thirst and AVP release as: (1) net water loss through absolute hypohydration or primary water depletion; and (2) a state of Na excess with no net water loss (relative dehydration), such as by hypertonic saline infusions. Although cerebral receptors regulate AVP secretion, substances equilibrating with the intracellular fluid (urea) do not stimulate AVP release. The principal determinant of extracellular fluid osmolality is Na, and plasma hyperosmolality during absolute hypohydration is characterized by hypernatremia. When further increases in plasma osmolality and AVP can no longer increase water conservation, thirst stimulates water intake at a plasma osmolality of approximately 295 or an average water deficit of 2–3%.

F. BLOOD VOLUME

Andersson[3] suggested that thirst may develop when the fluid volume of the body is reduced without any appreciable change in extracellular Na or tonicity. A baroreceptor mechanism composed of stretch receptors in the cardiac atria, aortic arch, and carotid sinuses responds to changes in blood volume or pressure by altering the tonic inhibition of AVP release.[52] Blood loss also stimulates an elevation of angiotensin II (Ang II);[79] both Ang II and isoproterenol[79] stimulate water consumption markedly. Attenuated renal blood flow stimulates renin release and thirst without change in overall water and salt balance.[39] Although Ang II is a potent dipsogen in experimental animals when injected intravenously (i.v.)[39] or intracerebroventricularly (i.c.v.),[36] the evidence in humans is less clear because most patients with high levels of plasma renin activity (PRA) and Ang II have no apparent abnormality in thirst.[106] Andersson[3] has proposed that Ang II increases the sensitivity of Na receptors. Thus, a volumetric mechanism mediated by the renal renin–angiotensin system could still have its final link in the Na receptors.

An alternative idea to Verney's osmoreceptor theory is a receptor/excitation mechanism sensitive to Na. Because certain substances known to stimulate Na-K-ATPase activity apparently interact with Na in eliciting AVP and thirst, this enzyme system may be essential for receptor excitation. For example, Gutman[58] injected an inhibitor of active Na transport and observed reduced drinking in response to a load of hypertonic saline in nephrectomized rats. Ouabain and glycerol injections had the same effect.[13] Because active Na extrusion is necessary for the maintenance of cell volume, any inhibition of the Na pump generally results in cell swelling. This could be an interesting interface between the osmoreceptor (cell shrinkage and thirst) and Na pump mechanisms (inhibition of the Na pump, cell swelling, and inhibited thirst) of osmoreceptor stimulation.

II. BEHAVIOR AND PHYSIOLOGY

A. DRINKING AND PALATIBILITY

Increasing water temperature dramatically reduced intake during both exercise and rest periods.[7,63,120] Because this effect predominated during the first 2–3 h of exercise (6 h total), other factors must eventually override acceptance when warm beverages are ultimately consumed. The earlier work in our lab showed that subjects exercising in the heat drank less warm water when dehydrated but more cool water even when less dehydrated, although increased plasma osmolality/Na or reduced plasma volume should have stimulated greater thirst and consumption in the hypohydrated subjects. This apparent paradox in consumption by the hypohydrated, hyperthermic individuals was explained by an enhanced displeasure for warm water.[63] During prolonged (6 h) intermittent exercise, consumption of both cool and warm water was enhanced when flavored.[63,121] Moreover, the flavor-induced increase in fluid consumption was more pronounced during exercise.[121]

B. THIRST, MISSING OSMOLS, AND REHYDRATION

As noted earlier, individuals working in the heat usually replace only two thirds of lost water. Despite decades of research and media awareness on the negative impact of dehydration/hypohydration on psychological and physiological performance, significant hypohydration is continually reported in endurance athletes, runners, bicyclists, military personnel, and industrial workers. During either passive or exertional dehydration in the heat, more water is lost from the extracellular space than other fluid compartments,[116] and this greater loss in plasma volume may be attributed to the concomitant loss of Na and chloride.[96]

Rothstein et al.[110] concluded that voluntary dehydration results from the inadequacy of thirst to stimulate sufficient drinking. To explain this inadequate thirst, Ladell[76] suggested that water cannot be retained, and thus rehydration will be incomplete until the solutes ("missing osmols") lost in sweat are replaced. In dehydrated exercising humans, food consumption elicited an increased fluid consumption during meals,[120] and with its attendant caloric and osmolar load, provided an impetus for further postprandial water consumption. Hubbard et al.[64] hypothesized that replacement of electrolytes is instrumental in ensuring adequate rehydration, and that regulation of extracellular Na via Na receptors and consumption will emerge as a plausible explanation for incomplete rehydration.

As early as 1933, Dill et al.[33] postulated that thirst was related to plasma Na, and Rothstein et al.[110] suggested that intake of enough salt to replace that lost in sweat might decrease voluntary dehydration. Nose et al.[95] demonstrated that rehydration with a NaCl solution prevented the fall in plasma Na associated with pure water intake, and speculated that voluntary dehydration may result from dilutional inhibition of drinking when only water is consumed. Nose and colleagues[93] subsequently reported that following exercise- or heat-induced dehydration in humans, a greater, albeit incomplete, fluid retention and plasma volume restoration were obtained with salt solutions vs. water, and concluded that the delay in drinking was probably caused by both an electrolyte deficit and removal of a volume-dependent drive by intravascular retention of fluid. While renal mechanisms can reduce both water and Na losses induced by exercise or dehydration, deficits can be fully restored only by drinking with electrolyte replacement.

C. OSMORECEPTORS AND SODIUM RECEPTORS

Verney's[127] classical study demonstrated the existence of cerebral receptors that respond to elevations in plasma osmolality mediated by hypertonic solutions of salt, sucrose, mannitol, and fructose by releasing AVP and stimulating thirst. However, Andersson[4] questioned the lack of AVP release and thirst when plasma osmolality was increased by substances such as urea and glucose. Andersson[4] suggested, and Hubbard et al.[64] repostulated, that extracellular Na and cerebral Na receptors may be crucial to the control of water balance. More recently, McKinley[87] proposed that both osmoreceptors and Na receptors are involved in thirst. Na appetite and excretion are blocked by two procedures: changing cerebrospinal Na concentration or ablating the periventricular tissue of the lateral terminalis, which also disrupts thirst and AVP secretion.[87]

Two cerebral receptors, redundant in eliciting effector actions, are not necessarily mutually exclusive, and provide a plausible explanation for the delayed (24 h) time period and osmolar replacement required for complete rehydration in hypohydrated, salt-depleted humans.[76] This dual receptor hypothesis can effectively explain the recent findings of Takamata et al.,[122] who observed an immediate thirst followed by a delayed Na preference and thirst in hypohydrated, Na-depleted subjects. We propose that the initially increased thirst and AVP secretion were in response to an elevated plasma osmolality, whereas the delayed (3 h rehydration) thirst as well as the increased salt preference and reduced urinary Na excretion were mediated by central Na receptors.

D. AGING

Elderly men and women have a reduced renal response to AVP[111] despite a normal osmoregulation of AVP secretion.[97] More importantly, both reduced thirst and intake are observed in elderly subjects following either water deprivation[27] or thermal dehydration and rehydration.[83]

Mack et al.[83] conjectured that the hyperosmotic hypovolemic state observed in the elderly is probably not a water deficit, but more likely represents a shift in the operating point for fluid volume control. The mechanisms for reduced thirst and drinking in elderly individuals are unknown but reduced palatability of beverages,[102] changes in oropharyngeal sensors[101] and decreased mouth dryness,[103] reduced baroreceptor sensitivity,[20] increased basal levels of atrial natriuretic peptide (ANP),[98] and age-related morphological changes in the supraoptic and paraventricular nuclei[60] have all been proposed. Exogenously administered ANP inhibits both thirst and AVP secretion in young adults,[17] but only AVP release in the elderly.[19]

III. HORMONAL INTEGRATION

A. ATRIAL NATRIURETIC PEPTIDE

In the past 15 years much information has accumulated on the role of ANP in the regulation of body fluids, especially with respect to renal and cardiovascular hemodynamics; for an excellent and exhaustive review, see Ruskoaho.[113] DeBold et al.[31] were among the first to suggest a role for ANP in the control of body fluid regulation. This hormone generally countermands the secretion of renin and its vasoconstrictor actions, reduces aldosterone (Ald) biosynthesis and release, and promotes diuresis and natriuresis;[78] consequently, its secretion and circulating levels are usually depressed during dehydration.[66]

Review of the literature indicates that acute bouts of exercise are accompanied by rapidly resolving increases in ANP.[40] Freund et al.[51] have concluded that multiple forms of exercise, exercise duration, and exercise intensity can all influence the response of ANP. Increments in circulating levels of ANP may be related to increased venous return,[75] pressor release,[81] as well as elevated heart rate and blood pressure.[50] Euhydration[42] and heat acclimation[75] may attenuate the acute exercise-induced elevations in circulating ANP.

In humans, hypohydration,[88] lower body negative pressure,[89] and increased G forces[99] are generally associated with lowered levels of circulating ANP. Miller et al.[89] also noted that the deactivation of cardiopulmonary baroreceptors by the lower body negative pressure may also have reduced the natriuretic and diuretic effects of ANP via the glomerular filtration rate. Moreover, when central blood volume was increased by head-out water immersion and this was followed by cycle ergometry, ANP was increased at an exercise intensity of 40% of maximal aerobic capacity;[117] head-out water immersion is ordinarily accompanied by natriuresis and diuresis, partially in response to increased central blood volume and concomitantly increased plasma ANP levels.[53] Indeed, when Kanstrup et al.[67] expanded blood volume (5.22 -> 5.71l) by administration of 6% dextran, ANP levels were significantly increased during exercise and subsequent to elevated cardiac output, cardiac filling, and stroke volume.

While Kraemer et al.[75] have reported that levels of ANP were unchanged in humans even when exercise intensity was considerable ($\approx$70% $\dot{V}O_2$ max), Goodman et al.[54] reported that after 150 min of exercise, ANP levels remained at 150% of control (pre-exercise) levels. Freund et al.[51] reported that during a marathon run elevated (fivefold) ANP levels at 10km were attenuated toward completion of the race, and attributed the decrease to decrements in venous return. The same workers[50] observed no effects of training on the ANP response to exercise, while Rogers[108] reported reductions in ANP following endurance training.

It is clear that further investigations are warranted under both acute and more protracted exercise scenarios; additional studies with hyper-, eu-, and hypohydrated volunteers would be useful if the effects of these manipulations on plasma volume were determined prior to, during, and upon completion of the exercise interval and compared to ANP responses. Additional controlled studies monitoring rehydration, water balance, electrolyte balance, other clinical indices of hydration, and ANP during exercise especially in the cold and at altitude as well as moderate and hot environments would shed further light on the role of ANP in the control of water balance during exercise. Of particular interest would be careful quantification of ANP levels in conditions of excessive rehydration and symptomatic hyponatremia;[5,92] it would be extremely important to determine whether inappropriate ANP responses contribute to water intoxication.

B. AVP, PLASMA RENIN ACTIVITY, AND ALDOSTERONE

There are literally hundreds of reports documenting in humans the effects on circulating levels of AVP, PRA (Ang I and II), and Ald during and subsequent to exercise under various environmental conditions (for reviews, see Francesconi,[43] Viru,[128] and Fallo[37]). Generally, exercise stimulates elevated circulating levels of these humoral factors. For example, increased synthesis and release or decreased catabolism of AVP can be attributed to a variety of effects of exercise including increased plasma osmolality,[130] reduced intravascular volume,[57] elevated extracellular Na,[82] thirst,[17] elevated circulating Ang II levels,[80] increased core temperature,[23] and increased sympathetic nervous system activity.[1] Similarly, both acute and prolonged exercise elicits increased circulating levels of Ang I and II and Ald, often through similar mechanisms including increased sympathetic activity,[84] decreased plasma volume,[107] increased plasma osmolality,[15] hypohydration,[48] decrements in renal blood flow, perfusion pressure, or clearance,[12] elevations in circulating potassium (K) concentrations[56] and hyperthermia.[41] Convertino et al.[23] demonstrated a correlation between the intensity of the exercise and the elevation in circulating levels of these hormones. Although Convertino et al.[24] demonstrated an effect of training (cycle, 2h/d, 8d, 65% VO_2 max) in reducing AVP and PRA increments during exercise, other reports illustrated no significant effects of training.[56] It is likely that the increased blood volume commonly seen in endurance-trained individuals[22] is partially related to increased sensitivity of renal collecting tubules to Ald.[21]

Heat acclimation regimens ordinarily combine an exercise intensity and heat stress that are sufficient to induce elevations in PRA and Ald[6] as well as AVP.[56] Moveover, Finberg and Berlyne[38] demonstrated that natural heat acclimatization induced by normal exposure to the heat of summer reduced the responses of plasma PRA and Ald to an exercise/heat stress (50°C ambient, minimal 40 min, bicycle ergometry, or level treadmill) regimen. Upon completion of a heat acclimation regimen,[47] elevations in circulating PRA and Ald as a result of exercise in the heat were attenuated.

When we[44] recently evaluated the ability of young adult male volunteers to become heat acclimated while consuming only 4 g/d of NaCl, we observed an exacerbated increase in circulating levels of PRA and Ald especially during the early phases of heat acclimation. The implications of these observations are apparent: Acute exercise in the heat is accompanied by significant elevations in AVP, PRA, and Ald designed to attenuate renal and sweat gland Na losses as well as renal fluid loss. As the process of heat acclimation progresses with attendant isotonic increments in total body water, extracellular fluid, and plasma volume,[55] then these elevations may be attenuated. Moreover, the ability of individuals to acclimate successfully to a rigorous and recurrent heat/exercise regimen while consuming a diet that delivered only 4 g/d of NaCl was accompanied by exacerbated increments in PRA and Ald during the early (day 1–4) acclimation stages. We had hypothesized that these adaptive hormonal responses were critical to the acquisition of complete acclimation while on the Na-restricted diet. Further, the intensity of the response may be directly related to the level of stress and inversely associated with Na availability.

Much additional information on the hormonal regulation of fluid/electrolyte balance during exercise has come from studies that have assessed these responses during single bouts of exercise in the heat or heat acclimation without fluid replacement, with water replacement, or with isotonic or hypertonic fluid replacement. For example, when Brandenberger et al.[15] used no fluid, water, or an isotonic sucrose solution to rehydrate men subjected to 3 h of intermittent exercise in the heat, they reported that intercurrent fluid replacement during exercise blunted the responses of AVP, PRA, and Ald with marginal differences between the water and isotonic solutions. However, they also reported[16] that rehydration with an isotonic electrolyte solution effectively neutralized the increment in Ald during cycle ergometry (85W) in the heat (34°C, 4 h). Moreover, Deuster et al.[32] reported that pre- and rehydration with a glucose–polymer beverage attenuated the elevation in AVP observed during 2 h of exercise (60–65% VO_2 max) when the increment was compared with a water rehydration trial. Earlier, Francis and MacGregor[49] concluded that during exercise in the heat (32°C, 50% VO_2 max, 2 h), replacement of sweat losses with an electrolyte solution moderated the increments in PRA and Ald that did occur during identical trials with water replacement.

Davies et al.[30] documented that during an 11-d acclimation program, increments in PRA and Ald were attenuated when 1% saline was used regularly (0.75 l/d) as a replacement beverage when compared to a second acclimation interval during which no supplemental saline was provided. Likewise, Griswell et al.[57] noted that plasma Ald levels were reduced during 115 min of cycle ergometry (65% VO_2 max) when a glucose–electrolyte drink was provided prior to and during the exercise regimen. Alternatively, when Nose et al.[94] compared the effects of rehydration with tap water or a 0.45% NaCl solution on hormonal responses subsequent to heat/exercise-induced dehydration (2.3% of original body weight), they observed no significant differences in circulating levels of PRA and Ald. Barr et al.[10] concluded that plasma Ald responses were similar during 6-h exercise trials (ergometry, 55% $\dot{V}O_2$ max) when water or saline (25 mmol/l) was used as the replacement beverage while plasma Ald was more than doubled when no replacement fluid was given. Generally, the data indicate that significant dehydration due to hypotonic sweat secretion with inadequate fluid replacement results in a hypernatremic hypovolemia, in which case the volume deficit may be the dominant factor in affecting hormonal responses. These responses could be exacerbated in hyponatremic hypovolemia, a situation that may arise during exercise in the heat with insufficient dietary Na intake.

Further conclusions may be drawn concerning the control of body fluids during exercise by examining the integrated responses of the fluid regulatory hormones when experimental manipulations increase the water content of the fluid compartments. Although fewer of these investigations have been reported, insights into integrated hormonal control of fluids are intriguing. For example, when Sheldahl et al.[117] used head-out water immersion to increase central blood volume, plasma AVP and Ald responses were attenuated following maximal exercise. Griswell et al.[57] provided 675 ml of beverage before and 275 ml at 15-min intervals during exercise (115 min), and careful examination of the data indicate that AVP levels were unaffected or even lowered during the first 60 min of exercise. Therminarias et al.[123] studied exercise to exhaustion at ambient temperatures of 30°C and 10°C, and reported that at 10°C the response of PRA was significantly reduced. They attributed this effect to cold-induced vasoconstriction with concomitant increments in central blood volume.

In a report with significant implications to the etiology of acute mountain sickness (AMS), Bartsch et al.[11] noted that ergonometric exercise (148 W) at high altitude (4559 m) induced exacerbated increases in AVP and Ald in a group of volunteers who developed AMS. Fluid retention, of course, may be an etiologic factor in the symptomatology of AMS, and certainly the more serious high-altitude pulmonary edema. In a study in which plasma volume was expanded by approximately 9% by i.v. administration of hyperoncotic albumin solution,[62] we demonstrated attenuated responses of PRA and Ald to exercise (40% $\dot{V}O_2$ max) in the heat (45°C).[46] When autologous red blood cells (600 ml) were infused prior to (48 h) exercise in the heat (1.56 m/s, 6%, 35°C), we[45] observed no effects of erythrocythemia on responses of PRA or Ald, both of which were increased by exercise in the heat. However, it is important to note that in the latter study, total blood volume was unaffected by erythrocyte infusion.[114]

Acknowledging the nominal inconsistencies probably engendered by the myriad of independent experimental variables applied, certain conclusions on the integrated hormonal control of body fluids during exercise are warranted. Acute or protracted exercise ordinarily results in elevations of AVP, PRA, and Ald, and these increments may be tempered, for example, by training, acclimation, euhydration or hyperhydration, electrolyte supplementation, increased central blood volume, increased sensitivity of receptors, and increased renal blood flow. These endocrinological adaptations during acute exercise contribute to sustaining plasma volume and total body water, and during recurrent exercise may be partially responsible for training-induced increases in plasma volume, extracellular fluid, and total body water.

IV. HEPATIC, RENAL, AND CNS RECEPTORS

A. HEPATIC AND PORTAL OSMORECEPTORS

Much of our knowledge of the integrated role of the liver, kidney, and central nervous system in responding to and regulating osmoeffectors comes from electrophysiological, physiological, and behavioral studies in animal models. Although the important role of hypothalamic osmoreceptors and intravascular stretch receptors in the regulation of fluid homeostasis is well documented, debate on the existence and significance of peripheral osmoreceptors persists.

Evidence for peripheral osmoreceptors was first provided by Haberich,[59] who reported that small amounts of either water or hypertonic saline infused into the portal vein produced a diuresis or antidiuresis, respectively, in rats. He further postulated[59] that hypotonicity is an adequate stimulus for portal osmoreceptors. Daly et al.[28] reported that infusion of hypertonic saline into the portal vein increased urinary flow and Na excretion more than an infusion into a systemic (femoral) vein. Subsequent studies have both supported and negated the existence of hepatic osmoreceptors (see Lang et al.[77]) Although disparate results suggest a species specificity,[77] Baertschi et al.[8] and Vallet and Baertschi[125] proposed that cannulation sites and procedures may explain negative findings because the osmoreceptors are probably located in the hepatic portal vein, and not the liver itself or hepatic veins. Furthermore, several studies in humans[69] have paralleled the observations in animals of an osmoreceptor in the splanchnic circulation. Adachi et al.[2] used intraportal infusion of hypertonic and hypotonic Ringer's solution in rats to demonstrate the presence of two classes of hepatic osmoreceptors that respond to hyper- and hypoosmotic stimuli, respectively. Electrophysiological studies favoring the existence of a hepatic osmoreceptor responding to changes in plasma osmolarity were reported by Niijima.[91]

B. CNS AND PERIPHERAL INTERACTIONS

Rogers et al.[109] and Vallet and Baertschi[126] concluded that a spinal afferent pathway exists between the parabrachial nucleus, ventrobasal complex, and the solitary tract nucleus and the supraoptic region of the hypothalamus, and it was later confirmed that this pathway is osmotically stimulated[71] and capable of releasing AVP.

Indeed, Baertschi et al.[8] clearly demonstrated that brief osmotic (NaCl) pulses to the portal vein of rats elicited significant increases in plasma AVP, supporting previous reports[18] that these peripheral osmoreceptors sense dynamic changes and not steady-state levels in plasma osmolality, with less than 1% change in portal blood osmolality eliciting a response.[59] Moreover, the central osmoreceptors that sense and affect the secretion of AVP following intracarotid infusion of hypertonic saline appear to be primarily involved in the steady-state osmoregulation of fluid balance.

Stoppini and Baertschi[119] perfused the portal vein of rats with 4% NaCl after treatment with verapamil, a calcium channel blocker, and atropine, an anticholinergic, and concluded that acetylcholine release by portal osmoreceptors activates afferents in response to hyperosmolarity. Tordoff et al.[124] confirmed that although infusion of 0.5M saline into the hepatic portal vein reduced subsequent salt intake,[14] similar intrajugular infusions did not. Using more physiological solutions Kobashi and Adachi[72] infused either water, 0.9% saline, or 1.8% saline into the hepatic portal or jugular vein and studied subsequent water intake in 24-h water-deprived rats. They observed that when water, but not 0.9% or 1.8% saline, was infused into the portal vein, rats consumed less water than those receiving water in the jugular vein. Koga et al.[73] studied the effects of intrahepatoportal stimulation with 3% NaCl–9% mannitol on hypothalamic thermoreceptors and concluded that changes in both tonicity and blood pressure affected the firing rate of thermosensitive neurons. They further theorized that the confluence of osmotic, baroreceptor, and thermosensitive pathways provides a mechanism for the interaction of nonthermal (osmotic) and thermoregulatory changes.

Using vagotomized and baroreceptor denervated rabbits, Ishiki et al.[65] reported that intraportal infusion of three hypertonic solutions each significantly decreased renal sympathetic nerve activity by 30% while both femoral arterial infusions and infusions subsequent to section of the hepatic nerve had no effects on renal nerve activity. Increased portal vein perfusion pressure reportedly enhanced renal hepatic afferent nerve activity,[74] and provided evidence for a hepatorenal reflex. Lang et al.[77] concluded that this hepatorenal reflex was stimulated by intrahepatic pressure and attenuated renal blood flow, glomerular filtration, and urinary flow.

There appear to be several implications of these observations for the integrated control of body fluids during exercise in humans. Under euhydrated or hyperhydrated conditions, hepatoportal receptors that respond to hypoosmotic stimuli contribute to reductions in circulating AVP through direct afferent input to the preoptic area of the hypothalamus. Alternatively, hypohydration or elevated Na concentrations would stimulate hepatoportal hyperosmoreceptors and induce the supraoptic nuclei to increase the biosynthesis and release of AVP. Moreover, direct effects on renal water and Na conservation or loss would also be anticipated. That is, hyperosmolarity would downregulate renal sympathetic nerve activity, probably moderate the release of renin and thus Ald, and promote the excretion of Na.

In the larger scheme of the multiple factors regulating fluid and electrolytes during exercise, these mechanisms would probably be more prominent, effective, and a focal point of interest if the exercise is accompanied by recurrent rehydration with replacement volumes of water or electrolyte beverages of known and varied tonicities. The hepatic osmoreceptors afford a mechanism whereby rapid changes in osmotic pressure mediated by intestinal absorption of water and electrolytes can be locally monitored and controlled via activation of the hypothalamo-neurohypophysial system and release of AVP. For example, suppression of warm-sensitive neurons in the preoptic area and anterior hypothalamus by central and peripheral osmotic stimuli may explain why dehydrated animals display a reduction in evaporative heat loss. Thus, the control of body temperature appears to be intimately associated with salt and water balance, and this interaction is clearly seen in a variety of heat illnesses.[61]

C. INTESTINAL OSMORECEPTORS AND EFFECTS

The intestines are an important and probably underacknowledged site for body fluid and electrolyte regulation. Stimulation of the volume receptors in the carotid sinus, thoracic aorta, and atria not only tonically inhibits the vasomotor center, but also contributes to the sympathetic input of the intestines.[118] Under pathophysiological conditions such as nonhypotensive hemorrhage, Na depletion, extracellular volume depletion, and dehydration, sympathetic input to the intestines is increased, mediating a reduction in intestinal transit while increasing contact time in the lumen, thereby resulting in an upregulation of electrolytes and fluid absorption from the intestinal lumen into the intravascular space.[26] Renin release mediated by this enhanced sympathetic activity can initiate further water conservation by the kidneys and colon. ANP has been shown either to inhibit Na and water absorption in isolated intestinal segments[115] or to have no effect on fluid movement.[68] More recently, Matsushita et al.[85] demonstrated in conscious dogs that circulating ANP is absorbed by the gut, reduces splanchnic blood flow, and suppresses net absorption of water and salt across the jejunum.

Blood flow to the intestines is often compromised to provide adequate flow to other regions.[112] Increased sympathetic activity due to exercise, increased exercise duration or intensity, or increased body temperature attenuates splanchnic blood flow in proportion to the increase in heart rate.[112] Although reductions in splanchnic flow inhibit absorption across the small intestine and reduced gastric emptying and intestinal absorption occur during exercise,[9,86] the mechanisms are unclear but may be related to reduced flow, ANP release, and/or changes in intestinal transit and contact time.

V. CONCLUSION

There can be little doubt that the integrated control of body fluid balance during exercise is an extremely complex and daunting example of physiological homeostasis. Indeed, with the possible exception of the skeletal system, every major organ system of the human body appears to play a significant, if not critical, role in the regulation of the body fluid compartments during exercise or, indeed, at rest. The chapters of this monograph will no doubt contribute to our understanding of the remarkable physiological responses that maintain the integrity, volume, and function of the intracellular, interstitial, and intravascular fluid compartments during exercise.

ACKNOWLEDGMENTS

The authors express their deep appreciation to Mrs. Diane Danielski for excellent word processing support and to Sgt. Michael Koratich for his expertise in the creation of automated reference files.

REFERENCES

1. Abraham, W.T. and Schrier, R.W. Body fluid volume regulation in health and disease. *Adv. Int. Med.* 39: 23–47, 1994.
2. Adachi, A., Niijima, A., and Jacobs, H.L. An hepatic osmoreceptor mechanism in the rat: Electrophysiological and behavioral studies. *Am. J. Physiol.* 231: 1043–1049, 1976.
3. Andersson, B. Thirst and brain control of water balance. *Am. Sci.* 59: 408–415, 1971.
4. Andersson, B. Regulation of water intake. *Physiol. Rev.* 58: 582–603, 1978.
5. Armstrong, L.E., Curtis, W.C., Hubbard, R.W., Francesconi, R.P., Moore, R., and Askew, E.W. Symptomatic hyponatremia during prolonged exercise in the heat. *Med. Sci. Sports Exer.* 25: 543–549, 1993.
6. Armstrong, L.E., Francesconi, R.P., Kraemer, W.J., Leva, N.M., DeLuca, J.P., and Hubbard, R.W. Plasma cortisol, renin and aldosterone during an intense heat acclimation program. *Int. J. Sports Med.* 10: 38–42, 1989.
7. Armstrong, L.E., Hubbard, R.W., Szlyk, P.C., Matthew, W.T., and Sils, I.V. Voluntary dehydration and electrolyte losses during prolonged exercise in the heat. *Aviat. Space Environ. Med.* 56: 765–770, 1985.
8. Baertschi, A.J., Massy, Y., and Kwon, S. Vasopressin responses to peripheral and central osmotic pulse stimulation. *Peptides* 6: 1131–1135, 1985.
9. Barclay, G.R. and Turnberg, L.A. Effect of moderate exercise on salt and water transport in the human jejunum. *Gut* 29: 816–820, 1988.
10. Barr, S.I., Costill, D.L., and Fink, W.J. Fluid replacement during prolonged exercise: Effects of water, saline or no fluid. *Med. Sci. Sports Exer.* 23: 811–817, 1991.
11. Bartsch, P., Maggiorini, M., Schobersberger, W., Shaw, S., Rascher, W., Girard, J., Weidmann, P., and Oelz, O. Enhanced exercise-induced rise of aldosterone and vasopressin preceding mountain sickness. *J. Appl. Physiol.* 71: 136–143, 1991.
12. Bello-Reuss, E. Pathophysiology of volume regulation and sodium metabolism. *The Kidney and Body Fluids in Health and Disease*, Klahr, S., Ed. Plenum Press, New York, 1983, 93–118.
13. Bergman, F., Costin, A., Chaimovitz, M., and Banzakein, F. The effect of ouabain on water consumption in the rat. *Experientia* 22: 700–701, 1967.
14. Blake, W.D. and Lin, K.K. Hepatic portal vein infusion of glucose and sodium solutions in the control of saline drinking in the rat. *J. Physiol. London* 274: 129–139, 1978.

15. Brandenberger, G., Candas, V., Follenius, M., and Kahn, J.M. The influence of the initial state of hydration on endocrine responses to exercise in the heat. *Eur. J. Appl. Physiol.* 58: 674–679, 1989.
16. Brandenberger, G., Candas, V., Follenius, M., Libert, J.P., and Kahn, J.M. Vascular fluid shifts and endocrine responses to exercise in the heat. *Eur. J. Appl. Physiol.* 55: 123–129, 1986.
17. Burrell, L., Lambert, H.J., and Baylis, P.H. Effect of atrial natriuretic peptide on thirst and arginine vasopressin release in humans. *Am. J. Physiol.* 260: R475–R479, 1991.
18. Chwalbinska–Moneta, J. Role of hepatic portal osmoreception in the control of ADH release. *Am. J. Physiol.* 236: E603–E609, 1979.
19. Clark, B.A., Elahi, D., Fish, L., McAloon-Dyke, N., Davis, K., Minaker, K.L., and Epstein, F.H. Atrial natriuretic peptides depress osmostimulated vasopressin release in young and elderly humans. *Am. J. Physiol.* 261: E252–E256, 1991.
20. Cleroux, J., Giannattasio, C., Grassi, G., Seravalle, G., Sanpieri, L., Cusipidi, C., Bolla, G., Valsecchi, M., Mazzola, C., and Mancia, G. Effects of aging on the cardiopulmonary receptor reflex in normotensive humans. *J. Hypertens.* 6 (Suppl. 4): S141–S144, 1989.
21. Convertino, V.A. Blood volume: Its adaptation to endurance training. *Med. Sci. Sports Exer.* 23: 1338–1348, 1991.
22. Convertino, V.A., Greenleaf, J.E., and Bernauer, E.M. Role of thermal and exercise factors in the mechanism of hypervolemia. *J. Appl. Physiol.* 48: 657–664, 1980.
23. Convertino, V.A., Keil, L.C., Bernauer, E.M., and Greenleaf, J.E. Plasma volume, osmolality, vasopressin, and renin activity during graded exercise in man. *J. Appl. Physiol.* 50: 123–128, 1981.
24. Convertino, V.A., Keil, L.C., and Greenleaf, J.E. Plasma volume, renin, and vasopressin responses to graded exercise after training. *J. Appl. Physiol.* 54: 508–514, 1983.
25. Conway, E.J. and McCormack, J.I. The total intracellular concentration of mammalian tissues compared with that of the extracellular fluid. *J. Physiol.* 120: 1–14, 1953.
26. Cooke, H.J. Role of the little brain in the gut in water and electrolyte homeostasis. *FASEB J.* 3: 127–138, 1989.
27. Crowe, M.J., Forsling, M.L., Rolls, B.J., Phillips, P.A., Ledingham, J.G.G., and Smith, R.F. Altered water excretion in healthy elderly men. *Age Ageing* 16: 285–293, 1987.
28. Daly, J.J., Roe, J.W., and Horrocks, P.A. A comparison of sodium excretion following the infusion of saline into systemic and portal veins in the dog: Evidence for a hepatic role in the control of sodium excretion. *Clin. Sci.* 33: 481–487, 1967.
29. Davenport, H.W. *Physiology of the Digestive Tract.* Year Book Medical Publishers, Chicago, 1982.
30. Davies, J.A., Harrison, M.H., Cochrane, L.A., Edwards, R.J., and Gibson, T.M. Effect of saline loading during heat acclimatization on adrenocortical hormone levels. *J. Appl. Physiol.* 50: 605–612, 1981.
31. DeBold, A.J., Borenstein, H.B., Veress, A.T., and Sonnenberg, H.A. A rapid and potent natriuretic response to intravenous injection of atrial myocardial extract in rats. *Life Sci.* 28: 89–94, 1981.
32. Deuster, P.A., Singh, A., Hoffman, A., Moses, F.M., and Chrousos, G.C. Hormonal responses to ingesting water or a carbohydrate beverage during a 2h run. *Med. Sci. Sports Exer.* 24: 72–79, 1992.
33. Dill, D.B., Bock, A.V., and Edward, H.T. Mechanism for dissipating heat in man and dog. *Am. J. Physiol.* 104: 36–43, 1933.
34. Elkinton, J.R., Danowski, T.S., and Winkler, A.W. Hemodynamic changes in salt depletion and in dehydration. *J. Clin. Invest.* 25: 120–129, 1946.
35. Elkinton, J.R., Winkler, A.W., and Danowski, T.S. Transfers of cell sodium and potassium in experimental and clinical conditions. *J. Clin. Invest.* 27: 74–81, 1948.

36. Epstein, A.N., Fitzsimons, J.T., and Rolls, B.J. Drinking induced by injection of angiotensin into the brain of the rat. *J. Physiol.* 210: 457–474, 1970.
37. Fallo, F. Renin–angiotensin–aldosterone system and physical exercise. *J. Sports Med. Phys. Fitness* 33: 306–312, 1993.
38. Finberg, J.P.M. and Berlyne, G.M. Modification of renin and aldosterone response to heat by acclimatization in man. *J. Appl. Physiol.* 42: 554–558, 1977.
39. Fitzsimons, J.T. The role of a renal thirst factor in drinking induced by extracellular stimuli. *J. Physiol. London* 201: 349–368, 1969.
40. Follenius, M. and Brandenberger, G. Increase in atrial natriuretic peptide in response to physical exercise. *Eur. J. Appl. Physiol.* 57: 159–162, 1988.
41. Follenius, M., Brandenberger, G., Reinhardt, B., and Simeoni, M. Plasma aldosterone, renin activity and cortisol responses to heat exposure in sodium depleted and repleted subjects. *Eur. J. Appl. Physiol.* 41: 41–50, 1979.
42. Follenius, M., Candas, V., Bothorel, B., and Brandenberger, G. Effect of rehydration on atrial natriuretic peptide release during exercise in the heat. *J. Appl. Physiol.* 66: 2516–2521, 1989.
43. Francesconi, R.P. Endocrinological responses to exercise in stressful environments. In: *Exercise and Sports Sciences Reviews*, Pandolf, K.B., Ed. Macmillan, New York, 1988, 255–284.
44. Francesconi, R.P., Armstrong, L., Leva, N., Moore, R., Szlyk, P., Matthew, W., Curtis, W., Hubbard, R., and Askew, E.W. Endocrinological responses to dietary salt restriction during heat acclimation. *Nutritional Needs in Hot Environments*, Marriott, B.M., Ed. National Academy Press, Washington, DC, 1993, 259–275.
45. Francesconi, R.P., Sawka, M.N., Dennis, R.C., Gonzalez, R.R., Young, A.J., and Valeri, C.R. Autologous red blood cell reinfusion: Effects on stress and fluid regulatory hormones during exercise in the heat. *Aviat. Space Environ. Med.* 59: 133–137, 1988.
46. Francesconi, R.P., Sawka, M.N., Hubbard, R.W., and Mager, M. Acute albumin-induced plasma volume expansion and exercise in the heat: Effects on hormonal responses in men. *Eur. J. Appl. Physiol.* 51: 121–128, 1983.
47. Francesconi, R.P., Sawka, M.N., and Pandolf, K.B. Hypohydration and heat acclimation: Plasma renin and aldosterone during exercise. *J. Appl. Physiol.* 55: 1790–1794, 1983.
48. Francesconi, R.P., Sawka, M.N., Pandolf, K.B., Hubbard, R.W., Young, A.J., and Muza, S. Plasma hormonal responses at graded hypohydration levels during exercise-heat stress. *J. Appl. Physiol.* 59: 1855–1860, 1985.
49. Francis, K.T. and MacGregor, R. Effect of exercise in the heat on plasma renin and aldosterone with either water or a potassium-rich electrolyte solution. *Aviat. Space Environ. Med.* 49: 461–465, 1979.
50. Freund, B.J., Claybaugh, J.R., Dice, M.S., and Hashiro, G.M. Hormonal and vascular fluid responses to maximal exercise in trained and untrained males. *J. Appl. Physiol.* 63: 669–675, 1987.
51. Freund, B.J., Wade, C.E., and Claybaugh, J.R. Effects of exercise on atrial natriuretic factor. *Sports Med.* 6: 364–376, 1988.
52. Gauer, O.H., Henry, J.P., Sicker, H.O., and Wendt, W.E. Heart and lungs as a receptor region controlling blood volume. *Am. J. Physiol.* 167: 786–787, 1951.
53. Gilmore, J.P. Neural control of extracellular volume in the human and non-human primate. In: *Handbook of Physiology, The Cardiovascular System III*, Shepherd, J.T. and Abboud, F.M., Eds. American Physiological Society, Bethesda, MD, 1983, 885–915.
54. Goodman, J.M., Logan, A.G., McLaughlin, P.R., Laprade, A., and Liu, P.P. Atrial natriuretic peptide duirng acute and prolonged exercise in well-trained men. *Int. J. Sports Med.* 14: 185–190, 1993.
55. Greenleaf, J.E., Brock, P.J., Keil, L.C., and Morse, J.T. Drinking and water balance during exercise and heat acclimation. *J. Appl. Physiol.* 54: 414–419, 1983.

56. Greenleaf, J.E., Sciaraffa, D., Shvartz, E., Keil, L.C., and Brock, P.J. Exercise training hypotension: implications for plasma volume, renin, and vasopressin. *J. Appl. Physiol.* 51: 298–305, 1981.
57. Griswell, D., Renshler, K., Powers, S.K., Tulley, R., Cicale, M., and Wheeler, K. Fluid replacement beverages and maintenance of plasma volume during exercise: Role of aldosterone and vasopressin. *Eur. J. Appl. Physiol.* 65: 445–451, 1992.
58. Gutman, J. An extrarenal effect of hydrochlorothiazide. *Experientia* 19: 544–545, 1963.
59. Haberich, F.J. Osmoreception in the portal circulation. *Fed. Proc.* 27: 1137–1141, 1968.
60. Hoogendijk, J.E., Fliers, E., Swaag, D.V., and Verwer, R.W.H. Activation of vasopressin neurons in the human supraoptic and paraventricular nucleus in senescence and senile dementia. *J. Neurol. Sci.* 69: 291–299, 1989.
61. Hubbard, R.W. and Armstrong, L.E. The heat illnesses: Biochemical, ultrastructural, and fluid-electrolyte considerations. In: *Human Performance Physiology and Environmental Medicine at Terrestrial Extremes*, Pandolf, K.B., Sawka, N.M., and Gonzalez, R.R., Eds. Benchmark Press, Indianapolis, 1988, 305–359.
62. Hubbard, R.W., Matthew, W.T., Horstman, D., Francesconi, R., Mager, M., and Sawka, M.N. Albumin-induced plasma volume expansion: Diurnal and temperature effects. *J. Appl. Physiol.* 56: 1361–1368, 1984.
63. Hubbard, R.W., Sandick, B.L., Matthew, W.T., Francesconi, R.P., Sampson, J.B., Durkot, M.J., Maller, O., and Engell, D.B. Voluntary dehydration and alliesthesia for water. *J. Appl. Physiol.* 57: 868–875, 1984.
64. Hubbard, R.W., Szlyk, P.C., and Armstrong, L.E. Influence of thirst and fluid palatability on fluid ingestion during exercise. In: *Perspectives in Exercise Science and Sports Medicine, Vol. 3, Fluid Homeostasis During Exercise*, Gisolfi, C.V. and Lamb, D.R., Eds. Benchmark Press, Carmel, IN, 1990, 39–95.
65. Ishiki, K., Morita, H., and Hosomi, H. Reflex control of renal nerve activity originating from the osmoreceptors in the hepatoportal region. *J. Auton. Nerv. Syst.* 36: 139–148, 1991.
66. Januszewicz, P., Thibault, G., Gutkowska, J., Garcia, R., Mercure, C., Jolicoeur, F., Genest, J., and Cantin, M. Atrial natriuretic factor and vasopressin during dehydration and rehydration in rats. *Am. J. Physiol.* 251: E497–E501, 1986.
67. Kanstrup, I.L., Marving, J., and Hoilund-Carlsen, P.F. Acute plasma expansion: Left ventricular hemodynamics and endocrine function during exercise. *J. Appl. Physiol.* 73: 1791–1796, 1992.
68. Kaufman, S. and Monckton, E. Influence of right atrial stretch and atrial natriuretic factor on rat intestinal fluid content. *J. Physiol. London* 402: 1–8, 1988.
69. Kiil, J. and Andersen, D. Evidence of a gastro-hepatic osmoregulation in humans and the influence of vagotomy on its activity. *Scand. J. Gastroent.* 7: 575–581, 1972.
70. Kleeman, C.R., Epstein, F.H., and White, C. Effect of variations in solute excretion and glomerular filtration on water diuresis. *J. Clin. Invest.* 35: 749–756, 1956.
71. Kobashi, M. and Adachi, A. A direct hepatic osmoreceptive afferent projection from nucleus tractus solitarius to dorsal hypothalamus. *Brain Res. Bull.* 20: 487–492, 1988.
72. Kobashi, M. and Adachi, A. Effect of hepatic portal infusion of water on water intake by water deprived rats. *Physiol. Behav.* 52: 885–888, 1992.
73. Koga, H., Hori, T., Inoue, T., Kiyohara, T., and Nakashima, T. Convergence of hepatoportal osmotic and cardiovascular signals on preoptic thermosensitive neurons. *Brain Res. Bull.* 19: 109–113, 1987.
74. Kostreva, D.R., Castaner, A., and Kampine, J.P. Reflex effects of hepatic baroreceptors on renal and cardiac sympathetic nerve activity. *Am. J. Physiol.* 238: R390–R394, 1980.
75. Kraemer, W.J., Armstrong, L.E., Hubbard, R.W., Marchitelli, L.J., Leva, N., Rock, P.B., and Dziados, J.E. Responses of plasma human atrial natriuretic factor to high intensity submaximal exercise in the heat. *Eur. J. Appl. Physiol.* 57: 399–403, 1988.
76. Ladell, W.S. Water and salt (sodium chloride) intakes. *The Physiology of Human Survival*, Edholm, O. and Bacharach, A., Eds., Academic Press, New York, 1965, 235–299.

77. Lang, F., Tschernko, E., and Haussinger, D. Hepatic regulation of renal function. *Exp. Physiol.* 77: 663–673, 1992.
78. Laragh, J.H. The endocrine control of blood volume, blood pressure, and sodium balance: Atrial hormone and renin system interactions. *J. Hypertens.* 4: 143–156, 1986.
79. Lee, M.C., Thrasher, T.N., and Ramsay, D.J. Is angiotensin essential in drinking induced by water deprivation and caval ligation?. *Am. J. Physiol.* 240: R75–R80, 1981.
80. Lees, K.R., MacFadyen, R.J., Doig, J.K., and Reid, J.L. Role of angiotensin in the extravascular system. *J. Hum. Hypertens.* 7: S7–S12, 1993.
81. Leppaluoto, J., Arjamaa, O., Vuoltecnaho, O., and Rushkoaho, H. Passive heat exposure leads to delayed increase in plasma levels of atrial natriuretic peptide in humans. *J. Appl. Physiol.* 71: 716–720, 1991.
82. Liard, J.F., Dolci, W., and Vallotton, M.B. Plasma vasopressin levels after infusions of hypertonic saline solutions into the renal, portal, carotid, or systemic circulation in conscious dogs. *Endocrinology* 114: 986–991, 1984.
83. Mack, G.W., Weseman, C.A., Langhans, G.W., and Scherzer, W. Body fluid balance in dehydrated healthy older men: Thirst and renal osmoregulation. *J. Appl. Physiol.* 76: 1615–1623, 1994.
84. Manhem, P. and Hokfelt, B. Prolonged clonidine treatment: Catecholamines, renin activity, and aldosterone following exercise in hypertensives. *Acta Med. Scand.* 209: 253–260, 1981.
85. Matsushita, K., Nishhida, Y., Hosomi, H., and Tanaka, S. Effects of atrial natriuretic peptide on water and NaCl absorption across the intestine. *Am. J. Physiol.* 260: R6–R12, 1991.
86. Maughan, R.J., Leiper, J.B., and McGaw, B.A. Effects of exercise intensity on absorption of ingested fluids in man. *Exp. Physiol.* 75: 419–421, 1990.
87. McKinley, M.J. Common aspects of the cerebral regulation of thirst and renal sodium excretion. *Kidney Int. (Suppl.)* 37: S102–S106, 1992.
88. Melin, B., Cure, M., Jimenez, C., Allevard, A.M., Geelen, G., and Gharib, C. Plasma atrial natriuretic peptide and vasopressin during thermal dehydration in supine posture. *Acta Physiol. Scand.* 141: 227–230, 1991.
89. Miller, J.A., Floras, J.S., Skorecki, K.L., Blendis, L.M., and Logan, A.G. Renal and humoral responses to sustained cardiopulmonary baroreceptor deactivation in humans. *Am. J. Physiol.* 260: R642–R648, 1991.
90. Moses, A.M. and Clayton, B. Impairment of osmotically stimulated AVP release in patients with primary polydipsia. *Am. J. Physiol.* 265: R1247–R1252, 1993.
91. Niijima, A. Afferent discharges from osmoreceptors in the liver of the guinea-pig. *Science* 166: 1519–1520, 1969.
92. Noakes, T.D. The hyponatremia of exercise. *Int. J. Sport Nutr.* 2: 205–228, 1992.
93. Nose, H., Mack, G.W., Shi, X., and Nadel, E.R. Role of osmolality and plasma volume during rehydration in humans. *J. Appl. Physiol.* 65: 325–331, 1988.
94. Nose, H., Mack, G.W., Shi, X., and Nadel, E.R. Involvement of sodium retention hormones during rehydration in humans. *J. Appl. Physiol.* 65: 322–336, 1988.
95. Nose, H., Morita, M., Yawata, T., and Morimoto, T. Recovery of blood volume and osmolarity after thermal dehydration in rats. *Am. J. Physiol.* 251: R492–R498, 1986.
96. Nose, H., Yawata, T., and Morimoto, T. Osmotic factors in restitution from thermal dehydration in rats. *Am. J. Physiol.* 249: R166–R171, 1985.
97. O'Neill, P.A. and McLean, K.A. Water homeostasis and ageing. *Med. Lab. Sci.* 49: 291–298, 1992.
98. Ohashi, M., Fujio, N., Nawata, H., Kato, K., Ibayashi, H., Kangawa, K., and Matsuo, H. High plasma concentrations of human atrial natriuretic polypeptide in aged men. *J. Clin. Endocrinol.* 64: 81–85, 1987.
99. Park, J.K., Seul, K.H., Park, B.O., Kim, S.H., and Cho, C.W. Effects of positive acceleration on atrial natriuretic peptide in humans. *Aviat. Space Environ. Med.* 65: 51–54, 1994.

100. Peters, J.P. Water exchange. *Physiol. Rev.* 24: 491–531, 1944.
101. Phillips, P.A., Bretherton, M., Risvanis, J., Casley, D., Johnston, C., and Gray, L. Effects of drinking on thirst and vasopressin in dehydrated elderly men. *Am. J. Physiol.* 264: R877–R881, 1993.
102. Phillips, P.A., Johnson, C.I., and Johnson, G.L. Disturbed fluid and electrolyte homeostasis following dehydration in elderly people. *Age Ageing* 22: 26–33, 1993.
103. Phillips, P.A., Rolls, B.J., Ledingham, J.G.G., Forsling, M.L., Morton, J.J., Crowe, M.J., and Wollner, L. Reduced thirst after water deprivation in healthy elderly men. *New Engl. J. Med.* 311: 753–759, 1984.
104. Pitts, G.C., Johnson, R.E., and Consolazio, F.C. Work in the heat as affected by intake of water, salt and glucose. *Am. J. Physiol.* 142: 253–259, 1944.
105. Ramsay, D.J., Rolls, B.J., and Wood, R.J. Thirst following water deprivation in dogs. *Am. J. Physiol.* 232: R93–R100, 1977.
106. Robertson, G.L. and Berl, T. Water metabolism. In: *The Kidney*, Brenner, B.M. and Rector, F.C., Jr., Eds. W.B. Saunders, Philadelphia, 1986, 385–432.
107. Roecker, L., Kirsch, K.A., Heyduck, B., and Altenkirch, H.U. Influence of prolonged physical exercise on plasma volume, plasma proteins, electrolytes, and fluid-regulating hormones. *Int. J. Sports Med.* 10: 270–274, 1989.
108. Rogers, P.J. Exercise induced increases in atrial natriuretic factor are increased by endurance training. *J. Am. Coll. Cardiol.* 18: 1236–1241, 1991.
109. Rogers, R.C., Novin, P., and Butcher, L.L. Hepatic sodium and osmoreceptors activate neurons in the ventrobasal thalamus. *Brain Res.* 168: 398–403, 1979.
110. Rothstein, A., Adolph, E.F., and Wills, J.H. Voluntary dehydration. *Physiology of Man in the Desert*, Adolph, E.F., Ed. Interscience, New York, 1947, 254–270.
111. Rowe, J.W., Shock, N.W., and DeFronzo, R.A. The influence of age on the renal response to water deprivation in man. *Nephron* 17: 270–278, 1976.
112. Rowell, L.B. *Human Circulation Regulation During Physical Stress*. Oxford University Press, New York, 1986.
113. Ruskoaho, H. Atrial natriuretic peptide: Synthesis, release and metabolism. *Pharmacol. Rev.* 44: 479–602, 1992.
114. Sawka, M.N., Gonzalez, R.R., Young, A.J., Muza, S.R., Pandolf, K.B., Latzka, W.A., Dennis, R.C., and Valeri, C.R. Polycythemia and hydration: Effects on thermoregulation and blood volume during exercise-heat stress. *Am. J. Physiol.* 255: R456–R463, 1988.
115. Seeber, A.M., Vical, N.A., Carchio, S.M., and Karara, A.L. Inhibition of water-sodium intestinal absorption by atrial extract. *Can. J. Physiol. Pharmacol.* 64: 244–247, 1986.
116. Senay, L.C., Jr. Effects of exercise in the heat on body fluid distribution. *Med. Sci. Sports* 11: 42–48, 1979.
117. Sheldahl, L.M., Tristani, F.E., Connelly, T.P., Levandoski, S.G., Skelton, M.M., and Cowley, A.W., Jr. Fluid regulatory hormones during exercise when central blood volume is increased by water immersion. *Am. J. Physiol.* 262: R779–R785, 1992.
118. Sjovall, H. Sympathetic control of jejunal fluid and electrolyte transport. An experimental study of cats and rats. *Acta Physiol. Scand. Suppl.* 535: 1–63, 1984.
119. Stoppini, L. and Baertschi, A.J. Activation of portal-hepatic osmoreceptors in rats: Role of calcium, acetycholine, and cyclic AMP. *J. Auton. Nerv. Syst.* 11: 297–308, 1984.
120. Szlyk, P.C., Sils, I.V., Francesconi, R.P., and Hubbard, R.W. Patterns of human drinking: Effects of exercise, water temperature, and food consumption. *Aviat. Space Environ. Med.* 61: 43–48, 1990.
121. Szlyk, P.C., Sils, I.V., Francesconi, R.P., Hubbard, R.W., and Armstrong, L.E. Effects of water temperature and flavoring on voluntary dehydration in men. *Physiol. Behav.* 45: 639–647, 1989.
122. Takamata, A., Mack, G.W., Gillen, C.M., and Nadel, E.R. Sodium appetite, thirst, and body fluid regulation in humans during rehydration without sodium replacement. *Am. J. Physiol.* 266: R1493–R1502, 1994.

123. Therminarias, A., Flore, P., Oddou-Chirpaz, M.F., Gharib, C., and Gauquelin, G. Hormonal responses to exercise during moderate cold exposure in young vs. middle-aged subjects. *J. Appl. Physiol.* 73: 1564–1571, 1992.
124. Tordoff, M.G., Schulkin, J., and Friedman, M.I. Further evidence for hepatic control of salt intake in rats. *Am. J. Physiol.* 253: R444–R449, 1987.
125. Vallet, P. and Baertschi, A.J. Sodium-chloride sensitive receptors located in hepatic portal vein of the rat. *Neurosci. Lett.* 17: 283–288, 1980.
126. Vallet, P.G. and Baertschi, A.J. Spinal afferents for peripheral osmoreceptors in the rat. *Brain Res.* 239: 271–274, 1982.
127. Verney, E.B. The antidiuretic hormone and factors which determine its release. *Proc. R. Soc. London Ser. B.* 135: 25–106, 1947.
128. Viru, A. Plasma hormones and physical exercises: A review. *Int. J. Sports Med.* 13: 201–209, 1992.
129. Vokes, T. Water homeostasis. *Annu. Rev. Nutr.* 7: 383–406, 1987.
130. Wade, C.E. and Claybaugh, J.R. Plasma renin activity, vasopressin concentration, and urinary excretory responses to exercise in man. *J. Appl. Physiol.* 49: 930–936, 1980.
131. Welt, L.G. and Nelson, W.P. Excretion of water by normal subjects. *J. Appl. Physiol.* 4: 709–714, 1952.

Part II

ENVIRONMENTAL INFLUENCES ON BODY FLUID BALANCE DURING EXERCISE

Chapter 7

BODY FLUID BALANCE DURING EXERCISE–HEAT EXPOSURE

Michael N. Sawka
Scott J. Montain
William A. Latzka

CONTENTS

I. Introduction..139

II. Body Water Loss 140

III. Exercise Performance and Tolerance.........................142
    A. Muscular Strength and Endurance 142
    B. Aerobic Exercise......................................145

IV. Temperature Regulation 147

V. Hyperhydration..150

VI. Summary..152

References 153

I. INTRODUCTION

A person performing exercise in the heat will often incur a body water deficit. Generally, the person dehydrates during exercise because of fluid nonavailability or a mismatch between thirst and body water requirements. In these instances, the person starts to exercise as euhydrated but incurs an exercise–heat-mediated dehydration over a prolonged period. This scenario is common for many athletic and occupational settings; however, in the military, particularly during combat, people may start exercise while already hypohydrated.[20] There are also several sports (e.g., boxing, power lifting, wrestling) in which athletes will purposely achieve hypohydration prior to competition.[91] These athletes want to compete in a lower weight class to gain a size advantage over competitors.

If dehydrated persons exercise in the heat, they will incur significant adverse effects. Dehydration will increase physiologic strain,[50] decrease exercise performance,[5,88] and negate the thermoregulatory advantages conferred by high aerobic fitness[11,12] and heat acclimation.[11,72] In addition, devastating medical consequences can occur if dehydrated persons perform strenuous exercise in the heat. For example, Massachusetts State Police recruits were limited access to water during training sessions in the summer of 1988, and 11 of 50 class members were hospitalized with serious heat injuries; two underwent kidney dialysis, and one required a liver transplant and later died.[16] Another example is that dehydration-induced heat stroke is believed responsible for 20,000 deaths among Egyptian troops during the 1967 Six-Day War with Israel.[38]

This chapter will review human hydration status and temperature regulation during exercise in the heat. Throughout this chapter, "euhydration" will refer to normal body water content, "hypohydration" will refer to body water deficit, and "dehydration" will refer to the loss of body water.

II. BODY WATER LOSS

Physical exercise routinely increases total body metabolism by 5–15 times resting levels to support skeletal muscle contraction. Approximately 70 to 90% of this energy is released as heat and needs to be dissipated to achieve body heat balance. Depending on the climatic conditions, the relative contributions of evaporative and dry (radiative and conductive) heat exchange to the total heat loss will vary. The hotter the climate, the greater the dependence on evaporative heat loss, and thus on sweating. Therefore, a substantial volume of body water may be lost via sweating to enable evaporative cooling in hot climates.[71]

A person's sweating rate is dependent on climatic conditions, clothing worn, and exercise intensity. Soldiers in the desert often have sweating rates of 0.3 to 1.2 l/h while performing military activities.[1,49] Persons wearing protective clothing often have sweating rates of 1 to 2 l/h while performing light-intensity exercise.[44,81] Likewise, athletes performing high-intensity exercise commonly have sweating rates of 1 to 2.5 l/h while in the heat.[71] During these situations, a principal problem is to match fluid consumption with sweat loss. Because thirst provides a poor index of body water needs, people will dehydrate by 2 to 8% of their body weight during situations of prolonged high sweat loss.[30]

Water is the largest component of the human body, comprising 45 to 70% of body weight. The average male (75 kg) is composed of about 45 l of water, which corresponds to about 60% of body weight. Adipose tissue is about 10% water and muscle tissue is about 75% water, so a person's total body water depends on body composition.[71] In addition, muscle water and glycogen content parallel each other, probably because of the osmotic pressure exerted by glycogen granules within the muscle's sarcoplasm.[54] As a result, trained athletes have a relatively greater total body water than their sedentary counterparts, by virtue of a smaller percentage body fat and a higher skeletal muscle glycogen concentration.

The water contained in body tissues is distributed between the intracellular and extracellular fluid spaces. Dehydration mediated by sweating will influence each fluid space as a consequence of free fluid exchange. Nose and colleagues[60] determined the distribution of body water loss among the fluid spaces as well as among different body organs. They thermally dehydrated rats by 10% of body weight, and after the animals regained their normal core temperature, the body water measurements were obtained. The water deficit was apportioned between the intracellular (41%) and extracellular (59%) spaces; and among the organs, 40% from muscle, 30% from skin, 14% from viscera, and 14% from bone. Neither the brain nor liver lost significant water content. They concluded that hypohydration results in water redistribution largely from the intra- and extracellular spaces of muscle and skin in order to maintain blood volume.

Figure 1 presents resting plasma volume and osmolality values for heat-acclimated persons when hypohydrated at various levels of body water loss. Sweat-induced dehydration will decrease plasma volume and increase plasma osmotic pressure in proportion to the level of fluid loss. Plasma volume decreases because it provides the precursor fluid for sweat, and osmolality increases because sweat is ordinarily hypotonic relative to plasma.[42,76] Sodium and chloride are primarily responsible for the elevated plasma osmolality.[76] It is the plasma hyperosmolality that mobilizes fluid from the intracellular to the extracellular space to enable plasma volume defense in hypohydrated subjects.

Some athletes use diuretics to reduce their body weight. Diuretics increase the rate of urine formation and generally result in the loss of solute.[90] Commonly used diuretics include thiazide (e.g., Diuril), carbonic anhydrase inhibitors (e.g., Diamox), and furosemide (e.g., Lasix). Diuretic-induced hypohydration generally results in an isoosmotic hypovolemia, with a much greater ratio of plasma loss to body water loss than either exercise- or heat-induced hypohydration.[37] Relatively less intracellular fluid is lost after diuretic administration because there is not an extracellular solute excess to stimulate redistribution of body water.

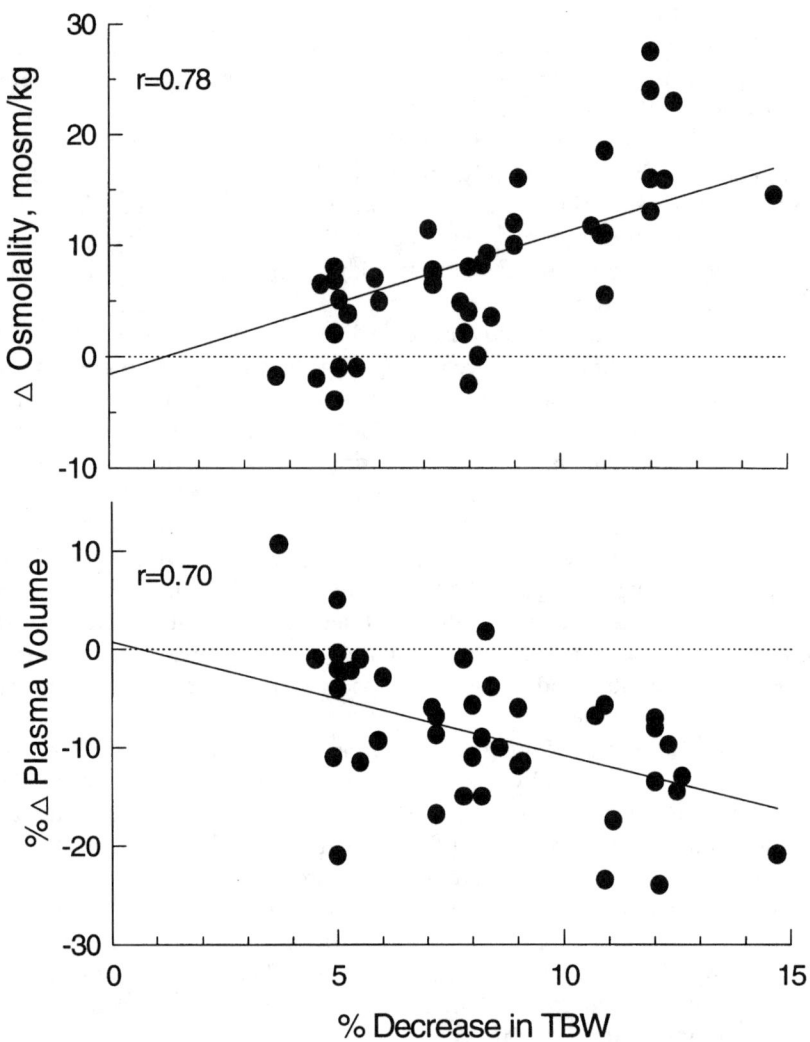

FIGURE 1 Body water loss effects on plasma osmolality and plasma volume. TBW, total body water. (From Sawka, M.N., et al., *J. Appl. Physiol.* 59:1394–1401, 1985, and Montain, S.J., et al., *J. Appl. Physiol.* 79: 1434–1439, 1995. With permission.)

III. EXERCISE PERFORMANCE AND TOLERANCE

A. MUSCULAR STRENGTH AND ENDURANCE

Muscular strength has been examined in 13 studies, of which 4 demonstrated a strength reduction after dehydration (see Table 1). Of the four studies that demonstrated strength reductions, hypohydration was achieved by fluid restriction in three[8,9,36] and by a combination of exercise and heat exposure in the fourth.[89] Therefore, prolonged fluid restriction, perhaps accompanied by a caloric deficit,[8,9,36] was the dehydration method that most often reduced muscular strength. The magnitude of water deficit appeared to influence the frequency with which muscular strength reductions were reported. Of seven studies that involved less than a 5% reduction in body weight, only one[9] reported a strength reduction; of six studies that involved a 5 to 8% reduction in body weight, three reported strength reductions.

Table 1   Influence of Hypohydration on Muscular Strength and Endurance

Dehydration Procedure	ΔWeight	Method	Strength	Endurance/ Power	Ref.
Sauna & exercise	–2kg	Back leg lifts	NC	—	2
Exercise in heat	–3%	Isometric	NC	—	30
Fluid restriction	–3%	Isometric	↓(11%)	—	9
Exercise in heat	–3%	Isometric	NC	↓	6
Fluid restriction	–4%	Isometric	NC	—	31
Sauna, exercise in heat, exercise	–4%	Isometric Arm cranking	NC —	— ↓(13 to 37%)	65
Sauna	–4%	Isometric, isotonic	— —	↓(31%) ↓(29%)	86
?	–4%	Isokinetic	NC	NC	48
Exercise & heat	–5%	Isometric	NC	—	87
Heat	–5%	Wingate test	—	NC	39
?	–5%	Isometric	NC	NC	78
Exercise in heat, sauna	–5%	Wingate test	NC in leg strength, ↓(7%) in shoulder and chest strength	↓(21%) peak power, ↓(10%) average power	89
Fluid restriction	–6%	Isometric, isotonic	↓(3%) —	— ↓	8
?	–7%	Isometric	NC	—	80
Fluid restriction	–8%	Isokinetic, Supramax. run	↓(11%) —	— NC	36

Note: NC = No change from euhydration.

Muscular endurance has been evaluated in six studies, of which four[6,8,65,86] reported reductions after hypohydration. The two studies that found no change in muscular endurance did not report their dehydration procedure,[48,78] but the other studies used fluid restriction,[8] stress,[65,86] and exercise and heat[6,65,86] to dehydrate volunteers. There were no systematic differences among these studies in the magnitude of water deficit, muscle group tested, or test methodology.

Saltin[65] examined the time to fatigue during maximal-effort arm cranking after losing 4% of body weight by sauna or exercise–heat exposure. Time to fatigue was reduced 13 and 37% after sauna and exercise–heat exposure, respectively. Hypohydration did not appear to affect neural activation of muscle, as muscle strength was unchanged by hypohydration. Differences in muscle glycogen were also unlikely, as the arm muscles were not used during the exercise dehydration procedures. The author speculated that the cause of the premature fatigue must be within muscle.

The mechanisms by which hypohydration increases skeletal muscle fatiguability have been little studied. Hypohydration does not appear to accelerate the rate of glycolysis, inasmuch as hypohydration does not increase muscle glycogen use during exercise[17,55] and blood lactate concentration is usually similar or lower during exercise when hypohydrated compared to euhydrated.[4,10,17,65,89] However, hypohydration could accelerate depletion of ATP and creatine phosphate concentration, or impair the ability to buffer the hydrogen and inorganic phosphate ions produced during exercise.

Torranin et al.[86] evaluated the isometric endurance of a small muscle group (hand grip) and the isotonic endurance of large muscle groups (arm and leg). Despite the use of very diverse methodology, they found a consistent 30% reduction in muscular endurance when hypohydrated. They speculated that during the hypohydration experiments, a greater muscle temperature might have mediated the reduced muscular endurance. The muscular endurance experiments were conducted approximately 1 h after the subjects had finished dehydrating in an 80°C sauna.

Bijlani and Sharma[6] performed muscular endurance experiments either immediately after or within 30 min of dehydrating subjects in a 41°C environment. In addition, all muscular testing (when euhydrated and hypohydrated) was conducted in a warm (30°C) environment. They present a figure demonstrating an inverse relationship between the control (euhydration) muscular endurance values and the dry bulb temperature. Therefore, an elevated muscle temperature could have mediated the reduced muscular endurance during the hypohydration experiments.[21,61]

Anaerobic exercise performance has been evaluated in three studies, of which two employed Wingate-type tests,[39,89] and one study employed a supramaximal endurance test.[36] Jacobs[39] performed a comprehensive evaluation of anaerobic exercise performance (Wingate test) when subjects euhydrated and when they were hypohydrated by 2, 4, and 5% of their initial body weight. This investigator found that hypohydration did not alter anaerobic exercise performance or postexercise blood lactate values. On the other hand, Webster and colleagues[89] reported that hypohydration (5% body weight) resulted in a 21% reduction in peak power and a 10% reduction in average power during a 40-s Wingate test. Both of these studies used similar methodologies, so their disparate results are not easily explained. Houston et al.[36] examined whether hypohydration (8% of body weight) affected endurance time for a supramaximal treadmill run. Dehydration was achieved by fluid and food restriction over several days, and the subjects were not exposed to heat stress. The authors reported the endurance time (56 vs. 55 s) was similar whether euhydrated or hypohydrated.

B. AEROBIC EXERCISE

Table 2 presents a summary of studies that examined the influence of hypohydration on maximal aerobic power and physical work capacity. In a temperate environment, a body water deficit of less than 3% body weight did not alter maximal aerobic power. Maximal aerobic power was decreased[11,13,89] in three of the five studies when hypohydration equaled or exceeded 3% body weight. Therefore, a critical water deficit (3% body weight) might exist before hypohydration reduces maximal aerobic power in a temperate environment. In a hot environment, Craig and Cummings[18] demonstrated that small (2% body weight) to moderate (4% body weight) water deficits resulted in large reduction of maximal aerobic power. Likewise, their data indicate a disproportionately larger decrease in maximal aerobic power with an increased magnitude of body water deficit. It seems that environmental heat stress has a potentiating effect on the reduction of maximal aerobic power elicited by hypohydration.

TABLE 2 Effect of Hypohydration on Maximal Aerobic Power and Physical Work Capacity

Dehydration Procedure	Weight Loss	Climate	Exercise Mode	Maximal Aerobic Power	Physical Work Capacity	Ref.
Diuretics	1%	Neutral	TM	NC	↓(6.2%)	4
Exercise, diuretics, sauna	2%	Neutral	CY	NC	↓(7W)	13
	3%	Neutral	CY	↓(8%)	↓(21 W)	
	4%	Neutral	CY	↓(4%)	↓(23 W)	
Fluid restriction	1%	Hot	CY	—	↓(6%)	62
	2%	Hot	CY	—	↓(8%)	
	3%	Hot	CY	—	↓(20%)	
Diuretics, sauna, exercise	–3%	Neutral	CY	—	↓(18%)	58
	–3%	Neutral	CY	—	↓(35%)	
	–3%	Neutral	CY	—	↓(44%)	
Sauna, heat, exercise, diuretics	4%	Neutral	CY	NC	↓(?)	65
Exercise & fluid restriction	3%	Neutral	Rowing	NC	↓(5%)	10
Heat	2%	Hot	TM	↓(10%)	↓(22%)	18
	4%	Hot	TM	↓(27%)	↓(48%)	
Exercise, heat	5%	Neutral	TM	↓(0.22 L/min)	—	11
Exercise, eat, sauna	5%	Neutral	TM	↓(7%)	↓(12%)	89
Fluid restriction	8%	Neutral	TM	NC	—	36

Note: NC = No change from euhydration, TM = treadmill exercise, CY = cycling exercise.

The physical work capacity for high-intensity aerobic exercise was decreased when hypohydrated. Physical work capacity was decreased by marginal (1 – 2% body weight) water deficits that did not alter maximal aerobic power,[4,13] and the reduction was larger with increasing water deficit. Clearly, hypohydration resulted in much larger decrements of physical work capacity in hot as compared to temperate environments.[18] It appears that the thermoregulatory system, perhaps via increased body temperatures, has an important role in the reduced exercise performance mediated by a body water deficit.

A reduced maximal cardiac output might be the physiological mechanism by which hypohydration decreases an individual's maximal aerobic power and physical work capacity. Hypohydration is associated with a decreased blood (plasma) volume during both rest and exercise. A decreased blood volume increases blood viscosity and can reduce venous return. During maximal exercise, viscosity-mediated increased resistance and reduced cardiac filling could both decrease stroke volume and cardiac output. Several investigators[3,66,82] have reported a tendency for reduced cardiac output when hypohydrated during short-term, moderate-intensity exercise.

It is not surprising that environmental heat stress potentiates the hypohydration mediated reduction in maximal aerobic power. For euhydrated individuals, environmental heat stress alone decreases maximal aerobic power by ~7%.[73] A hypohydrated person would be attempting the same exercise challenge with an already compromised vascular volume. In the heat, the superficial skin veins reflexively dilate to increase cutaneous blood flow and volume. The redirection of blood flow to the cutaneous vasculature could decrease maximal aerobic power by (1) reducing the portion of cardiac output perfusing contracting muscles, or (2) decreasing the effective central blood volume and central venous pressure, thus reducing venous return and cardiac output. A substantial volume of blood can be redirected to the skin, therefore being removed from the effective central circulation and not available to perfuse the skeletal muscles.[64] As a result, both environmental heat stress and hypohydration can act independently to limit cardiac output, and therefore oxygen delivery, during maximal exercise.

Studies have demonstrated that moderate levels of hypohydration can impair endurance exercise performance. Armstrong and colleagues[4] studied the effects of a body water deficit on competitive distance-running performance. They had athletes compete in 1500-, 5000- and 10,000-m races when euhydrated and when hypohydrated. Hypohydration was achieved by diuretic administration (furosemide), which decreased body weight by 2% and plasma volume by 11%. Running performance was impaired at all race distances, but to a greater extent in the longer races (~5% for the 5000 and 10,000 m) than the shorter race (3% for 1500 m). Burge et al.[10] recently examined whether hypohydration (3% body weight loss) affected simulated 2,000 m rowing performance. They found that on average, it took 22 s longer to complete the task when hypohydrated compared to when euhydrated. Average power was reduced 5% by hypohydration.

Two recent studies examined the benefits of drinking fluids during moderately intense aerobic exercise. In both studies, high-intensity performance tests were performed immediately after 50 to 60 min of cycling during which volunteers either drank nothing or drank sufficient fluid to replace sweat losses. Walsh et al.[88] reported that time to fatigue when cycling at 90% $\dot{V}O_2$ max was

51% longer (6.5 vs. 9.8 min) when subjects drank sufficient fluids to prevent dehydration. Below et al.[5] found that cyclists performed a performance ride 6.5% faster if they drank fluids during exercise. The results of these studies clearly demonstrate the detrimental effects of dehydration on endurance athletic performance.

Several studies have documented the detrimental effects of dehydration on human tolerance to submaximal exercise in the heat. Adolph and associates[1] performed experiments in the California deserts during 1942 and 1943. In those experiments, subjects attempted endurance (2 to 23 h) walks (at 4 to 6.5 km/h) in the desert ($T_a \sim 38°C$) and either were allowed to drink water ad libitum or refrained from drinking. They reported that 1 of 59 (2%) and 11 of 70 soldiers (16%) suffered exhaustion from heat strain during a desert walk when they did or did not drink, respectively. In subsequent experiments, they reported that 1 of 59 subjects (2%) and 15 of 70 subjects (21%) suffered exhaustion from heat strain during an attempted 8-h desert walk when they did and did not drink, respectively. The subjects' magnitude of dehydration was not provided in either set of experiments. Ladell[43] had subjects attempt a 140-min walk in a hot ($T_a = 38°C$) environment while ingesting different combinations of salt and water. They reported that exhaustion from heat strain occurred in 9 of 12 (75%) experiments when receiving neither water or salt, and 3 of 41 (7%) experiments when receiving only water. Sawka and colleagues[74] had subjects attempt treadmill walks (~25% $\dot{V}O_2$ max for 140 min) in a hot, dry ($T_a = 49°C$, rh = 20%) environment when euhydrated and when hypohydrated by 3, 5, and 7% of their body weight. All 8 subjects completed the euhydration and 3% hypohydration experiments, and 7 subjects completed the 5% hypohydration experiments. For the 7% hypohydration experiments, 6 subjects discontinued after completing only (mean) 64 min. Clearly, dehydration increases the incidence of exhaustion from heat strain.

To address whether hypohydration alters heat tolerance, Sawka et al.[75] had subjects walk to voluntary exhaustion when either euhydrated or hypohydrated (8% of total body water). The experiments were designed so that the combined environment ($T_a = 49°C$, relative humidity = 20%) and exercise intensity (47% $\dot{V}O_2$ max) would not allow thermal equilibrium, and heat exhaustion would eventually occur. Hypohydration reduced tolerance time from 121 to 55 min, but more importantly, hypohydration reduced the core temperature that a person could tolerate. Heat exhaustion occurred at a core temperature ~0.4°C lower when hypohydrated than when euhydrated. These findings suggest that hypohydration not only impairs exercise performance, but also reduces tolerance to heat strain.

IV. TEMPERATURE REGULATION

Hypohydration increases core temperature responses during exercise in temperate[12,29] and hot[74] climates. A critical deficit of 1% of body weight elevates core temperature during exercise.[22] As the magnitude of water deficit increases, there is a concomitant graded elevation of core temperature during exercise heat stress.[50,74] Changing the pattern of drinking, and the timing of dehydration, does not alter the close coupling between body water and core temperature during exercise.[51] Figure 2 illustrates relationships between body water loss and core temperature elevations reported by studies that examined several water deficit levels. The magnitude of core temperature elevation ranges from 0.1 to 0.23°C for every percent of body weight lost.[1,50,74,83] These studies suggest that the core temperature elevation, for a given water deficit, becomes greater with increased exercise intensity. If true, the physiological consequences of dehydration are accentuated for endurance athletes compared to persons performing industrial and occupational tasks. Hypohydration also negates the thermoregulatory advantages conferred by high aerobic fitness and heat acclimation for exercise in the heat.[11,12,72]

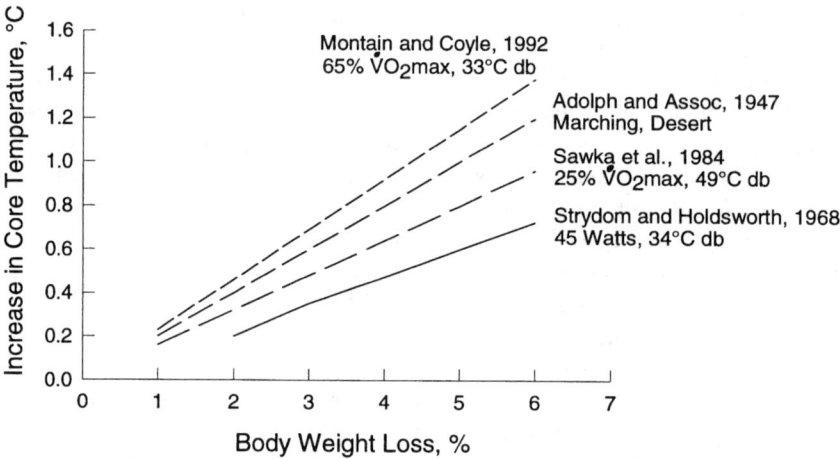

FIGURE 2 Relationships for the elevation in core temperature (above euhydration) at a given body water loss.

Hypohydration is associated with both reduced[52,76,83] and unchanged[15,84,85] sweating rates during exercise at a given metabolic rate. However, investigators reporting no change in sweating rate usually observed an elevated core temperature. Figure 3A shows with increased hypohydration levels a systematic reduction in total body sweating rate for a given core temperature during exercise in the heat.[74] Likewise, Figure 3B presents the local sweating response to hypohydration (5% body weight) during exercise in the heat.[69] This figure suggests that hypohydration increases the threshold temperature for the onset of sweating, but does not alter the sensitivity (slope) of the sweating response to increases in body temperature.

The physiological mechanisms mediating the altered control of sweating when hypohydrated are not clearly defined. Both the singular and combined

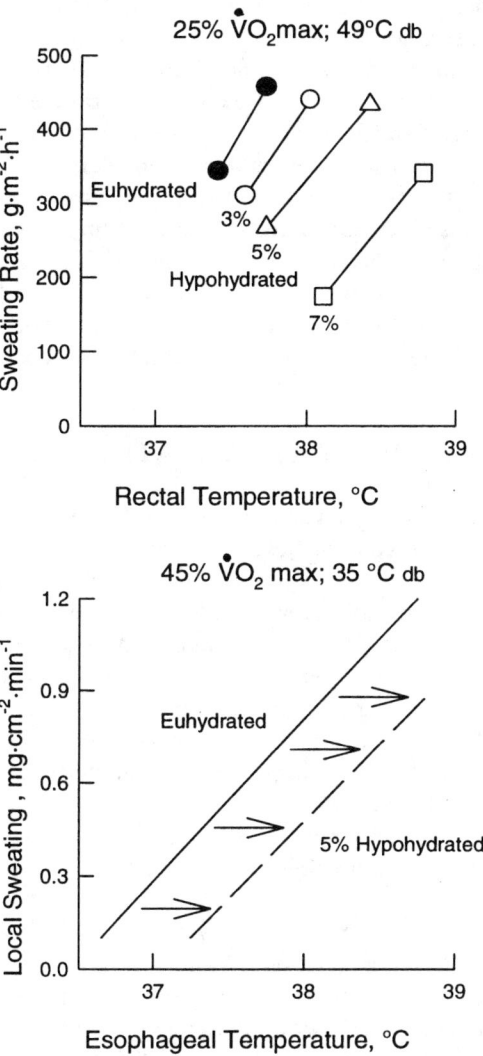

FIGURE 3 Whole body (top) and local (bottom) sweating response to core temperature during euhydration and hypohydration exercise–heat stress. (From Sawka, M.N., et al., *J. Appl. Physiol.* 59:1394–1401, 1985, and Sawka, M.N., et al., *Am. J. Physiol.* 257:R311–R316, 1989. With permission.)

effects of plasma hyperosmolality and hypovolemia have been suggested as mediating the reduced sweating response during exercise–heat stress.[67] Plasma osmolality changes may relate to tonicity changes in the extracellular fluid bathing the hypothalamic neurons.[41,77] Silva and Boulant[79] have demonstrated that in rat brain slices, there are preoptic-anterior hypothalamic neurons that are both thermosensitive and osmosensitive. Such data suggest a central interaction between thermoregulation and body water regulation.[35]

Isotonic hypohydration alone can impair heat loss and increase core temperature during exercise–heat exposure.[15,23,53] Studies[24,53] have reported that isotonic hypohydration reduces skin blood flow for a given core temperature, and therefore the potential for dry heat exchange. Fortney et al.[24] have provided a rationale as to why an isoosmotic hypohydration might reduce skin blood flow and sweating rate. They theorized that hypovolemia might reduce cardiac preload and alter the activity of atrial baroreceptors that have afferent input to the hypothalamus. Therefore, a reduced atrial filling pressure might modify neural information to the hypothalamic thermoregulatory centers that control skin blood flow and sweating. Subsequent studies[27,47] have demonstrated that acute unloading of atrial baroreceptors during exercise with periods of lower body negative pressure impairs heat loss and increases core temperature.

V. HYPERHYDRATION

Hyperhydration, or greater than normal body water, has been suggested to improve, above euhydration levels, thermoregulation and exercise–heat performance. The concept that hyperhydration might be beneficial for exercise performance arose from the adverse consequences of hypohydration. It was theorized that body water expansion might reduce the cardiovascular and thermal strain of exercise by expanding blood volume and reducing blood tonicity, thereby improving exercise performance. Studies that have directly expanded blood volume (e.g., infusion) have usually reported decreased cardiovascular strain[34,59,70] during exercise, but disparate results on heat dissipation[19,59,70] and exercise–heat performance.[19,45] Studies that have attenuated plasma hyperosmolality during exercise–heat stress generally report improved heat dissipation,[25,33,56,68] but have not addressed exercise performance.

Table 3 provides a chronological review of studies evaluating hyperhydration effects on thermoregulation. Generally, most studies reported lower core temperatures during exercise after hyperhydration. The magnitude of the core temperature reduction, however, was relatively small. Three of the seven studies[46,52,56] reported higher sweating rates with hyperhydration. In all cases, heart rate was lower during exercise with hyperhydration. Together, these findings support the notion that hyperhydration can reduce the thermal and cardiovascular strain of exercise.

The mechanism or mechanisms responsible for the lower exercise core temperatures when hyperhydrated remain unclear. In several studies,[52,57] overdrinking before exercise lowered body core temperature prior to exercise. This was likely due to the caloric cost of warming the ingested fluid. Exercise per se did not exacerbate the difference that existed prior to exercise. Hyperhydration in these studies, therefore, apparently did not improve heat dissipation during the exercise period. However, other studies[46,52,56] reported greater exercise sweating rates during hyperhydration. Grucza et al.[32] found that sweating was initiated earlier during hyperhydration. The findings of these latter studies suggest that hyperhydration may improve heat dissipation during exercise–heat stress.

TABLE 3 Hyperhydration Effects on Thermoregulation

Year	Pre-Exercise Hydration Treatments	Exercise-Environmental Conditions	Temperature Core	Temperature Skin	Sweat Rate	Ref.
1965	2 l water vs. no water	90 min treadmill (Ta = 49°C)	↓(0.3°C)	—	↑	52
1971	1.5 l water vs. no water or 1.0 l 2% saline	60 min cycle (~50% V̇O$_2$max) (Ta = 20°C)	↓(0.5°C) ↑(0.3°C)	—	—	57
1971	2.5–3.0 l water vs. ad libitum	70 min cycle (~50% V̇O$_2$max) (Ta = 24°C)	NC NC	NC	NC	30
1974	1.5 l water vs. no water vs. 1.5 l 2–3% saline	60 min cycle (45% V̇O$_2$max) (Ta = 30°C)	↓ ↑	—	↑ ↓	56
1974	1 l water vs. no water vs. 1 l with rehydration	120 min treadmill (75% V̇O$_2$max) (Ta = 33°C)	↓(0.2°C) ↓(0.8°C)	—	NC NC	28
1980	2.0 l water with ADH vs. euhydration	30 min cycle (55% V̇O$_2$max) (Ta = 35°C)	NC	—	—	53
1987	2.0 l water vs. euhydration	45 min cycle (~52% V̇O$_2$max) (Ta = 23°C)	↓(0.4°C) ↓(Δ0.2°C)	NC	↓	32
1988	0.5 l isotonic solution vs. euhydration	4 h intermittent cycle (70 W) (Ta = 36°C)	NC	NC	NC	14
1990	1.5 l water vs. 1.5 l water with glycerol or ad libitum	90 min treadmill (~60% V̇O$_2$max) (Ta = 42°C)	↓(0.7°C) NC	—	↑ NC	46

Note: NC = No change from euhydration.
Ta = ambient temperature.

The believed thermal benefits of hyperhydration do not appear dependent on acclimation state. Moroff and Bass[52] examined the effect of hyperhydration on the heat acclimation response. Repeated hyperhydration prior to exercise during 9 d of exercise–heat stress did not affect the acclimation response. Furthermore, overdrinking produced similar effects on core temperature, heart rate, and sweating whether hyperhydration was induced before or after the heat acclimation protocol.

Although many studies have attempted to induce hyperhydration by overdrinking water or water–electrolyte solutions, these approaches have produced only transient expansion of body water. One problem often encountered is that much of the fluid overload is rapidly excreted. Recently, evidence has accrued that greater fluid retention can be achieved with an aqueous solution containing glycerol. Riedesel et al.[63] reported that following hyperhydration with a glycerol solution compared to water alone, subjects excreted significantly less of the water load. Improved fluid retention after hyperhydration with glycerol solutions has been confirmed by others,[26,46] and there are reports that hyperhydration can be maintained for prolonged periods with repeated glycerol intake.[40]

Lyons et al.[46] examined whether glycerol-mediated hyperhydration improved thermoregulatory responses to exercise–heat stress. Subjects completed three trials in which they exercised in a hot (42°C) climate. For one trial, fluid ingestion was restricted to 5.4 ml/kg body weight, and in the other two trials subjects ingested water (21.4 ml/kg) with or without a bolus of glycerol (1 g/kg). Ninety minutes after this hyperhydration period, subjects began exercise. Glycerol ingestion increased fluid retention 30% compared to drinking water alone. During exercise, glycerol hyperhydration produced a higher sweating rate and substantially lower core temperatures (0.7°C) compared to control conditions and water hyperhydration.

Few studies have examined whether hyperhydration improves exercise performance or heat tolerance. Blyth and Burt[7] were the first to report the effects of hyperhydration on performance during exercise–heat stress. Their subjects ran to exhaustion in a hot climate (49°C) when normally hydrated and when hyperhydrated by drinking 2 l of fluid 30 min prior to exercise. When hyperhydrated, 13 of 18 subjects ran longer before exhaustion. The average time to exhaustion (17.3 vs. 16.9 min) did not, however, reach statistical significance. More recently, Luetkemeier and Thomas[45] examined whether hypervolemia improved cycling performance. They reported that blood volume expansion (+450/500 ml) increased simulated time trial performance 10% (81 vs. 90 min). No study to date has examined whether hyperhydration improves exercise–heat tolerance.

VI. SUMMARY

During exercise, sweat output often exceeds water intake, thus producing a body water deficit, or hypohydration. The water deficit affects both intracellular and extracellular volume. It also results in plasma hypertonicity and hypovolemia. Muscular strength is generally maintained when hypohydrated, but muscular endurance can be reduced. Aerobic exercise tasks are likely to be adversely affected by hypohydration, and the potential is greater in warm environments. Hypohydration increases heat storage and reduces one's ability to tolerate heat strain. The increased heat storage is mediated by reduced sweating rate and reduced skin blood flow for a given core temperature. Hyperhydration has been suggested to reduce thermal strain during exercise in the heat; however, data supporting that notion are not robust.

REFERENCES

1. Adolph, E. F., et al. *Physiology of Man in the Desert,* Interscience Publishers, 1947.
2. Ahlman, K. and Karvonen, M. J. Weight reduction by sweating in wrestlers, and its effect on physical fitness, *J. Sports Med. Phys. Fitness,* 1:58–62, 1961.
3. Allen, T. E., Smith, D. P., and Miller, D. K. Hemodynamic response to submaximal exercise after dehydration and rehydration in high school wrestlers, *Med. Sci. Sports,* 9:159–163, 1977.
4. Armstrong, L. E., Costill, D. L., and Fink, W. J. Influence of diuretic-induced dehydration on competitive running performance, *Med. Sci. Sports Exer.* 17:456–461, 1985.
5. Below, P. R., Mora-Rodríguez, R., González-Alonso, J., and Coyle, E. F. Fluid and carbohydrate ingestion independently improve performance during 1 h of intense exercise, *Med. Sci. Sports Exer.* 27:200–210, 1995.
6. Bijlani, R. L. and Sharma, K. N. Effect of dehydration and a few regimes of rehydration on human performance, *Ind. J. Physiol. Pharmacol.* 24:255–266, 1980.
7. Blyth, C. S. and Burt, J. J. Effect of water balance on ability to perform in high ambient temperatures, *Res. Q. Exer. Sport,* 3:301–307, 1932.
8. Bosco, J. S., Greenleaf, J. E., Bernauer, E. M., and Card, D. H. Effects of acute dehydration and starvation on muscular stength and endurance, *Acta Physiol. Pol.* 25:411–421, 1974.
9. Bosco, J. S., Terjung, R. L., and Greenleaf, J. E. Effects of progressive hypohydration on maximal isometric muscular strength, *J. Sports Med. Phys. Fitness,* 8:81–86, 1968.
10. Burge, C. M., Carey, M. F., and Payne, W. R. Rowing performance, fluid balance, and metabolic function following dehydration and rehydration, *Med. Sci. Sports Exer.* 25:1358–1364, 1993.
11. Buskirk, E. R., Iampietro, P. F., and Bass, D. E. Work performance after dehydration: Effects of physical conditioning and heat acclimatization, *J. Appl. Physiol.* 12:189–194, 1958.
12. Cadarette, B. S., Sawka, M. N., Toner, M. M., and Pandolf, K. B. Aerobic fitness and the hypohydration response to exercise-heat stress, *Aviat. Space Environ. Med.* 55:507–512, 1984.
13. Caldwell, J. E., Ahonen, E., and Nousiainen, U. Differential effects of sauna-, diuretic-, and exercise-induced hypohydration, *J. Appl. Physiol.* 57:1018–1023, 1984.
14. Candas, V., Libert, J.-P., Brandenberger, G., Sagot, J.-C., and Kahn, J.-M. Thermal and circulatory responses during prolonged exercise at different levels of hydration, *J. Physiol. Paris,* 83:11–18, 1988.
15. Claremont, A. D., Costill, D. L., Fink, W., and Van Handel, P. Heat tolerance following diuretic induced dehydration, *Med. Sci. Sports,* 8:239–243, 1976.
16. Commonwealth of Massachusetts, *The Report of the Investigation of Attorney General James M. Shannon of the Class 12 Experience at the Edward W. Connelly Criminal Justice Training Center, Agawam, Massachusetts,* Department of the Attorney General, Boston, 1988.
17. Costill, D. L. and Saltin, B. Muscle glycogen and electrolytes following exercise and thermal dehydration, in *Biochemistry of Exercise II,* University Park Press, Baltimore, 1975, 352–360.
18. Craig, F. N. and Cummings, E. G. Dehydration and muscular work, *J. Appl. Physiol.* 21:670–674, 1966.
19. Deschamps, A., Levy, R. D., Cosio, M. G., Marliss, E. B., and Magder, S. Effect of saline infusion on body temperature and endurance during heavy exercise, *J. Appl. Physiol.* 66:2799–2804, 1989.
20. Draper, E. S. and Lombardi, J. J. *Combined Arms in a Nuclear/Chemical Environment: Force Development Testing and Experimentation. Summary Evaluation Report Phase I,* U.S. Army Chemical School, Ft. McClellan, AR, 1986.

21. Edwards, R. H. T., Harris, R. C., Hultman, E., Kaizer, L., Koh, D., and Nordesjo, L. Effect of temperature on muscle energy metabolism and endurance during successive isometric contractions, sustained to fatigue, of the quadriceps muscle in man, *J. Physiol.* 220:335–352, 1972.
22. Ekblom, B., Greenleaf, C. J., Greenleaf, J. E., and Hermansen, L. Temperature regulation during exercise dehydration in man, *Acta Physiol. Scand.* 79:475–483, 1970.
23. Fortney, S. M., et al. Effect of acute alterations of blood volume on circulatory performance in humans, *J. Appl. Physiol.* 50:292–298, 1981.
24. Fortney, S. M., Nadel, E. R., Wenger, C. B., and Bove, J. R. Effect of blood volume on sweating rate and body fluids in exercising humans, *J. Appl. Physiol.* 51:1594–1600, 1981.
25. Fortney, S. M., Wenger, C. B., Bove, J. R., and Nadel, E. R. Effect of hyperosmolality on control of blood flow and sweating, *J. Appl. Physiol.* 57:1688–1695, 1984.
26. Freund, B. J., Montain, S. J., Young, A. J., Sawka, M. N., DeLuca, J. P., Pandolf, K. B., and Valeri, C. R. Glycerol hyperhydration: Hormonal, renal, and vascular fluid responses, *J. Appl. Physiol.* 79:2069–2077, 1995.
27. Gaddis, G. M. and Elizondo, R. S. Effect of central blood volume decrease upon thermoregulation responses to exercise in the heat, *Fed. Proc.* 43:627, 1984.
28. Gisolfi, C. V. and Copping, J. R. Thermal effects of prolonged treadmill exercise in the heat, *Med. Sci. Sports*, 6:108–113, 1974.
29. Grande, F., Monagle, J. E., Buskirk, E. R., and Taylor, H. L. Body temperature responses to exercise in man on restricted food and water intake, *J. Appl. Physiol.* 14:194–198, 1959.
30. Greenleaf, J. E. and Castle, B. L. Exercise temperature regulation in man during hypohydration and hyperhydration, *J. Appl. Physiol.* 30:847–853, 1971.
31. Greenleaf, J. E., Matter, M., Jr., Bosco, J. S., Douglas, L. G., and Averkin, E. G. Effects of hypohydration on work performance and tolerance to +Gz acceleration in man, *Aerosp. Med.* 37:34–39, 1966.
32. Grucza, R., Szcypaczewska, M., and Kozlowski, S. Thermoregulation in hyperhydrated men during physical exercise, *Eur. J. Appl. Physiol.* 56:603–607, 1987.
33. Harrison, M. H., Edwards, R. J., and Fennessy, P. A. Intravascular volume and tonicity as factors in the regulation of body temperature, *J. Appl. Physiol.* 44:69–75, 1978.
34. Hopper, M. K., Coggan, A. R., and Coyle, E. F. Exercise stroke volume relative to plasma-volume expansion, *J. Appl. Physiol.* 64:404–408, 1988.
35. Hori, T., Nakashima, T., Koga, A., Kiyohama, T., and Inoue, T. Convergence of thermal, osmotic and cardiovascular signals on preoptic and anterial hypothalamic neurons in the rat, *Brain Res. Bull.* 20:879–885, 1988.
36. Houston, M. E., Marrin, D. A., Green, H. J., and Thomson, J. A. The effect of rapid weight loss on physiological functions in wrestlers, *Physician Sportsmed.* 9:73–78, 1981.
37. Hubbard, R. W. and Armstrong, L. E. The heat illnesses: Biochemical, ultrastructural, and fluid-electrolyte considerations, in *Human Performance Physiology and Environmental Medicine at Terrestrial Extremes,* Pandolf, K. B., Sawka, M. N., and Gonzalez, R. R., Eds., Benchmark Press, Indianapolis, 1988, 305–359.
38. Hubbard, R. W., Mager, M., and Kerstein, M. Water as a tactical weapon: A doctrine for preventing heat casualties, *Army Sci. Conf. Proc.*125–139, 1982.
39. Jacobs, I. The effects of thermal dehydration on performance of the Wingate Anaerobic Test. *Int. J. Sports Med.* 1:21–24, 1980.
40. Koeningsberg, P., Lyons, T. P., Nagy, R., and Riedesel, M. L. 40 hour glycerol-induced hyperhydration, *Fed. Proc.* 5:A768, 1991. (Abstract).
41. Kozlowski, S., Greenleaf, J. E., Turlejska, E., and Nazar, K. Extracellular hyperosmolality and body temperature during physical exercise in dogs, *Am. J. Physiol.* 239:R180–R183, 1980.
42. Kubica, R., Neilsen, B., Bonnesen, A., Rasmussen, I. B., Stoklosa, J., and Wilk, B. Relationship between plasma volume reduction and plasma electrolyte changes after prolonged bicycle exercise, passive heating and diuretic dehydration, *Acta Physiol. Pol.* 34:569–580, 1983.

43. Ladell, W. S. S. The effects of water and salt intake upon the performance of men working in hot and humid environments, *J. Physiol.* 127:11–46, 1955.
44. Levine, L., Quigley, M. D., Cadarette, B. S., Sawka, M. N., and Pandolf, K. B. Physiological strain associated with wearing toxic-environment protective systems during exercise in the heat, in *Advances in Industrial Ergonomics and Safety II,* Das, B., Ed., Taylor & Francis, London, 1990, 897–904.
45. Luetkemeier, M. J. and Thomas, E. L. Hypervolemia and cycling time trial performance, *Med. Sci. Sports Exer.* 26:503–509, 1994.
46. Lyons, T. P., Riedesel, M. L., Meuli, L. E., and Chick, T. W. Effects of glycerol-induced hyperhydration prior to exercise in the heat on sweating and core temperature, *Med. Sci. Sports Exer.* 22:477–483, 1990.
47. Mack, G., Nose, H., and Nadel, E. R. Role of cardiopulmonary baroreflexes during dynamic exercise, *J. Appl. Physiol.* 65:1827–1832, 1988.
48. Mnatzakian, P. A. and Vaccaro, P. Effects of 4% dehydration and rehydration on hematological profiles, urinary profiles and muscular endurance of college wrestlers, *Med. Sci. Sports Exer.* 14:117, 1982. (Abstract).
49. Molnar, G. W., Towbin, E. J., Gosselin, R. E., Brown, A. H., and Adolph, E. F. A comparative study of water, salt, and heat exchanges of men in tropical and desert environments, *Am. J. Hyg.* 44:411–433, 1946.
50. Montain, S. J. and Coyle, E. F. Influence of graded dehydration on hyperthermia and cardiovascular drift during exercise, *J. Appl. Physiol.* 73:1340–1350, 1992.
51. Montain, S. J. and Coyle, E. F. Influence of the timing of fluid ingestion on temperature regulation during exercise, *J. Appl. Physiol.* 75:688–695, 1993.
52. Moroff, S. V. and Bass, D. E. Effects of overhydration on man's physiological responses to work in the heat, *J. Appl. Physiol.* 20:267–270, 1965.
53. Nadel, E. R., et al. Effect of hydration state on circulatory and thermal regulations, *J. Appl. Physiol.* 49:715–721, 1980.
54. Neufer, P. D., Sawka, M. N., Young, A. J., Quigley, M. D., Latzka, W. A., and Levine, L. Hypohydration does not impair skeletal muscle glycogen resynthesis after exercise, *J. Appl. Physiol.* 70:1490–1494, 1991.
55. Neufer, P. D., Young, A. J., Sawka, M. N., Quigley, M. D., Levine, L., and Latzka, W. A. Substrate levels and muscle metabolism while hypohydrated, *FASEB J.* 3(Abstr.):A990, 1989.
56. Nielsen, B. Effects of changes in plasma volume and osmolality on thermoregulation during exercise, *Acta Physiol. Scand.* 90:725–730, 1974.
57. Nielsen, B., Hansen, G., Jorgensen, S. O., and Nielsen, E. Thermoregulation in exercising man during dehydration and hyperhydration with water and saline, *Int. J. Biometeorol.* 15:195–200, 1971.
58. Nielsen, B., Kubica, R., Bonnesen, A., Rasmussen, I. B., Stoklosa, J., and Wilk, B. Physical work capacity after dehydration and hyperthermia, *Scand. J. Sports Sci.* 3:2–10, 1981.
59. Nose, H., Mack, G. W., Shi, X., Morimoto, K., and Nadel, E. R. Effect of saline infusion during exercise on thermal and circulatory regulations, *J. Appl. Physiol.* 69:609–616, 1990.
60. Nose, H., Morimoto, T., and Ogura, K. Distribution of water losses among fluid compartments of tissues under thermal dehydration in the rat, *Jpn. J. Physiol.* 33:1019–1029, 1983.
61. Petrofsky, J. S. and Lind, A. R. The relationship of body fat content to deep muscle temperature and isometric endurance in man, *Clin. Sci. Mol. Med.* 48:405–412, 1975.
62. Pinchan, G., Gauttam, R. K., Tomar, O. S., and Bajaj, A. C. Effects of primary hypohydration on physical work capacity, *Int. J. Biometeorol.* 32:176–180, 1988.
63. Riedesel, M. L., Allen, D. Y., Peake, G. T., and Al-Qattan, K. Hyperhydration with glycerol solutions, *J. Appl. Physiol.* 63:2262–2268, 1987.
64. Rowell, L. B. *Human Circulation: Regulation During Physical Stress,* Oxford University Press, New York, 1986.
65. Saltin, B. Aerobic and anaerobic work capacity after dehydration, *J. Appl. Physiol.* 19:1114–1118, 1964.

66. Saltin, B. Circulatory response to submaximal and maximal exercise after thermal dehydration, *J. Appl. Physiol.* 19:1125–1132, 1964.
67. Sawka, M. N. Physiological consequences of hypohydration: Exercise performance and thermoregulation, *Med. Sci. Sports Exer.* 24:657–670, 1992.
68. Sawka, M. N., Gonzalez, R. R., Young, A. J., Dennis, R. C., Valeri, C. R., and Pandolf, K. B. Control of thermoregulatory sweating during exercise in the heat, *Am. J. Physiol.* 257:R311–R316, 1989.
69. Sawka, M. N., Gonzalez, R. R., Young, A. J., Muza, S. R., Pandolf, K. B., Latzka, W. A., Dennis, R. C., and Valeri, C. R. Polycythemia and hydration: Effects on thermoregulation and blood volume during exercise-heat stress, *Am. J. Physiol.* 255:R456–R463, 1988.
70. Sawka, M. N., Hubbard, R. W., Francesconi, R. P., and Horstman, D. H. Effects of acute plasma volume expansion on altering exercise-heat performance, *Eur. J. Appl. Physiol.* 51:303–312, 1983.
71. Sawka, M. N. and Pandolf, K. B. Effects of body water loss on exercise performance and physiological functions, in *Fluid Homeostasis During Exercise, Vol. 3,* Gisolfi, C. V. and Lamb, D. R., Eds., Benchmark Press, Indianapolis, 1990, 1–38.
72. Sawka, M. N., Toner, M. M., Francesconi, R. P., and Pandolf, K. B. Hypohydration and exercise: Effects of heat acclimation, gender, and environment, *J. Appl. Physiol.* 55:1147–1153, 1983.
73. Sawka, M. N., Young, A. J., Cadarette, B. S., Levine, L., and Pandolf, K. B. Influence of heat stress and acclimation on maximal aerobic power, *Eur. J. Appl. Physiol.* 53:294–298, 1985.
74. Sawka, M. N., Young, A. J., Francesconi, R. P., Muza, S. R., and Pandolf, K. B. Thermoregulatory and blood responses during exercise at graded hypohydration levels, *J. Appl. Physiol.* 59:1394–1401, 1985.
75. Sawka, M. N., Young, A. J., Latzka, W. A., Neufer, P. D., Quigley, M. D., and Pandolf, K. B. Human tolerance to heat strain during exercise: Influence of hydration, *J. Appl. Physiol.* 73:368–375, 1992.
76. Senay, L. C., Jr. Relationship of evaporative rates to serum [Na$^+$], [K$^+$], and osmolarity in acute heat stress, *J. Appl. Physiol.* 25:149–152, 1968.
77. Senay, L. C., Jr. Temperature regulation and hypohydration: A singular view, *J. Appl. Physiol.* 47:1–7, 1979.
78. Serfass, R. C., Stull, G. A., Alexander, J. F., and Ewing, J. L. The effects of rapid weight loss and attempted rehydration on strength and endurance of the handgripping muscles in college wrestlers, *Res. Q. Exer. Sport,* 55:46–52, 1968.
79. Silva, N. L. and Boulant, J. A. Effects of osmotic pressure, glucose, and temperature on neurons in preoptic tissue slices, *Am. J. Physiol.* 247:R335–R345, 1984.
80. Singer, R. N. and Weiss, S. A. Effects of weight reduction on several anthropometric, physical, and performance measures of wrestlers, *Res. Q. Exer. Sport,* 39:361–369, 1968.
81. Speckman, K. L., Allan, A. E., Sawka, M. N., Young, A. J., Muza, S. R., and Pandolf, K. B. Perspectives in microclimate cooling involving protective clothing in hot environments, *Int. J. Indus. Ergonomics,* 3:121–147, 1988.
82. Sproles, C. B., Smith, D. P., Byrd, R. J., and Allen, T. E. Circulatory responses to submaximal exercise after dehydration and rehydration, *J. Sports Med.* 16:98–105, 1976.
83. Strydom, N. B. and Holdsworth, L. D. The effects of different levels of water deficit on physiological responses during heat stress, *Int. Z. Angew. Physiol. Einschl. Arbeitsphysiol.* 26:95–102, 1968.
84. Strydom, N. B., Wyndham, C. H., van Graan, C. H., Holdsworth, L. D., and Morrison, J. F. The influence of water restriction on the performance of men during a prolonged march, *S. Afr. Med. J.* 40:539–544, 1966.
85. Swamy, W., Pichan, G., and Nayar, H. S. Effects of body dehydration on soldiers during military operations in heat, in *Proc. 13th Commonwealth Defence Conference on Operational Clothing and Combat Equipment,* 1981, 1–8.

86. Torranin, C., Smith, D. P., and Byrd, R. J. The effect of acute thermal dehydration and rapid rehydration on isometric and isotonic endurance, *J. Sports Med. Phys. Fitness*, 19:1–9, 1979.
87. Tuttle, W. W. The effect of weight loss by dehydration and the withholding of food on the physiologic responses of wrestlers, *Res. Q. Exer. Sport*, 14:159–166, 1943.
88. Walsh, R. M., Noakes, T. D., Hawley, J. A., and Dennis, S. C. Impaired high-intensity cycling performance time at low levels of dehydration, *Int. J. Sports Med.* 15:392–398, 1994.
89. Webster, S., Rutt, R., and Weltman, A. Physiological effects of a weight loss regimen practiced by college wrestlers, *Med. Sci. Sports Exer.* 22:229–234, 1990.
90. Weiner, I. M. and Mudge, G. H. Diuretics and other agents employed in the mobilization of edema fluid, in *The Pharmacological Basis of Therapeutics,* Gilman, A. G., Goodman, L. S., Rall, T. W., and Murad, F., Eds., MacMillan, New York, 1985, 887–907.
91. Zambraski, E. J., Foster, D. T., Gross, P. M., and Tipton, C. M. Iowa wrestling study: Weight loss and urinary profiles of collegiate wrestlers, *Med. Sci. Sports*, 8:105–108, 1976.

Chapter **8**

ENVIRONMENTAL INFLUENCES ON BODY FLUID BALANCE DURING EXERCISE: COLD EXPOSURE

Beau J. Freund
Andrew J. Young

CONTENTS

I. Introduction..160

II. Overview: Human Heat Balance During Rest and Exercise
   in the Cold 160
   A. Biophysical Factors....................................161
   B. Thermoregulatory Responses 162
   C. Exercise and Heat Balance in the Cold 162
   D. Individual Modifying Factors 164
      1. Body Morphology 164
      2. Physical Fitness 165
      3. Age 165
      4. Gender 165
      5. Nutrition Status 166
      6. Acclimatization....................................166
      7. Clothing 166

III. Challenges to Fluid Balance During Cold Exposure............167
   A. Factors Increasing Fluid Losses in the Cold 167
      1. Cold-Induced Diuresis 167
      2. Respiratory Fluid Losses 169
      3. Cold-Weather Clothing.............................170
      4. Metabolic Cost of Movement in Cold Terrain 171
   B. Factors Limiting Fluid Intake in the Cold 171
      1. Fluid Availability 172
      2. "Voluntary" Dehydration 173

IV. Dehydration Effects in the Cold..............................174
   A. Physical and Cognitive Performance 174
   B. Dehydration and Cold Injury Susceptibility.................175

V. Countermeasures: Maintaining Euhydration 176

VI. Summary...177

References 177

I. INTRODUCTION

Physical work, mental stress, and exposure to climatic extremes, alone or in concert, can markedly disrupt body fluid balance. This is as true in cold as in hot climates. For example, soldiers conducting cold-weather operations are often dehydrated by 3–8% of their body weight.[11,64] This dehydration is similar to the magnitude experienced by people in hot climates. Few studies have investigated cold effects on body water regulation or the influence of dehydration on exercise capacity, thermoregulation or cold-injury susceptibility during cold weather.

Some 60% of the earth's land has January low temperature below 0°C and more than 25% of the earth's land experiences January lows below –18°C.[6] However, cold weather need not deter outdoor exercise. People can exercise safely even in extreme cold if they wear clothing adequate to maintain body core temperature and protect the skin from peripheral cold injury. However, cold weather and wearing cold-weather protective clothing can affect body fluid balance and, in turn, degrade physical performance and increase susceptibility to cold injury. This section will briefly review the physiological responses to defend body temperature in cold environments and then consider in detail: (1) factors affecting fluid balance in cold climates; (2) the effects of dehydration on exercise in the cold; and (3) possible countermeasures to minimize dehydration in the cold.

II. OVERVIEW: HUMAN HEAT BALANCE DURING REST AND EXERCISE IN THE COLD

Humans protect themselves against the cold first by behavioral thermoregulation. That is, they wear clothing, remain in shelters and use various heat-

---

The views, opinions, and findings in this report are those of the authors and should not be construed as official Department of the Army position, policy, or decision unless so designated by other official documentation.

generating devices. However, when behavioral strategies alone fail to defend body temperature homeostasis, physiological responses are elicited. Besides protecting against the cold effects and playing a role in the etiology of cold injuries, these physiological responses may alter metabolism and fluid balance of persons living and working in cold climates.

A. BIOPHYSICAL FACTORS

The biophysics of human thermal balance is considered in detail elsewhere (Chapter 3), so only a brief summary will be presented here.[66]

Body temperature reflects the net effects of internal heat production and heat transfers between the body and ambient environment. The heat balance equation describes the relationship:

$$S = M - (\pm W_k) \pm E \pm R \pm C \pm K \; [W/m^2]$$

M represents metabolic heat production and W_k represents energy leaving (positive for concentric work) or entering (negative for eccentric work) the body as external work. Heat exchange between the body and environment occurs via evaporation (E), radiation (R), convection (C), and conduction (K). The sum of these processes is body heat storage (S), which represents heat gain if positive or heat loss if negative.

In environments colder than body temperature, heat flows from the body core toward the environment, primarily via dry heat-loss exchange (i.e., conduction and convection). Wind increases convective heat loss from the body surface,[66] thus providing the basis for the concept of wind chill[70] (Table 1). Water has a much higher thermal conductivity than air. Therefore, convective heat transfer is greater (perhaps 70-fold) during water immersion than during exposure to air of the same temperature.[32] Clothing insulates the body from the environment, limiting convective and conductive heat loss — although wet clothing provides considerably less insulation than dry.

Another environmental factor influencing physiological function is atmospheric air's water content. Saturation vapor pressure of air decreases as air temperature falls. Therefore, as air temperature falls, so too does atmospheric moisture content, even if the relative humidity is high. Fluid is transferred from the body to air via evaporation as it comes in contact with skin and with respiration as water-saturated air is exhaled. The potential for fluid loss from the body is inversely related to the inspired air's water content; therefore, greater fluid losses generally occur with cold air, which is relatively dry.[66] Thus, environmental characteristics besides temperature influence the potential for body heat and water loss and the resulting physiological strain of defending homeostasis.

B. THERMOREGULATORY RESPONSES

Humans respond to cold in two principal ways: (1) vasomotor responses reduce dry heat loss, and (2) metabolic heat production increases.

Cold exposure elicits vasoconstriction, which reduces peripheral blood flow. The vasoconstrictor response is not limited to the extremities, but is widespread throughout the peripheral shell. The decrease in peripheral blood flow reduces convective heat transfer between the body's core and shell (skin, subcutaneous fat, and skeletal muscle), and increases body insulation. Heat is lost from the body surface faster than it is replaced. As a result, whole-body cold exposure causes a decline in skin temperature over the entire body. Thus, during cold exposure, core temperature is defended at the expense of declining skin temperature. The blood flow reduction and consequent fall in skin temperature contribute to the etiology of cold injuries.[59] The hands and fingers are particularly susceptible to cold injury[12] and a loss of manual dexterity because effects of cold-induced vasoconstriction are pronounced in those regions.[30]

The other mechanism to defend body temperature during cold exposure involves an increase in metabolic heat production. Muscle is the primary source of increased metabolic heat. Besides generating external force, muscle contractions also liberate considerable heat (approximately 70% of total energy expended). Thus, physical activity (work or exercise) increases metabolic heat production (exercise is considered next). When skin and/or core temperature are reduced, and exercise or physical activity are not initiated, shivering begins. Shivering is an involuntary pattern of repeated, rhythmic muscle contractions that may start immediately, or after several minutes of cold exposure; it usually begins in torso muscles, then spreads to the limbs.[38] Certain animals respond to cold exposure with an increase in metabolic heat production by noncontracting tissue — that is, nonshivering thermogenesis.[45] However, there is no clear evidence that humans share this mechanism.[74]

C. EXERCISE AND HEAT BALANCE IN THE COLD

Physical activity can increase metabolic heat production more than shivering. Whereas maximal shivering can elevate $\dot{V}O_2$ to about 2 l/min,[81] exercise can increase $\dot{V}O_2$ to 5 l/min or higher. However, exercise not only increases metabolic heat production, but also facilitates body heat loss by increasing skin and muscle blood flow. This enhances convective heat transfer from the body core to peripheral shell. Also, limb movement increases convective heat loss from body surfaces by disrupting the stationary layer of air, or water, that develops at the skin surface. Thus, while metabolic heat production increases progressively as exercise intensity increases, so too does heat loss due to rising muscle and skin blood flow. In cold air, metabolic heat production during exercise can be high enough to completely compensate for increased heat loss and allow core temperature to be maintained even when ambient temperature is extremely cold.[74] In contrast, increased heat loss during exercise in cold

TABLE 1 Wind Chill Chart

Wind Speed (Mi/h)	Actual Temperature (°F)									
	50	40	30	20	10	0	-10	-20	-30	-40	-50	-60
					Equivalent Chill Temperature (°F)							
Calm	50	40	30	20	10	0	-10	-20	-30	-40	-50	-60
5	48	37	27	16	6	-5	-15	-26	-36	-47	-57	-68
10	40	28	16	3	-9	-21	-33	-46	-58	-70	-83	-95
15	36	22	9	-5	-18	-32	-45	-58	-72	-85	-99	-112
20	32	18	4	-10	-25	-39	-53	-67	-82	-96	-110	-124
25	30	15	0	-15	-29	-44	-59	-74	-89	-104	-118	-133
30	28	13	-2	-18	-33	-48	-63	-79	-94	-109	-125	-140
35	27	11	-4	-20	-35	-51	-67	-82	-98	-113	-129	-145
40[a]	26	10	-6	-22	-37	-53	-69	-85	-101	-117	-132	-148
	Little Danger (In less than 5 h with dry skin. Greatest hazard from false sense of security.)				Increasing Danger (Exposed flesh may freeze within 1 min.)				Great Danger (Exposed flesh may freeze within 30 s.)			

[a] Wind speeds greater than 40 mi/h have little additional effect.

water can be so great that metabolic heat production, even during intense exercise, is insufficient to defend body core temperature.[74]

During submaximal exercise in the cold, $\dot{V}O_2$ can be higher than, or the same as, $\dot{V}O_2$ in temperate conditions, depending on the exercise intensity and clothing insulation.[82] At low intensities of exercise, when clothing is inadequate, $\dot{V}O_2$ is higher in cold than temperate conditions. In this case, metabolic heat production is insufficient to maintain core and skin temperatures high enough to prevent shivering. Thus, the increased $\dot{V}O_2$ represents the added oxygen requirement for shivering. As metabolic heat production rises with increasing exercise intensity, the stimulus for shivering declines, and at some point exercise metabolism is high enough to completely prevent shivering. At this intensity and higher, $\dot{V}O_2$ during exercise is the same in cold and temperate conditions. The exercise intensity at which metabolic heat production is sufficient to prevent shivering depends on the severity of cold stress. Further, that intensity will not necessarily be the same for all persons exposed to the same cold stress due to individual characteristics that may modify the magnitude of physiological responses. These individual modifying factors are discussed later.

Cold exposure can reduce maximal oxygen uptake ($\dot{V}O_2$ max), but not always.[82] Conditions must be severe enough to markedly reduce core or muscle temperature before $\dot{V}O_2$ max is reduced.[8,9,23,38,50] Exposure to conditions that lower core temperature less than 0.5°C do not significantly reduce $\dot{V}O_2$ max.[68] Lower body temperatures may impair myocardial contractility and limit maximal heart rate[8,9,23,38,50] sufficiently to limit maximal cardiac output, thus accounting for the reduced $\dot{V}O_2$ max.

D. INDIVIDUAL MODIFYING FACTORS
1. Body Morphology

Differences in body size, configuration, and composition explain much of the variability between individuals in their capability to defend body temperature during cold exposure. Inasmuch as the principal avenue of heat loss in humans exposed to cold is convective heat transfer at the skin surface, a large surface area favors greater heat loss than a smaller surface area. On the other hand, a large body mass favors maintenance of a constant temperature by virtue of a greater total heat content compared to a small body mass. Gonzalez[32] explains that the ratio of surface area to body mass governs heat loss. All other factors being equal (which is rarely the case), persons with a large surface area-to-mass ratio experience greater declines in body temperature during cold exposure than those with smaller surface area to mass ratios.[14,74]

Body fat is another anthropomorphic characteristic modifying the stress an individual experiences with cold exposure. Thermal resistivity of fat is greater than that of either skin or muscle.[74] Thus, thermal conductance decreases and insulation increases as subcutaneous fat thickens. Therefore, different persons exposed to the same cold conditions do not experience the same cold stress, or exhibit physiological responses of the same magnitude.

2. Physical Fitness

There is no consensus concerning the influence of physical fitness, particularly aerobic capacity, on thermoregulatory response to cold. Cross-sectional studies conclude that fit persons maintain warmer skin temperatures than less fit persons during rest in cold air.[10] However, the effect appeared due to thinner subcutaneous fat thickness and higher metabolic heat production in fit compared to less fit subjects, rather than to a fitness effect per se. Longitudinal studies indicate that endurance training strengthens cutaneous vasoconstrictor response to cold,[43,79] which therefore may provide a thermoregulatory advantage for persons exposed to cold.

3. Age

Aging is widely thought to compromise body temperature defense during cold exposure.[83] The incidence of hypothermia on admission to hospitals may be greater for persons age 60 or older.[44] However, overall incidence of hypothermia compared to other ailments resulting in hospital admission is low, and factors such as injury, illness, and alcohol or drug intoxication may confound these data.[16,42] Epidemiological surveys of body temperature of older persons while in their own homes do not indicate a large incidence of hypothermia.[17,24] Nevertheless, controlled laboratory comparisons show that older men may be less able than younger men to defend core temperature during cold exposures. The cutaneous vasoconstrictor response to cold may be slower, and cold-induced vasodilation is blunted in older men.[48] Shivering thermogenesis may also be less in older men.[83] The latter effect probably results from a loss of muscle mass, rather than an aging effect on thermoregulation per se.[48] These aging effects begin to be apparent after about 45 years of age in men.[83] Data from one study, however, indicated that older women defended core temperature during cold exposure as well as or better than younger women.[75] Here again, body composition changes with aging (the older women were much fatter than the younger women) probably accounted for the difference attributed to aging.

4. Gender

Gender-related differences in body size, shape, and composition, and hormonal effects associated with the menstrual cycle affect heat balance and thermoregulatory response to cold.[71] These differences contribute to a disparity in cold tolerance between men and women, which is particularly apparent in cold water. Generally, women have greater fat content and thicker subcutaneous fat thickness than men of comparable age. A thicker subcutaneous fat layer accounts for the greater maximal tissue insulation and lower critical water temperature (coldest water tolerated without shivering) observed in women as compared to men.[60] Despite this, greater fat content may not provide women with a thermoregulatory advantage over men.

When women and men of equivalent subcutaneous fat thickness are considered, the women usually have a greater surface area and smaller total body mass than men. Although insulation is equivalent, total heat loss is greater due to the larger surface area for convective heat flux. Body heat content is less in the women because of their smaller body mass. Therefore, body temperature falls more rapidly for any given thermal gradient and metabolic rate.[32,49,51] When men and women of equivalent subcutaneous fat thickness exercised in cold water at the same metabolic rate per unit surface area, both experienced similar core temperature changes.[49] Comparing men and women of equivalent total body mass still seems to put women at a disadvantage in the cold. At equal mass, women's greater fat content enhances insulation, and surface area differences between genders are less pronounced. Nevertheless, their smaller lean body mass — the source of metabolic heat production — limits capacity for heat production compared to men of comparable total body mass. Under cold conditions that stimulate shivering, especially maximal shivering, the limited thermogenic capacity will result in a more rapid core temperature decline in women than men of equivalent total body mass.

5. Nutrition Status

Both carbohydrate and fat are oxidized to meet the metabolic cost of shivering. The increase in plasma catecholamines that typically occurs with cold exposure facilitates mobilization of both glycogen and triglyceride stores.[75] Debate exists as to the importance of muscle glycogen as a substrate for shivering.[40,47,84] It is quite clear, however, persons who become hypoglycemic during cold exposure have a reduced tolerance to cold stress and are more susceptible to cold injury.[27,33,37] Hypoglycemia restricts or abolishes the shivering response to cold exposure and hence, significantly blunts metabolic heat production.[27,28,33,37] The effects of hypoglycemia on shivering may be mediated by the central nervous system.[27]

6. Acclimatization

Persons chronically exposed to cold exhibit adjustments in thermoregulation.[81] Habituation is, by far, the most common adjustment. Blunting of both shivering and cold-induced vasoconstriction are the hallmarks of habituation.[81] These adjustments enable skin to be kept warmer during cold exposure, but can exacerbate heat loss and the fall in core temperature. Besides habituation, cold acclimatization (natural environment) and cold acclimation (laboratory environment) can heighten responses to cold, or induce responses not apparent in the unacclimatized state. These adjustments follow two patterns. A more pronounced thermogenic response to cold characterizes metabolic acclimatization/acclimation.[81] Enhanced heat conservation mechanisms characterize the insulative acclimatization/acclimation pattern.[81] More rapid cutaneous vasoconstriction develops in some chronically cold-exposed persons. This adjustment may reflect enhanced sympathetic nervous system responses.[81] Although repeated cold exposure can cause measurable differences in human physiological responses to subsequent cold exposure, the importance of these adjustments in preserving thermal balance during cold exposure is limited. This is especially true in comparison to the marked improvements that occur with repeated exposures to hot environments.

7. Clothing

If too little clothing is worn, hypothermia and its consequences can occur. Wearing clothing with high insulation can effectively attenuate body heat loss during cold exposure even in extreme cold. For optimal effectiveness, the insulative value of the clothing should be balanced with metabolic heat production. As described earlier, heat production rises with increasing physical activity or exercise intensity. Excessive clothing insulation during exercise in the cold leads to increases in core temperature. This stimulates sweating. Sweating can wet clothing materials, thus degrading insulative properties and increasing risk for cold injury. It is generally recommended that persons wear several layers of clothing during cold exposure to enable clothing addition or removal as exercise intensity and weather conditions dictate.

III. CHALLENGES TO FLUID BALANCE DURING COLD EXPOSURE

Cold exposure can compromise fluid balance. Some effects result from increased fluid losses, others result from reduced fluid intake. Both physiological and physical mechanisms exert influences. This section describes some of the most significant factors challenging fluid balance during cold exposure.

A. FACTORS INCREASING FLUID LOSSES IN THE COLD
1. Cold-Induced Diuresis

Cold-induced diuresis (CID) is one area regarding fluid balance in cold that has received considerable attention. Debate exists with regard to: (1) the impact of CID; (2) the nature of the diuresis — that is, free water or osmotic; and (3) the physiological mechanism or mechanisms responsible for CID. Table 2 summarizes key studies regarding CID.

More than 200 years ago, Sutherland[72] first reported CID as an increased urine flow following cold-water bathing. Sutherland, however, made no mention or speculation about the possible influence of hydrostatic pressure effects vs. cold exposure per se. Not until 1909 did Gibson[31] demonstrate an increased urine flow as the direct result of cold exposure. In 1940, Bazett et al.[7] published

TABLE 2   Significant Studies Regarding Cold-Induced Diuresis

Authors/Year	Environment/Situation	Findings
Sutherland (1764)[a]	Cold-water bathing	↑Urine loses
Gibson (1909)[a]	Cold air (4–10°C)	↑Urine flow with ↓temperature
Bazett et al. (1940)[a]	2 weeks in cold climate	↑Urine flow, ↓B.V., ↓P.V.
Eliot et al. (1949)	Cold air (15°C)	↑Urine flow blocked by ADH
Bader et al. (1952)	Cold air (15°C)	Demonstrated confounding factors influence CID
Segar & Moore (1968)	Cold air (13°C)	↑Urine flow and ↓ADH
Lennquist et al. (1974)[a]	Cold air (15°C)	Examined mechanisms for CID concluded *not* ADH mechanism
Wallenberg et al. (1976)	Cold air (15°C)	Evidence CID *is* pressure natriuresis
Young et al. (1987), Muza et al. (1988)	Cold water (18°C) in cold-acclimated subjects	Evidence CID is *not* pressure diuresis
Various authors (1985–present)	Cold air and cold water	Conflicting findings regarding hormonally mediated or not, ADH, vs. ANF, vs. pressure

Note: ↑ = increase; ↓ = decrease; B.V. = blood volume; P.V. = plasma volume; ADH = antidiuretic hormone; CID = cold-induced diuresis; ANF = atrial natriuretic factor.

[a] = "field" studies or observations, others are laboratory experiments.

a field study that confirmed that cold exposure increased urine flow, and also reduced blood and plasma volume.

Confounding factors influence the magnitude of CID and whether or not a diuresis even occurs during cold exposure. Bader et al.[4] demonstrated that CID could be prevented by exercising moderately during cold exposure. It also appears CID can be influenced by: (1) intensity and duration of cold exposure; (2) hydration; (3) body posture; (4) exercise; (5) diet; (6) gender; (7) age; (8) body composition; and (9) time of day.[4,28,43,46]

Lennquist and associates[46] conducted a series of studies to determine the mechanisms responsible for CID; they concluded CID was not the result of a fall in antidiuretic hormone (ADH), as others had suggested.[4,21,69]

The hypothesis that CID was simply a pressure diuresis was favored by many. The logic for that explanation was that increased systemic arterial blood pressure would increase renal blood pressure and thereby reduce tubular reabsorption of both water and solute (i.e., electrolytes). In support, Wallenberg and Granberg[76] demonstrated that blood pressure increases during cold exposure correlated with sodium excretion (r ≈ 0.60). However, data from two other publications[55,80] suggests CID may not be a pressure diuresis. The two papers reported data from the same experiments in which subjects were immersed in cold water before and following a 5-week cold-water acclimation program. Mean arterial blood pressure markedly increased during the initial cold-water exposure before acclimation. However, following acclimation, blood pressure did not increase during cold exposure.[55] The CID response to cold-water immersion was not affected by cold acclimation; that is, the magnitude of diuresis was the same during the post-test as it was during the initial pretest despite the lower blood pressure response.[80] Together, these data provide evidence that CID and blood pressure responses can be disassociated. Hence, the validity of the pressure diuresis hypothesis is challenged.

With regard to CID, the following conclusions can be made: (1) the mechanisms remain undefined; (2) the central movement of fluid caused by peripheral vasoconstriction may be involved but other mechanisms should be explored; (3) if studies are to be meaningful, confounding factors must be controlled or specifically examined.

2. Respiratory Water Losses

Cold dry air is often credited as a contributor to fluid losses, particularly respiratory fluid loss, in cold environments. However, the actual magnitude of these losses is not usually measured or reported. Fluid loss via respiration depends on ventilatory volume and the water vapor content of the inspired air.[13] Respiratory water losses can be estimated from metabolic rate, inspired air temperature, and water vapor pressure. As mentioned earlier, despite high relative humidities (100% used for demonstration) cold air contains significantly less water than warmer air of even a lower relative humidity. The difference in water vapor pressure between the saturated air in the lung (water vapor 44 mm Hg) and ambient air determines the amount of respiratory water lost with each breath. Using predictive models,[13,53] respiratory fluid losses can be estimated.

Respiratory water loss rises with increasing metabolic rate. To determine the effect of cold air and metabolic rate on respiratory water loss, we predicted respiratory water losses during both rest and exercise at three ambient temperatures and water vapor pressures. A 24-h scenario was modeled in which a person rests for 8 h, performs moderate activity for 12 h, and performs strenuous work for 4 h. The models indicate that respiratory losses are 50% greater at −20 vs. 25°C (i.e., 1.02 vs. 0.68 l/24 h; see Table 3). Hence, respiratory water losses can contribute to dehydration in the cold. However, metabolic rate (i.e., sweating) appears to have a far greater impact than ambient temperature on respiratory fluid losses and hence, fluid requirements.

TABLE 3 Effects of Ambient Temperature on Respiratory Water Loss

Temperature (°C)	rh (%)	Water Vapor (mmHg)	Metabolic Rate (W)	Respiratory Water (ml/h)
25	65	15	Rest (100)	~10
0	100	5	Rest (100)	~13
−20	100	1	Rest (100)	~15
25	65	15	Light–moderate (300)	~30
0	100	5	Light–moderate (300)	~40
−20	100	1	Light–moderate (300)	~45
25	65	15	Moderate–heavy (600)	~60
0	100	5	Moderate–heavy (600)	~80
−20	100	1	Moderate–heavy (600)	~90

If 8 h Rest, 12 h Light–Moderate Activity, and 4 h Moderate–Heavy Activity

		Total Respiratory Loss
25	65	~680 ml/24h
0	100	~905 ml/24h
−20	100	~1020 ml/24h

Note: Effect of cold air itself could account for increased respiratory water losses as great as 340 ml/24h (i.e., 50% increase); rh = relative humidity; W = watts.

3. Cold-Weather Clothing

Heavy and cumbersome winter clothing also influences water losses in the cold. Significant metabolic heat can be generated and stored, stimulating sweating even in cold climates. Figure 1 demonstrates the relationship of total insulation and metabolic rate on thermal comfort of individuals exposed to different ambient temperatures.[32] A resting person requires considerably more total insulation to keep warm than persons performing moderate to heavy work/exercise. Note in Table 4 that a person dressed in the U.S. Army Extended Cold Weather Clothing System (insulation ~ 4.0 Clo) sweats little while resting in the cold. However, during strenuous exercise in that uniform an estimated 2.0 l/h of sweat would be lost. This clothing system allows little evaporation and would become sweat-soaked during heavy exercise. A wet uniform has serious implications for heat loss and subsequent cold injury susceptibility when the exercise/work is stopped. If the clothing system is altered to reduce total insulation to a Clo of 1.9, estimated sweating decreases by fivefold — that is, to about only 0.4 l/h (Table 4). Therefore, persons in cold climates should dress in layers that can be removed or replaced, allowing insulation to be matched to metabolic rate when work rates decrease and increase.

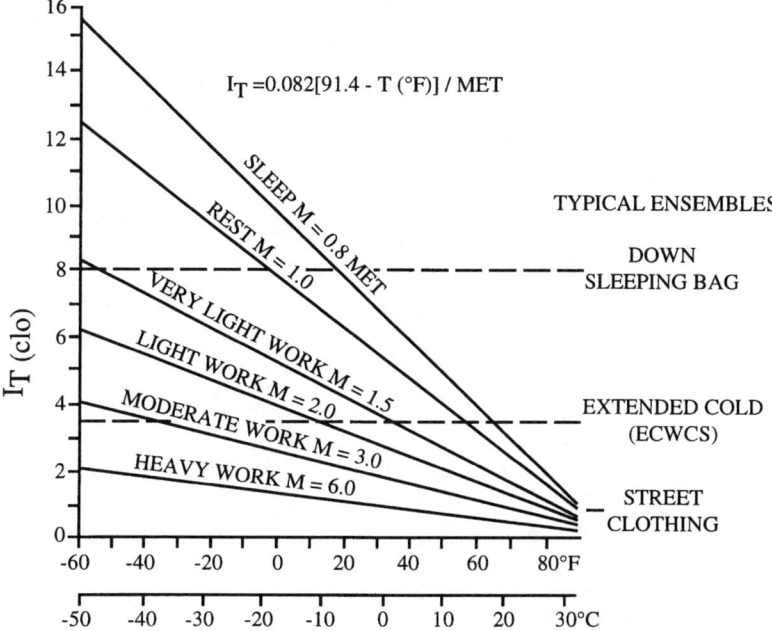

FIGURE 1 Total insulation (I_T, Clo) of clothing plus air necessary for comfort at various metabolic rates (1 met = 100 watts). ECWCS = U.S. Army Extended Cold Weather Clothing System. (From Gonzalez, R. R., in Pandolf et al., Eds., *Human Performance Physiology and Environmental Medicine at Terrestrial Extremes*, 1988, 45–95. With permission.)

4. Metabolic Cost of Movement in Cold Terrain

Figure 2 illustrates the effects of terrain type and cover associated with cold climates (e.g., snow) on the energy cost of movement.[57] The energy cost of walking 2.5 mi/h on a blacktop surface is ~ 150 W. However, deep snow increases metabolic rate for movement at the same speed by three- to fourfold. As discussed above, high metabolic rates can stimulate sweating and hence increase fluid replacement requirements. The hobbling effects of cumbersome cold-weather clothing increase the metabolic rate during physical activity by an additional 10–20%.[3,73] The magnitude of the hobbling effect on metabolic rate depends on the number of clothing layers as well as the exercise or work intensity.

B. FACTORS LIMITING FLUID INTAKE IN THE COLD

Cold-weather-related factors can constrain fluid intake in the cold. These effects become more significant with increasing duration of cold exposure. That is, constraints to drinking may be a simple inconvenience to a winter jogger, or a serious threat to health and performance to a winter hunter or hiker.

TABLE 4 Effects of Work and Clothing on Sweat Loss

Temperature (°C)	Clo	Metabolic Rate (W)	Sweat Loss (ml/h)
0	4.0[a]	Rest (100)	100
−20	4.0	Rest (100)	100
0	4.0	Light–moderate (300)	1100
−20	4.0	Light–moderate (300)	800
0	4.0	Moderate–heavy (600)	1900
−20	4.0	Moderate–heavy (600)	1900
0	1.9[b]	Moderate–heavy (600)	900
−20	1.9	Moderate–heavy (600)	400

Note: 1 Clo unit represents the insulation of a business suit; W = watts.

[a] = approximate Clo for U.S. Army Extended Cold Weather Clothing System (ECWCS)
[b] = approximate Clo for ECWCS parka with field coat liner over Woodland Battle Dress Uniform

1. Fluid Availability

Fluid availability can constrain fluid intake in the cold. Individual and bulk water supplies often freeze during cold weather, and to thaw frozen containers can take several hours. Care must be given to ensure that sufficient water supplies are protected from freezing. During outdoor competitions, fluid supplies at water points should be kept warm in vehicles or tents. Individuals carrying their own water supplies during winter should wear personal water bottles or canteens close to the body, inside clothing (or sleeping bags, at night). Although snow or ice might be available, hunters, hikers, and campers should not plan to rely on such sources for drinking water. Orth[56] has observed: "In experiments conducted last winter, it was found that at −50°F and an altitude of approximately 600 feet, using a Coleman stove it took 200 ml of fuel (gasoline) and 30–45 minutes to melt enough snow to give 600 ml of water. It was determined it would take more than six hours per day and a half a gallon of gasoline to get sufficient water for one man." Clearly, the time and fuel required to use snow and ice as a major drinking water source are prohibitive for most outdoor recreationists. In addition, snow is often contaminated. Therefore, drinking water must be carried or supplied at regular intervals.

Another factor constraining fluid intake during cold weather concerns the fluid content of foods. This is more of a problem for people whose activity entails prolonged periods of outdoor exposure than for people who live indoors and spend relatively short periods outside for activity and

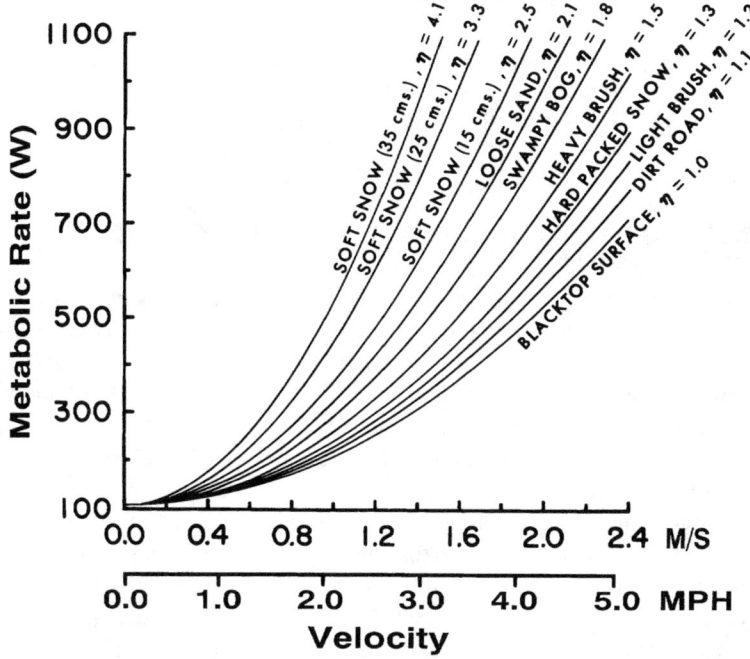

FIGURE 2 Predicted energy expenditure for walking at various speeds considering the type of terrain. (Modified from Pandolf et al., *J. Appl. Physiol.: Respir. Environ. Exer. Physiol.*, 43:577–581, 1977. With permission.)

exercise. The light-weight packaged food used by most hikers and campers, especially types formulated for winter use, contain little fluid. Many packaged foods are dehydrated and require considerable fluid to rehydrate the various components. High-water-content food items such as fruits and vegetables are often avoided during cold weather because they may freeze.

2. Voluntary Dehydration

A blunted thirst sensation can also contribute to reduced fluid intake.[1] This condition, termed "voluntary dehydration,"[36] occurs in hot climates, but may be even more pronounced in the cold.[64,77] Rogers et al.[64] reported that during survival experiments in the subarctic, despite marked dehydration thirst was not displayed or reported until individuals came inside and warmed. Afferent stimulation from cold skin and/or a reduced body core temperature may modify thirst sensation. In addition, persons in cold climates sometimes consciously choose to restrict fluid intake, despite thirst sensations. For example, women may avoid drinking if sheltered bathrooms are unavailable, in order to minimize the need to disrobe to urinate outdoors in the cold. Both men and women often limit drinking late in the day to avoid having to leave a warm tent or sleeping bag during the night to urinate.

IV. DEHYDRATION EFFECTS IN THE COLD

Dehydration adversely affects physical performance in hot climates and these same dehydration effects would probably also be observed in cold weather. However, few studies have investigated dehydration effects in the cold.

A. DEHYDRATION AND PHYSICAL AND COGNITIVE PERFORMANCE

Numerous studies report physical performance decrements during cold exposure. The decrements include reductions in manual dexterity and coordination,[52,78] muscular strength,[18,39,41] maximal power output, jumping and sprint performance,[9] submaximal and maximal exercise performance,[2,22,58] and maximal aerobic work capacity.[8,19] However, other studies report no reduction in submaximal performance[62] or maximal aerobic power.[58,63,65] Upon close examination, the discrepancy between studies can be explained by considering the effects of cold on body core and/or muscle temperature. In the studies finding no effect of cold exposure on performance,[58,62,63,65] exposures were too short or protective clothing too effective for body temperature to fall. When muscle temperature falls, maximal muscle tension during voluntary sustained contractions decreases significantly, as does peak power output.[15,20] Therefore, cold exposure only reduces performance when muscle temperatures are markedly lowered.

The preceding studies do not address dehydration effects on physical performance in the cold. Lennquist et al.[46] concluded that CID and the resulting negative water balance reduced physical work capacity. However, Lennquist et al. failed to include a cold-exposed, euhydrated group for comparison, so it is difficult to determine the direct effects of hypohydration per se. It could be argued that their performance decrements might have resulted from muscle cooling.

Roberts et al.[62] examined dehydration effects on physical performance in the cold. In this study, one group of subjects were maintained euhydrated, while a second subject group dehydrated by 3.5% of body weight (exercise and fluid restriction). Subjects then performed two 30-min cycle exercise tests at 75% of maximal oxygen consumption. One exercise test was performed in a temperate environment (24°C) and one during cold air (0°C) exposure. There was no significant effect of cold or hypohydration on submaximal exercise performance. However, exercise duration and/or intensity were too short or too low to really evaluate effects of hydration and temperature.

Many studies report that cold exposure reduces cognitive performance. However, only one controlled study examined dehydration effects on cognitive performance in the cold. Banderet et al.[5] studied two groups of 18 subjects. One maintained euhydration while the other dehydrated by 2.5% body weight (exercise and fluid restriction). Hypohydration degraded cognitive performance as assessed by performance measures of coding, number comparison, computer interaction, pattern comparison, and grammatical reasoning. However, effects were no different from what would be expected in warm conditions.

B. DEHYDRATION AND COLD INJURY SUSCEPTIBILITY

Dehydration by as little as 1% body weight degrades exercise thermoregulation.[35] It is well known that dehydrated persons are more susceptible to heat exhaustion.[67] Furthermore, Adolf and associates[1] indicated that body fluid losses in excess of 10% body weight are life threatening. Much less is known about the effect of dehydration on susceptibility to cold injuries.

A variety of mechanisms account for the effects of dehydration on thermoregulation in the heat.[67] A delayed onset of sweating, as well as reduced sweating rate during hypohydration, constrains evaporative heat loss.[67] This results in additional heat storage and a greater rise in body core temperature, which has important implications for physical performance and for thermal injury/illness as well. Dehydration also appears to affect a person's perception of effort. Montain and Coyle[54] demonstrated significantly higher ratings of perceived exertion during exercise in the heat when little or no water was ingested compared to trials in which large or moderate amounts of fluid were ingested.

The overall effect of dehydration on thermoregulation in the cold depends on a combination of factors that determine whether an overall gain or loss in body heat storage will occur. For example, in moderately cold climates when individuals are wearing heavy clothing and performing heavy work or exercise, dehydration could exacerbate the core temperature rise and increase heat strain. On the other hand, in severe cold, or when work rates are low and body heat losses exceed heat production, dehydration may accentuate peripheral cooling (see below).

Dehydration is often suggested to increase susceptibility to peripheral cold injuries.[29] Numerous case reports indicate that patients suffering from peripheral cold injury are often dehydrated. However, little direct evidence demonstrates that dehydration itself significantly increases the risk for peripheral cold injury.

Roberts and Berberich[61] assessed hydration effects on peripheral and central body cooling during cold exposure. Two groups of subjects, one maintained euhydrated and the other dehydrated by 4.6% of body weight (exercise and fluid restriction), were exposed to cold air on 2 days prior to dehydration and 2 days following dehydration. Subjects wore standard military cold weather clothing and after 15 min cold exposure they removed their gloves and glove liners. Rectal temperature responses were similar. While finger temperature responses were similar across trials, the skin temperature of the back of the hand in the dehydration group was significantly colder following dehydration. The control group showed no differences in response across trials. These data indicate that dehydration may increase the susceptibility to cold injury. However, the large variability between groups and trials suggests that caution be exercised when interpreting these data.

Another study of dehydration effects on thermoregulation during cold exposure was conducted by Roberts and colleagues.[62] Two groups of subjects, both provided a complete complement of arctic clothing, lived in an environmentally controlled chamber for 5 d (temperature range −25 to 0°C). During this period, one group was provided 3 l of fluid/d while the other group received only 1.5 l/d. During an initial pretest in the cold before dehydration and twice during the 5-d experiments, cooling responses were studied during 90-min cold air exposures (0°C), during which one glove was removed. Temperatures over time cooling curves for each digit were obtained and the area under the curve was calculated. Results indicated that the group receiving only 1.5 l of water per day were dehydrated by approximately 2.5% of total body weight while the other group's body weight remained essentially unchanged. There were no changes in finger-cooling responses in the group receiving adequate fluid while the group on restricted fluid showed "decreases in the average temperature over time." However, closer examination of the data indicates that the difference between groups was accounted for by an apparent increase in mean finger temperature per unit time of the euhydrated group rather than a greater fall in temperature in the dehydrated group. Although the authors suggest the data supports the hypothesis that dehydration increases susceptibility to peripheral cold injury, additional work is clearly merited.

V. COUNTERMEASURES: MAINTAINING EUHYDRATION IN THE COLD

To prevent dehydration, ensure adequate fluid ingestion. However, due to various factors that cause dehydration in cold environments, this is not easily accomplished. Recent efforts have been made to investigate potential countermeasures to prevent or blunt cold-induced dehydration and hence the related decrements to performance and health. Glycerol, a nontoxic, naturally occurring metabolic by-product and food additive, improved fluid retention over standard electrolyte beverages or water alone. Our laboratory[25] demonstrated that 3 h after drinking approximately 1.75 l of water in an attempt to achieve hyperhydration, only 33% of the fluid was retained. The rest was eliminated by the kidney. When the same volume of water was consumed with approximately 70 g of glycerol added, nearly a doubling in fluid retention occurred — that is, 59%.[25] The experiments were done in temperate conditions so they were repeated during cold air exposure. Again, greater fluid retention was found following the ingestion of glycerol and water vs. water alone.[26] Differences in fluid retention with glycerol resulted from a blunted increase in urine flow. Importantly, the differences in urine flow were entirely accounted for by differences in free water and not osmotic clearance.[25,26] Although further study is required, these studies provide evidence that differences in the antidiuretic hormone response may be responsible for the improved fluid retention with glycerol containing solutions. In addition to improving fluid retention and adding calories, glycerol also reduces a fluid's freezing point (e.g., a 30% glycerol solution reduces the freezing point 9°C below water). Hence, adding glycerol might also be effective in preventing drinking water from freezing.

VI. SUMMARY

Body fluid losses in cold climates can be similar to those in hot environments. Fluid loss results from sweating and increased respiratory water losses as well as CID. Additional studies are needed to further document the magnitude of cold-induced dehydration as well as the specific distribution of these losses throughout various body water compartments. Fluid intake in cold environments can be reduced as a result of logistical constraints in fluid delivery, problems with water freezing, reduced thirst sensation, and voluntary fluid restriction. Dehydration negatively influences physical and cognitive performance as well as thermoregulation and possible susceptibility to peripheral cold injury. More research is needed to determine the direct effects of cold-induced dehydration on thermoregulatory responses to cold and susceptibility to peripheral cold injury. Recent experimental findings suggest that ingestion of glycerol in drinking water might be an effective countermeasure to reduce or delay cold-induced dehydration and the associated decrements to performance. Additional countermeasures and aids for maintaining hydration during cold exposure should be explored.

REFERENCES

1. Adolph, E. F. et al., *Physiology of Man in the Desert*. Interscience, New York, 1947.
2. Adolph, E. F. and Molnar, G. W., Exchanges of heat and tolerances to cold in men exposed to outdoor weather, *Am. J. Physiol.*, 146:507–537, 1946.
3. Amor, A. F., Vogel, J. A., and Worsley, D. E., The Energy Cost of Wearing Multilayer Clothing, APRE Report, (TM) 18/73, Farnborough, U.K., 1973.
4. Bader, R. A., Eliot, J. W., and Bass, D. E., Hormonal and renal mechanisms of cold diuresis, *J. Appl. Physiol.*, 4:649–658, 1952.
5. Banderet, L. E., MacDougall, D. M., Roberts, D. E., Tappan, D., Jacey, M., and Gray, P., Effects of Hypohydration or Cold Exposure and Restricted Fluid Intake Upon Cognitive Performance, Technical Note T15/86, U.S. Army Research Institute of Environmental Medicine, Natick, MA, 1986.
6. Bates, R. E. and Bilello, M. A., Defining the Cold Regions of the Northern Hemisphere, Technical Report 178, Cold Regions Research & Engineering Laboratory, Hanover, NH, 1966.
7. Bazett, H. C., Sunderman, F. W., Dupe, J., and Scott, J. C., Climatic effects on the volume and composition of blood in man, *Am. J. Physiol.*, 129:69–83, 1940.
8. Bergh, U. and Ekblom, B., Physical performance and peak aerobic power at different body temperatures, *J. Appl. Physiol.*, 46:885–889, 1979.
9. Bergh, U. and Ekblom, B., Influence of muscle temperature on maximal muscle strength and power output in human skeletal muscles, *Acta Physiol. Scand.*, 107:33–37, 1979.

10. Bittel, J. H. M., Nonott-Varly, C., Livecchi-Gonnot, G. H., Savourey, G. L. M. J., and Hanniquet, A. M., Physical fitness and thermoregulatory reactions in a cold environment in men, *J. Appl. Physiol.*, 65:1984–1989, 1988.
11. Bly, C. G., Johnson, R. E., Kark, R. M., Consolazio, C. F. Swain, H. L., Laudani, A., Maloney, M. M., Figueroa, W. G., and Imperiale, L. E., Survival in the cold, *U.S. Armed Forces Med. J.*, 1:615–628, 1950.
12. Boswick, J. A., Thompson, J. D., and Jonas, R. A., The epidemiology of cold injuries, *Surg. Gynecol. Obstet.*, 149:326–332, 1979.
13. Brebbia, D. R., Goldman, R. F., and Buskirk, E. R., Water vapor loss from the respiratory tract during outdoor exercise in the cold, *J. Appl. Physiol.*, 11: 219–222, 1957.
14. Burton, A. C. and Edholm, O. G., Vascular reactions to cold, in *Man in a Cold Environment*, Bayliss, L. E., Feldberg, W., and Hodgkin, A. L., Eds., Edward Arnold, London, 1955, 129–147.
15. Clarke, R. S. J., Hellon, R. F., and Lind, A. R., The duration of sustained contractions of the human forearm at different muscle temperatures, *J. Physiol. London*, 143:454–473, 1958.
16. Coleshaw, S. R. K., Easton, J. C., Keatinge, W. R., Floyer, M. A., and Garrard, J., Hypothermia in emergency admissions in cold weather, *Clin. Sci.*, 70:93, 1986.
17. Collins, K. J., Dore, C., Exton-Smith, A. N., Fox, R. H., and Macdonald, I. C., Accidental hypothermia and impaired temperature homeostasis in the elderly, *Br. Med. J.*, 1:353–356, 1977.
18. Coppin, E. G., Livingstone, S. D., and Kuehn, L. A., Effects on handgrip strength due to arm immersion in a 10°C water bath, *Aviat. Space Environ. Med.*, 49:1322–1326, 1978.
19. Craig, F. N. and Cummings, E. C., Dehydration and muscular work, *J. Appl. Physiol.*, 21:670–674, 1966.
20. Davies, C. T. M. and Young, K., Effect of temperature on the contractile properties and muscle power of triceps surae in humans, *J. Appl. Physiol.*, 55:191–195, 1983.
21. Eliot, J. W., Bader, R. A., and Bass, D. E., Blood changes associated with cold diuresis, *Fed. Proc.*, 8:41, 1949.
22. Faulkner, J. A., White, T. P., and Markley, J. M., The 1979 Canadian ski marathon: A natural experiment in hyperthermia, in *Exercise in Health and Disease* — Balke Symposium, Nagle, F. J. and Montoye, H. J., Eds., Charles C Thomas, Springfield, IL, 1981, 184–195.
23. Fortney, S. M. and Senay L. C., Effect of training and heat acclimation on exercise responses of sedentary females, *J. Appl. Physiol.*, 47:978–984, 1979.
24. Fox, R. H., Woodward, P. M., Exton-Smith, A. N., Green, M. F., Donnison, D. V., and Wicks, M. H., Body temperatures in the elderly: A national study of physiological, social, and environmental conditions, *Br. Med. J.*, 1:200–206, 1973.
25. Freund, B. J., Montain, S. J., Young, A. J., Sawka, M. N., DeLuca, J. P., Pandolf, K. B., and Valeri, C. R., Glycerol hyperhydration: Hormonal, renal and vascular fluid responses, *J. Appl. Physiol.*, 79:2069–2077, 1995.
26. Freund, B. J., McKay, J. M., Roberts, D. E., Laird, J. E., O'Brien, C., Shoda, G. R., Young, A. J., and Sawka, M. N., Glycerol hyperhydration reduces the diuresis induced by water alone during cold air exposure, *Med. Sci. Sports Exer.*, 26:S5, 1994.
27. Freund, B. J., O'Brien, C., and Young, A. J., Alcohol ingestion and temperature regulation during cold exposure, *Wildern. Med.*, 5:88–98, 1994.
28. Gale, E. A. M., Bennett, T., Green, J. H., and MacDonald, I. A., Hypoglycemia, hypothermia and shivering in man, *Clin. Sci.*, 61:463–469, 1981.
29. Gamble, W. B., Perspectives in frostbite and cold weather injuries, in *Advances in Plastic Surgery*, Vol. 10: Mosby-Year Book, St. Louis, MO, 1994, 21–71.
30. Gaydos, H. F., Effect on complex manual performance of cooling the body while maintaining the hands at normal temperatures, *J. Appl. Physiol.*, 12:373–376, 1958.
31. Gibson, A. G., On the diuresis of chill, *Q. J. Med.*, 3:52–60, 1909.

32. Gonzalez, R.R., Biophysics of heat transfer and clothing considerations, in *Human Performance Physiology and Environmental Medicine at Terrestrial Extremes*, Pandolf, K. B., Sawka, M. N., and Gonzalez, R. R., Eds., Benchmark Press, Indianapolis, 1988, 45–95.
33. Graham, T. and Dalton, J., Effect of alcohol on man's response to mild physical activity in a cold environment, *Aviat. Space Environ. Med.*, 51:793–796, 1980.
34. Greenleaf, J. E., Problem: Thirst, drinking behavior, and involuntary dehydration, *Med. Sci. Sport Exer.*, 24:645–656, 1992.
35. Greenleaf, J. E. and Harrison, M. H., Water and electrolytes, in *Nutrition and Aerobic Exercise*, Layman, D. K., Ed., American Chemical Society, Washington, DC, 1986, 107–124.
36. Greenleaf, J. E. and Sargent, F., II, Voluntary dehydration in man, *J. Appl. Physiol.*, 20:719–724, 1965.
37. Haight, J. S. J. and Keatinge, W. R., Failure of thermoregulation in the cold during hypoglycemia induced by exercise and ethanol, *J. Physiol.*, 229:87–97, 1973.
38. Horvath, S. M., Exercise in a cold environment, in *Exercise Sport Science Review*, Miller, D. I., Ed., Franklin Institute, Philadelphia, 1981, 221–263.
39. Horvath, S. M. and Freedman, A., The influence of cold upon the efficiency of man, *J. Aviat. Med.*, 18:158–164, 1947.
40. Jacobs, I., Tiit, T., and Kerrigan-Brown, D., Muscle glycogen depletion during exercise at 9°C and 21°C, *Eur. J. Appl. Physiol.*, 54:35–39, 1985.
41. Johnson, D. J. and Leider, F. E., Influence of cold bath on maximum handgrip strength, *Percept. Mot. Skills* 44:323–326, 1977.
42. Keatinge, W., Medical problems of cold weather, *J. R. Coll. Physicians London* 20:283–287, 1986.
43. Kollias, R. B. and Buskirk, E. R., Effects of physical condition in man on thermal responses to cold air, *Int. J. Biometeorol.*, 16:389–402, 1972.
44. LeBlanc, J., Cote, J., Dulac, S., and Dulong-Turcot, F., Effects of age, sex and physical fitness on responses to local cooling, *J. Appl. Physiol.*, 44:813–817, 1978.
45. LeBlanc, J., Robinson, D., Sharman, D. F., and Tousignant, P., Catecholamines and short-term adaptation to cold in mice, *Am. J. Physiol.*, 213:1419–1422, 1967.
46. Lennquist, S., Granberg, P. O., and Wedin, B., Fluid balance and physical work capacity in humans exposed to cold, *Arch. Environ. Health* 29:241–249, 1974.
47. Martineau, L. and Jacobs, I., Muscle glycogen utilization during shivering thermogenesis in humans, *J. Appl. Physiol.*, 65:2046–2050, 1988.
48. Mathew, L., Purkayastha, S. S., Singh, R., and Gupta, J. S., Influence of aging in the thermoregulatory efficiency of man, *Int. J. Biometeorol.*, 30:137–145, 1986.
49. McArdle, W. D., Magel, J. R., Gergley, T. J., Spina, R. J., and Toner, M. M., Thermal adjustment to cold-water exposure in resting men and women, *J. Appl. Physiol.*, 56:1565–1571, 1984.
50. McArdle, W. D., Magel, J. R., Lesmes, G. R., and Pechar, G. S., Metabolic and cardiovascular adjustment to work in air and water at 18, 25 and 33°C, *J. Appl. Physiol.*, 40:85–90, 1976.
51. McArdle, W. D., Magel, J. R., Spina, R. J., Gergley, T. J., and Toner, M. M., Thermal adjustment to cold-water exposure in exercising men and women, *J. Appl. Physiol.*, 56:1572–1577, 1984.
52. Meese, G. B., Kok, R., Lewis, M. I., and Wyon, D. P., The Effects of Moderate Cold and Heat Stress on the Potential Work Performance of Industrial Workers: Part 2. National Building Research Institute Council for Scientific and Industrial Research, Pretoria, South Africa, 1981.
53. Mitchell, J. W., Nadel, E. R., and Stolwijk, J. A. J., Respiratory weight losses during exercise, *J. Appl. Physiol.*, 22:474–476, 1972.

54. Montain, S. J. and Coyle, E. F., Influence of graded dehydration on hyperthermia and cardiovascular drift during exercise, *J. Appl. Physiol.*, 73:1340–1350, 1992.
55. Muza, S. R., Young, A. J., Sawka, M. N., Bogart, J. E., and Pandolf, K. B., Respiratory and cardiovascular responses to cold stress following repeated cold water immersion, *Undersea Biomed. Res.*, 15:165–178, 1988.
56. Orth, G. L., Food requirements in the arctic regions, *Mil. Surg.* March: 204–206, 1949.
57. Pandolf, K. B, Givoni, B., and Goldman, R. F., Predicting energy expenditure with loads while standing or walking very slowly, *J. Appl. Physiol.: Respir. Environ. Exer. Physiol.*, 43:577–581, 1977.
58. Patton, J. F. and Vogel, J. A., Effects of acute cold exposure on submaximal endurance performance, *Med. Sci. Sports Exer.*, 16:494–497, 1984.
59. Purdue, G. F. and Hunt, J. L., Cold injury: A collective review, *J. Burn Cancer Res.*, 7:331–341, 1986.
60. Rennie, D. W., Covino, B. G., Blair, M. R., and Rodahl, K., Physical regulation of temperature in Eskimos, *J. Appl. Physiol.*, 17:326–332, 1962.
61. Roberts, D. E. and Berberich, J. J., The role of hydration on peripheral response to cold, *Mil. Med.*, 12:605–608, 1988.
62. Roberts, D. E., Patton, J. R., Pennycook, J. W., Jacey, M. J., Tappan, D. V., Gray, P., and Heyder, E., Effects of Restricted Water Intake on Performance in a Cold Environment, Technical Note T2/84, U.S. Army Research Institute of Environmental Medicine, Natick, MA, 1984.
63. Rodahl, K., Horvath, S. M., Birkhead, N. C., and Issekutz, B., Jr., Effects of dietary protein on physical work capacity during severe cold stress, *J. Appl. Physiol.*, 17:763–767, 1962.
64. Rogers, T. A., Setliff, J. A., and Klopping, J. C., Energy cost, fluid and electrolyte balance in subarctic survival situations, *J. Appl. Physiol.*, 19:1–8, 1964.
65. Saltin, B., Cold work and altitude: Central circulatory aspects, Proceedings on the Symposia on Arctic Biology and Medicine IV. *The Physiology of Work in Cold and Altitude*, Arctic Aeromedical Laboratory, Fort Wainwright, AK, 1966, 313–360.
66. Santee, W. R. and Gonzalez, R. R., Characteristics of the thermal environment, in *Human Performance Physiology and Environmental Medicine at Terrestrial Extremes*, Pandolf, K. B., Sawka, M. N., and Gonzalez, R. R., Eds., Benchmark Press, Indianapolis, 1988, 1–43.
67. Sawka, M. N., Physiological consequences of hypohydration: Exercise performance and thermoregulation, *Med. Sci. Sport Exer.*, 24:657–670, 1992.
68. Schmidt, V. and Bruck, K., Effect of a precooling maneuver on body temperature and exercise performance, *J. Appl. Physiol.*, 50:772–778, 1981.
69. Segar, W. E. and Moore, W. W., The regulation of antidiuretic hormone release in man, *J. Clin. Invest.*, 47:2143–2150, 1968.
70. Siple, P. A. and Passel, C. R., Measurements of dry atmospheric cooling in subfreezing temperatures, *Proc. Am. Philos. Soc.*, 89:177–199, 1945.
71. Stephenson, L. A. and Kolka, M. A., Thermoregulation in women, in *Exercise Sports Science Review*, Holloszy, J. O., Ed., Williams & Wilkens, Baltimore, 1993, 231–262.
72. Sutherland, A., Of the Dropsy, in *An Attempt to Ascertain and Extend the Virtues of Bath and Bristol Waters*, 2nd ed., Frederick & Leake, 1764, 213–218.
73. Teitlebaum, A. and Goldman, R. F., Increased energy cost with multiple clothing layers, *J. Appl. Physiol.*, 32:743–744, 1972.
74. Toner, M. M. and McArdle, W. D., Physiological adjustments of man to the cold, in *Human Performance Physiology and Environmental Medicine at Terrestrial Extremes*, Pandolf, K. B., Sawka, M. N., and Gonzalez, R. R., Eds., Benchmark Press, Indianapolis, 1988, 361–399.
75. Wagner, J. A. and Horvath, S. M., Influences of age and gender on human thermoregulatory responses to cold exposures, *J. Appl. Physiol.*, 58:180–186, 1985.
76. Wallenberg, L. R. and Granberg, P. O., The relationship between cold-induced natriuresis and arterial blood pressure in man, *Scand. J. Clin. Lab. Invest.*, 34:225–231, 1974.

77. Wyant, K. W. and Caron, P. L., Water discipline and an arctic ration prototype, *Mil. Med.*, 148:435–439, 1983.
78. Wyon, D. P., Kok, R., Lewis, M. I., and Meese, G. B., Effects of moderate cold and heat stress on factory workers in Southern Africa., *S. Afr. J. Sci.*, 78:184–189, 1982.
79. Young, A. J., Sawka, M. N., Latzka, W. A., Gonzalez, R. R., and Pandolf, K. B., Effect of aerobic fitness on thermoregulation, *Med. Sci. Sports Exer.*, 25:S62, 1993.
80. Young, A. J., Muza, S. R., Sawka, M. N., and Pandolf, K. B., Human vascular fluid responses to cold stress are not altered by cold acclimatization, *Undersea Biomed. Res.*, 14:215–228, 1987.
81. Young, A. J., Human adaptation to cold, in *Human Performance Physiology and Environmental Medicine at Terrestrial Extremes*, Pandolf, K. B., Sawka, M. N., and Gonzalez, R. R., Eds., Benchmark Press, Indianapolis, 1988, 401–434.
82. Young, A. J., Energy substrate utilization during exercise in extreme environments, in *Exercise Sport Science Review*, Pandolf, K. B. and Holloszy, J. O., Eds., Williams & Wilkens, Baltimore, 1990, 65–117.
83. Young, A. J., Effects of aging on human cold tolerance, *Exp. Aging Res.*, 17:205–213, 1991.
84. Young, A. J., Sawka, M. N., Neufer, P. D., Muza, S. R., Askew, E. W., and Pandolf, K. B., Thermoregulation during cold water immersion is unimpaired by low muscle glycogen levels, *J. Appl Physiol.*, 66:1809, 1989.

Chapter 9

ENVIRONMENTAL INFLUENCES ON BODY FLUID BALANCE DURING EXERCISE: ALTITUDE

Reed W. Hoyt
Arnold Honig

CONTENTS

I. Hypohydration at Altitude 184

II. Energy and Water Balance in the Field 185
    A. Respiratory Evaporative Water Loss......................186
    B. Metabolic Water Production 187
    C. Cutaneous Evaporative Water Loss 187

III. Negative Water and Sodium Balance at Altitude................189
    A. Anorexia and Hypodipsia 189
    B. Diuretic and Natriuretic Effects of Altitude.................190
    C. Peripheral Arterial Chemoreceptors and Renal
       Excretory Function 190
    D. Special Conditions Influencing Body Fluid Homeostasis 191

IV. Summary...192

Acknowledgment 192

References 192

The opinions or assertions contained herein are the private views of the author and are not to be construed as official or reflecting the views of the Department of the Army or the Department of Defense.

Recreation at high altitude is becoming increasingly popular. North American Rocky Mountain recreational areas between 2000 and 3500 m elevation receive millions of visitors each year, while many thousands of mountaineers, hikers, and soldiers are exposed to altitudes over 4000 m.[24] Thermal stress, heavy physical activity, long workdays, and restricted food and water availability are common at altitude. However, adapting to decreased oxygen availability is often the foremost physiologic challenge faced by humans at high altitudes.

Although the amount of oxygen in the atmosphere remains constant at about 21%, barometric pressure (P_B) and the partial pressure of oxygen (PO_2) decrease curvilinearly with increasing elevation.[74] The PO_2 decreases with increasing elevation because the partial pressure of any gas is equal to the total P_B multiplied by the fractional concentration of that dry gas (Dalton's law). For example, the ambient partial pressure of oxygen decreases by half from sea level (P_B = 760 mm Hg; PO_2 = 160 mm Hg) to 5500 m or 18,000 ft elevation (P_B = 380 mm Hg; PO_2 = 80 mm Hg).

I. HYPOHYDRATION AT ALTITUDE

Hypohydration is a hallmark of successful adaptation to hypobaric hypoxia.[10,40,64] A loss of total body water (TBW) is evident in young resting mammals after exposure to moderate hypoxia (3000 to 5000 m) for 3 to 4 d.[10,40,42,45,56] This hypoxia-induced loss in TBW includes decreases in plasma volume, extracellular volume,[6,7,9,22,46,47] and calculated intracellular volume.[38,42,43,56,62,68] The decrease in plasma volume leads to increases in blood hemoglobin concentration and arterial oxygen content, and probably improves oxygen delivery to peripheral tissues.[40]

The increased urinary excretion of water and sodium underlying the loss of TBW at altitude is a physiologic response to hypoxemia — namely, decreased arterial PO_2.[40] Diuresis and natriuresis occur regardless of the means by which hypoxemia is produced, whether by ascent into the mountains, in a low pressure chamber, by breathing gases with a low oxygen content, etc. Hypobaria without hypoxia results in neither diuresis nor natriuresis.[17,18] In this chapter, hypoxia refers to hypoxic hypoxia that results in hypoxemia.

Various lines of research show that mammalian adaptation to moderate hypoxia is associated with the loss of TBW. Analysis of the carcasses of full-grown mice exposed to chronic hypoxia (4300 and 6300 m) revealed significantly decreased TBW.[27] In addition, indicator dilution studies of humans showed that exposure to 3500 to 4300 m elevation for 6 to 14 d resulted in reduced TBW and decreased calculated intracellular fluid volume[42,43,56,68] (Table 1). In these studies, TBW volume changes were estimated from equilibrium tracer concentrations after administration of D_2O[56] or ^3H_2O.[42,43,68]

Contradictory reports suggest that humans exposed for 8 to 14 d to 4300 m to 5334 m elevation exhibit little change in TBW (–2 to +3%) and an apparent increase in calculated intracellular volume.[21,28,29,70] In these studies, TBW

TABLE 1 Effect of Hypoxia on Human TBW, ECF, and ICF Volumes Estimated by Various Techniques

Subject No.	Altitude (m)	Duration (d)	Method	TBW	ICF	ECF	Ref.
12	4300	6	a,b	↓	↓	NC	56
9	3500	12	c,d	↓	↓	↓	42
19	3500	12	c,d	↓	↓	NC	43
10	3500	12	c,d	↓	↓	↓	68
4	4300	8	e	NC	NM	NM	70
9	4300	14	b,e,f	↑	↑	↓	28
9	4300	14	b,f	NC	↑	↓	29
8	5334	10	b,f	↓[a]	↑	↓	21

Note: Key for methods: a = equilibrium D_2O; b = thiocyanate; c = equilibrium ^3H_2O; d = radiosulfate, $Na^{35}SO_4$; e = bolus D_2O injection; f = bolus 4-aminoantipyrine injection. TBW = total body water; ICF = intracellular fluid; ECF = extracellular fluid; NC = no change; NM = no measurement.

[a] Relatively small 0.8 l, 2% decrease.

Modified from Hoyt, R. W., et al., *J. Appl. Physiol.* 71,509, 1991. With permission.

volume was estimated from the time course of tracer elimination after bolus injections of 4-aminoantipyrine[21,28,29] or D_2O.[28,70] However, the findings of these older studies are questionable. The 4-aminoantipyrine method apparently overestimates TBW at high altitude (Dr. J. P. Hannon, personal communication), and accurate determination of TBW by the bolus D_2O method is difficult.[28,70]

Water balance studies of humans at moderate altitude also provide evidence that hypohydration occurs in response to hypoxia.[10,13,45] In these studies, the difference between preformed dietary water intake and urine output was reduced at altitude, suggesting a decrease in TBW. This estimated loss of TBW does not account for any fluid lost due to increased respiratory evaporative water loss at altitude.[10]

II. ENERGY AND WATER BALANCE IN THE FIELD

In the following sections, the relationship of evaporative water loss to metabolic water gain is illustrated using data from two energy balance studies of soldiers at moderate altitudes.[38,39] In the first study,[38] 23 Marines were studied during a physically demanding, winter military training course at the Marine Corps Mountain Warfare Training Center, Bridgeport, California, at 2200 to 2550 m elevation. In the second study,[39] 6 soldiers were studied over 6 d of strenuous winter military training on Mt. Rainier, Washington, at elevations from 2550 to 3100 m.

The doubly labeled water (DLW) method of estimating total daily energy expenditure (TDEE), the methods of estimating food intake and body energy store use, and the calculations of metabolic water production are described elsewhere.[38,39] Briefly, the DLW method is based on the assumption that after an initial oral dose of stable $^2H_2O + H_2^{18}O$, deuterium (^2H) is eliminated from the body as water, whereas ^{18}O leaves as both water and exhaled carbon dioxide (CO_2).[67] The rate of CO_2 production ($\dot{V}CO_2$) can be calculated from the difference in elimination rates of the two isotopes. Energy expenditure is calculated from $\dot{V}CO_2$, using a metabolic fuel quotient that accounts for both macronutrient intake and body fuel store use, and conventional indirect calorimetric relationships.[57]

Metabolic water production was calculated from energy expenditure and substrate oxidation assuming: the change in fat free mass (FFM) was 27% protein and 73% water, with protein oxidation in g = [dietary intake + (0.27 × ΔFFM)]; all dietary carbohydrate was oxidized, with carbohydrate oxidation in g = dietary intake; fat oxidation was equal to the change in fat mass (FM) in grams where ΔFM = [(fat oxidation in kcal)/(9.4 kcal/g)], and fat oxidation in kcal = total energy expenditure − [(g of protein oxidized × 4.75 kcal/g) + (g of carbohydrate oxidized × 4.18 kcal/g)]; and metabolic water production = (0.41 g H_2O × g protein oxidized) + (0.60 g H_2O × g carbohydrate oxidized) + (1.07 g H_2O × g fat oxidized).[57] Changes in body composition were variously determined by isotope dilution, anthropometry, or hydrostatic weighing, while dietary intake was estimated from self-recorded dietary records.

Net respiratory evaporative water loss was calculated as the difference between respiratory water efflux and influx. Respiratory water efflux was estimated from pulmonary ventilation, and air temperature, and humidity using the equation of Ferrus et al.[19] Pulmonary ventilation was calculated from DLW estimates of oxygen consumption assuming a ventilation-to-oxygen consumption ($\dot{V}E/\dot{V}O_2$) ratio of 31:1.[63] Respiratory water influx was estimated from pulmonary ventilation and ambient absolute humidity.[20] Net cutaneous evaporative water loss was estimated using the computer simulation model of Kraning.[54] Body surface area (BSA) was calculated from height and weight.[16] Absolute humidity was estimated from the average of the daily high and low dry-bulb temperatures assuming 50% relative humidity. Meterologic data was recorded with a portable field weather station.[65] A total of 29 normal males (age, 28 ± 4 y; height, 178 ± 7 cm; weight, 79.5 ± 6.7 kg; percentage body fat, 19 ± 4%; BSA, 1.98 ± 0.12 m²) participated in these studies (Table 2).

A. RESPIRATORY EVAPORATIVE WATER LOSS

Inhalation of cold dry air and increases in pulmonary ventilation are generally thought to increase respiratory evaporative water loss at altitude. As noted by others,[60] the empirical equations of Ferrus and co-workers[19] suggest respiratory evaporative water loss may not always increase at altitude. On one hand, as inspired gas temperature decreases at altitude, expired gas temperature

TABLE 2   Field Study Characteristics

Subject Number	Duration (d)	Altitude (m)	Temp. (°C)	PaH$_2$O[a] (mm Hg)	TDEE[b] kcal/d (MJ/d)	Ref.
23	11	2200 to 2550	−15 to 13	4	4920 ± 911 (20.6 ± 3.8)	38
6	6	2550 to 3100	−14 to −7	2	4560 ± 566 (19.1 ± 2.4)	39

Note: 1 MJ = 239 kcal; values are means ± SD. Volunteers had ad libitum access to drinking water.

[a] PaH$_2$O = partial pressure of water vapor in the ambient air, estimated from mean of daily high and low dry-bulb temperatures assuming 50% relative humidity.
[b] TDEE = total daily energy expenditure.

and expired water loss decrease significantly. Also, as inspired water vapor pressure decreases, expired water vapor content decreases significantly. The amount of water vapor expired per liter of ventilated gas decreases negligibly with increases in ventilation.[19] On the other hand, increased ventilation, due to increases in the $\dot{V}E/\dot{V}O_2$ ratio at altitude, increases total respiratory water loss.

The effects of air temperature, humidity, and $\dot{V}E/\dot{V}O_2$ ratio on respiratory evaporative water loss at sea level, moderate altitude, and high altitude are illustrated in Figure 1. The estimates of net respiratory evaporative water loss at sea level and moderate altitudes were similar. Apparently, increases in respiratory water loss due to the moderate $\dot{V}E/\dot{V}O_2$ ratio were counterbalanced by decreases in expired water loss due to decreased inspired air temperature and humidity. However, a typical $\dot{V}E/\dot{V}O_2$ for 4300 m elevation results in about a 200 ml/d increase in respiratory evaporative water loss above that at moderate altitude or sea level.

B. METABOLIC WATER PRODUCTION

It is well known that fat oxidation, per gram, generates nearly twice the water of carbohydrate oxidation (1.07 vs. 0.6 g H$_2$O/g). However, on an energy basis, metabolic water produced by fat and carbohydrate oxidation is similar: 0.13 and 0.15 g H$_2$O/kcal or 31 and 36 g H$_2$O/MJ, respectively. Protein yields about 0.4 g H$_2$O/g oxidized, but is usually a minor fuel (<15% of total calories)[15] and consequently contributes minimally to metabolic water production (only about 50 g H$_2$O/d in the field studies). Notably, at sea level and at moderate altitude, but not at 4300 m, metabolic water production balances net respiratory water loss (Figure 1).

C. CUTANEOUS EVAPORATIVE WATER LOSS

Cutaneous evaporative water losses of the soldiers in the field studies,[38,39] were estimated using a computer simulation model.[54] Additional information

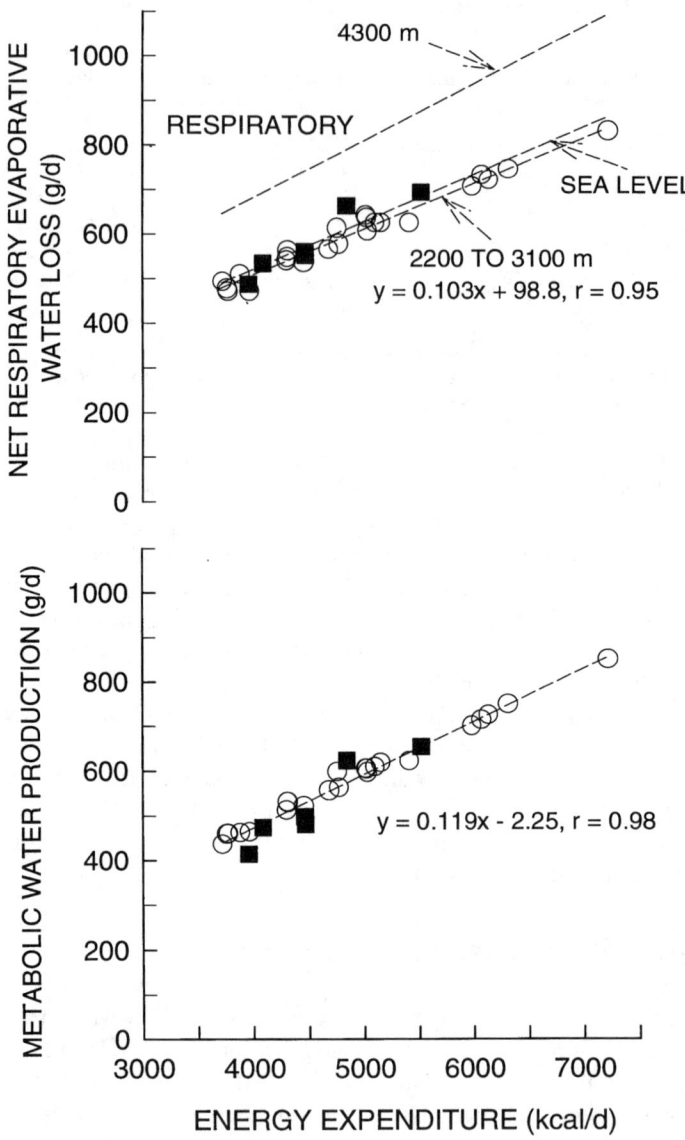

FIGURE 1 Net respiratory evaporative water loss and metabolic water production as functions of total daily energy expenditure. Filled squares (■) correspond to individual values (N = 6) in the study by Hoyt et al.[39] Open circles (○) correspond to individual values (N = 23) in an earlier study by Hoyt et al.[38] The sea-level regression (y = 0.107x + 92.2, r = 0.94) was calculated assuming ambient temperature = 20°C, PaH_2O = 9 mm Hg, and $\dot{V}E/\dot{V}O_2$ = 23. The regression for 4300 m elevation (y = 0.129x + 166.6, r = 0.97) was calculated from moderate altitude data using $\dot{V}E/\dot{V}O_2$ = 42.

about this model, weather data collection, and the biophysics of heat transfer and clothing is provided elsewhere.[32,54,65] Cutaneous evaporative water losses were calculated for the 12-h daylight period when radiant loads and air temperatures were elevated. Computer model inputs include subject age and physical characteristics (weight, height, percentage body fat, BSA), clothing insulation, and local weather conditions (air temperature, humidity, wind speed). Estimated clothing insulation ranged from 0.7 to 2.7 clo, but information about the time course of doffing and donning clothing was not collected. A working value of 1.0 clo during exercise was used, assuming that the soldiers adhered to training doctrine and removed or adjusted clothing to avoid overheating. Rates of energy expenditure during physical activity were estimated from DLW TDEE values and ambulatory activity monitor data.

The main factors determining cutaneous evaporative water loss in the specific scenario under consideration were ambient temperature and wind speed, and the rate of energy expenditure. Differences in BSA were less important due to the similarity in the physical characteristics of the subjects. In the first study,[38] estimated cutaneous evaporative water loss was 1.3 ± 0.6 l/d (range = 0.9 to 2.9 l/d). In the second study on Mount Rainier,[39] where wind speeds were higher and air temperatures lower, estimated cutaneous evaporative water loss averaged 0.3 l/d (range = 0 to 1 l/d). Using the field study data, the computer model suggested that with moderate rates of energy expenditure and low air temperatures, high rates of cutaneous evaporative water loss could be avoided by reducing clothing insulation. However, high levels of energy expenditure were associated with high rates of cutaneous evaporative water loss, even when air temperatures were low and overdressing was avoided.

III. NEGATIVE WATER AND SODIUM BALANCE AT ALTITUDE

Carcass analysis, indicator dilution, and water balance studies show that mammalian adaptation to moderate hypoxia is associated with the loss of TBW.[40] This physiologic loss of TBW is not prevented by overdrinking,[72] and eventually leads to a new steady state.[8,10,40] The decrease in TBW includes losses in plasma volume and extracellular fluid volume.[6,7,9,22,46,47] The loss of extracellular fluid volume requires negative water and sodium balances, either through reduced intake or increased excretion.

A. ANOREXIA AND HYPODIPSIA

Exposure to moderate hypoxia appears to be associated with reduced appetite and thirst in humans and many other mammals.[40] In resting rats, acute exposure to moderate hypoxia inhibits food and salt appetite as well as thirst, probably by independent mechanisms.[6,7,22,66] Food and water intakes are reduced in the first 1 to 4 d, while salt intake may be inhibited for a longer time. Reduced intestinal reabsorption of sodium and chloride might also contribute to negative sodium and water balance during moderate hypoxia.[75] In humans, a pattern of transiently reduced food and water intake is also evident at altitudes of 3500 to 4300 m. Significant reductions in spontaneous food intake may persist for one or more weeks,[13,45,70] with men apparently affected more than women.[31,32] A more transient reduction in the spontaneous water intake of resting individuals may also occur.[10] In poorly tolerated hypoxia, the general aversion to food, water, and salt may simply reflect altitude illness rather than an adaptive physiologic mechanism.

B. DIURETIC AND NATRIURETIC EFFECTS OF ALTITUDE

Mountaineers recognize copious urine production (Höhendiurese) as a sign of successful adaptation to altitude. In fact, exposure to acute moderate hypoxia (3000 m to 5000 m) results in diuresis and natriuresis in humans and many mammals.[2,3,9,11,35,51,53,61,69,71,73] In contrast, when hypoxia is poorly tolerated or severe, for example, above 5000 m or when arterial PO_2 is less than 40 mm Hg, renal water and salt excretion usually decrease.[35,36,51,69] The resulting fluid retention is often associated with acute mountain sickness and even cerebral and pulmonary edema.[4,25,26,68]

C. PERIPHERAL ARTERIAL CHEMORECEPTORS AND RENAL EXCRETORY FUNCTION

Peripheral arterial chemoreceptors, through stimulation by low oxygen pressures, are probably the principal sensors controlling renal salt and water excretion during acute hypoxia in humans and animals.[36,40] In normoxic mammals, arterial chemoreceptor stimulation, either by perfusion of isolated carotid bodies with hypoxic blood or by pharmacological means, increases absolute and fractional renal sodium and water excretion.[36,40] When brain or kidneys, but not the peripheral arterial chemoreceptors, are exposed to physiologic levels of hypoxia, diuresis and natriuresis are absent.[36]

The pathway for peripheral arterial chemoreceptor mediation of renal sodium and water excretion in response to hypoxia is unknown. Increased renal sodium and water excretion is: (1) not related to hyperventilation or hypocapnia, (2) not a pressure diuresis, and (3) not dependent on intact cardiovascular pressure or volume sensors.[3,36,40,49,50] However, removal of the nerves to the carotid body chemoreceptors, or carotid body deactivation, abolished the natriuretic response to hypoxia.[5,36,40] These results show that the stimulation of peripheral arterial chemoreceptors increases renal sodium excretion through specific reflex mechanisms.

In normoxic mammals, sodium excretion in response to arterial chemoreceptors stimulation results from decreased renal tubular sodium reabsorption.[36,40] This decreased renal sodium absorption occurs despite renal vasoconstriction that may decrease glomerular filtration rate and renal blood flow. Sectioning of renal nerves abolishes this vasoconstriction and facilitates natriuresis, suggesting that hypoxic natriuresis is hormonally mediated. However, all attempts to identify the endogenous natriuretic substance inhibiting renal tubular sodium reabsorption during peripheral arterial chemoreceptor stimulation have been unsuccessful.

Only a few studies of humans exist that demonstrate the role of the arterial chemoreceptors in the control of renal excretory function. One study demonstrated that almitrine bismesylate, a highly specific chemoreceptor stimulant, has a diuretic effect.[52] More recently, Swenson and co-workers[71] investigated whether people with a high ventilatory response to hypoxia — that is, a high peripheral chemoreceptor sensitivity — had a greater diuretic and natriuretic response to hypoxia than those with a lower ventilatory response. Diet was controlled for several days to reduce possible influences of variations in salt intake. They found that isocapnic hypoxic ventilatory drive, a measure of chemoreceptor sensitivity, was positively correlated with hypoxic diuresis and natriuresis, but not with bicarbonate excretion. Their findings suggest that (1) respiratory alkalosis is very probably not the cause of high-altitude natriuresis and diuresis, and (2) peripheral arterial chemoreceptors have a role in controlling renal salt and water excretion in humans during whole-body hypoxia.[71] These results are consistent with research suggesting that reduced chemoreceptor sensitivity may be a factor initiating maladaptation at altitude.[58] These results are also in complete agreement with results from animal experiments.[3,36,49,50]

D. SPECIAL CONDITIONS INFLUENCING BODY FLUID HOMEOSTASIS

In severe hypoxia, decreases in renal sodium and water excretion, associated with reductions in renal blood flow and glomerular filtration rate, can be attenuated by renal denervation.[35,36] Presumably, the antinatriuretic and antidiuretic effects of severe hypoxia are mediated through efferent renal sympathetic nerves activated in response to brain hypoxia.[35,36] Perhaps during arterial hypoxemia, all factors that impair oxygen transport would promote sympathetic nerve activation and decrease the natriuretic and diuretic responses to hypoxia. Such factors might include age,[14,41,48,55,59] anemia, hypovolemia, dehydration, or cardiorespiratory insufficiency. In addition, exercise at altitude can override the natriuretic and diuretic effects of hypoxia.[76]

The natriuretic effects of hypoxia also depend on normal blood volume and thus normal activation of the cardiovascular stretch and pressure receptors.[1,36] This interaction between chemoreceptor and stretch receptors would explain why the natriuresis induced by moderate hypoxia is transient.[36] To date, however, the interaction between baro- and chemoreceptors in the control of renal function has only been studied in animals.[49] Also, systematic studies of the basal, chemoreceptor-independent mechanisms that can influence salt and water metabolism during whole-body hypobaric hypoxia are needed.[34,36,40]

Other factors complicating the physiologic responses to hypoxia include growth,[27,37,66] predisposition to altitude illness,[4] speed of ascent,[44] diet,[12,33,45] and possibly gender. Women apparently acclimatize to altitude as well as men,[30] but research on the influence of the phase of the menstrual cycle is lacking. Diets high in carbohydrate appear to reduce the incidence of acute mountain sickness[12,33] — possibly because the end products of carbohydrate oxidation, CO_2 and water, have little impact on renal function, and the energy yield per liter of oxygen is higher for carbohydrate than for fat.[57]

IV. SUMMARY

A hallmark of successful adaptation to high altitude is a hypoxia-induced loss of TBW. The diuresis and natriuresis that underlie this physiologic loss of body fluid are, in part, due to arterial chemoreceptor influences on renal excretory function. However, factors such as exercise, abrupt ascent to altitude, excessive salt intake, inadequate water consumption, and elevated evaporative water losses can override the natriuretic and diuretic effects of hypoxia and lead to acute mountain sickness.

Respiratory water losses at sea level and moderate altitudes appear to be balanced by metabolic water production. But at high altitudes, where $\dot{V}E/\dot{V}O_2$ ratios are elevated, respiratory water loss can exceed metabolic water production and may contribute significantly to the loss of body water. In addition, strenuous exercise can be associated with high rates of cutaneous evaporative water loss, even when air temperatures are low and overdressing is avoided.

ACKNOWLEDGMENT

The authors thank Dr. K.K. Kraning II for his assistance in modeling rates of cutaneous evaporative water loss.

REFERENCES

1. Al-Obaidi, M., E. M. Whitaker, and F. Karim. The effect of discrete stimulation of carotid body chemoreceptors on atrial natriuretic peptide in anaesthetized dogs. *J. Physiol.* 443: 519–531, 1991.
2. Al-Obaidi, M. and F. Karim. Primary effects of carotid chemoreceptor stimulation on gracilis muscle and renal blood flow and renal function in dogs. *J. Physiol.* 455:73–88, 1992.
3. Bardsley, P. A., B. F. Johnson, A. G. Stewart, and G. R. Barer. Natriuresis secondary to carotid chemoreceptor stimulation with almitrine bismesylate in the rat: The effect on kidney function and the responses to renal denervation and deficiency of antidiuretic hormone. *Biomed. Biochim. Acta* 50: 175–182, 1991.

4. Bärtsch, P., N. Pluger, M. Audetat, S. Shaw, P. Weidmann, P. Vock, W. Vetter, D. Rennie, and O. Oelz. Effects of slow ascent to 4559 m on fluid homeostasis. *Aviat. Space Environ. Med.* 62:105–110, 1991.
5. Behm, R., H. Mewew, W. H. D. Keizer, T. Unger, and R. Rettig. Cardiovascular and renal effects of hypoxia in conscious carotid body-denervated rats. *J. Appl. Physiol.* 74:2795–2800, 1993.
6. Behm, R., A. Honig, M. Griethe, M. Schmidt, and P. Schneider. Sustained suppression of voluntary sodium intake of spontaneously hypertensive rats (SHR) in hypobaric hypoxia. *Biomed. Biochim. Acta* 43: 975–985, 1984.
7. Behm, R., B. Gerber, J.-O. Habeck, C. Huckstorf, and K. Ruckborn. Effect of hypobaric hypoxia and almitrine on voluntary salt and water intake in carotid body denervated spontaneously hypertensive rats. *Biomed. Biochim. Acta* 48: 689–695, 1989.
8. Butterfield, G. E., J. Gates, S. Fleming, G. A. Brooks, J. R. Sutton, and J. T. Reeves. Increased energy intake minimizes weight loss in men at high altitude. *J. Appl. Physiol.* 72: 1741–1748, 1992.
9. Christensen, B. M., H. L. Johnson, and A. V. Ross. Organ fluid changes and electrolyte excretion of rats exposed to high altitude. *Aviat. Space Environ. Med.* 46:16–20, 1975.
10. Claybaugh, J. R., C. E. Wade, and S. A. Cucinell. Fluid and electrolyte balance and hormonal response to the hypoxic environment. In: *Hormonal Regulation of Fluid and Electrolytes,* Claybaugh, J. R. and Wade, C. E., Eds. Plenum Press, New York, 1989, 187–214.
11. Colice, G., S. Yen, G. Ramirez, J. Dietz, and L.-C. Ou. Acute hypoxia-induced diuresis in rats. *Aviat. Space Environ. Med.* 62:551–554, 1991.
12. Consolazio, C. F., L. O. Matoush, H. L. Johnson, H. J. Krzywicki, T. A. Daws, and G. J. Isaac. Effects of high-carbohydrate diets on performance and clinical symptomatology after rapid ascent to high altitude. *Fed. Proc.* 28:937–943, 1969.
13. Consolazio, C. F., L. O. Matoush, H. L. Johnson, and T. A. Daws. Protein and water balances of young adults during prolonged exposure to high altitude (4300 m). *Am. J. Clin. Nutr.* 21:154–161, 1968.
14. Dill, D. B., F. G. Hall, K. D. Hall, C. Dawson, and J. L. Newton. Blood, plasma and red cell volumes: Age, exercise and environment. *J. Appl. Physiol.* 21:597–602, 1966.
15. Dohm, G. L., G. J. Kasperek, E. B. Tapscott, and H. A. Barakat. Protein metabolism during endurance exercise. *Fed. Proc.* 44:348–352, 1985.
16. Dubois D., and E. F. Dubois. A formula to estimate the approximate surface area if height and weight be known. *Arch. Intern. Med.* 17:863–871, 1916.
17. Epstein, M., and T. Saruta. Effects of simulated high altitude on renin-aldosterone and Na homeostasis in normal man. *J. Appl. Physiol.* 33:204–210, 1972.
18. Epstein, M. and T. Saruta. Effects of an hyperoxic hypobaric environment on renin-aldosterone in normal man. *J. Appl. Physiol.* 34:49–52, 1973.
19. Ferrus, L., D. Commenges, J. Gire, and P. Varène. Respiratory water loss as a function of ventilatory or environmental factors. *Respir. Physiol.* 56:11–20, 1984.
20. Fjeld, C. R., K. H. Brown, and D. A. Schoeller. Validation of the deuterium oxide method for measuring average daily milk intake in infants. *Am. J. Clin. Nutr.* 48:671–679, 1988.
21. Frayser, R., I. D. Rennie, G. W. Gray, and C. S. Houston. Hormonal and electrolyte response to exposure to 17,500 ft. *J. Appl. Physiol.* 38:636–642, 1975.
22. Fregly, M. J., E. L. Nelson, and P. E. Tyler. Water exchange in rats exposed to cold, hypoxia, and both combined. *Aviat. Space Environ. Med.* 47:600–607, 1976.
23. Gonzalez, R. R. (1988). Biophysics of heat transfer and clothing characteristics. In: *Human Performance Physiology and Environmental Medicine at Terrestrial Extremes.* Pandolf, K. B., Sawka, M. N., and Gonzalez, R. R., Eds. Benchmark Press, Indianapolis, 45-95.
24. Hackett, P. H., and R. C. Roach. High altitude medicine. In: *Wilderness Medicine.* 3rd ed. Auerbach, P. S., Ed. C.V. Mosby, Boston, 1–37.

25. Hackett, P. H., D. Rennie, S. E. Hofmeister, R. F. Grover, E. B. Grover, and J. T. Reeves. Fluid retention and relative hypoventilation in acute mountain sickness. *Respiration* 43:321–329, 1982.
26. Hamilton, A. J., A. Cymerman, and P. M. Black. High altitude cerebral edema. *Neurosurgery* 19:841–849, 1986.
27. Hannon, J. P. and G. B. Rogers. Body composition of mice following exposure to 4300 and 6100 meters. *Aviat. Space Environ. Med.* 46:1232–1235, 1975.
28. Hannon, J. P., K. S. K. Chinn, and J. L. Shields. Effects of acute high altitude exposure on body fluids. *Fed. Proc.* 38:1178–1184, 1969.
29. Hannon, J. P., K. S. K. Chinn, and J. L. Shields. Alterations in serum and extracellular electrolytes during high-altitude exposure. *J. Appl. Physiol.* 31:266–273, 1971.
30. Hannon, J. P. Comparative altitude adaptability of young men and women. In: *Environmental Stress: Individual Human Adaptations*. Folinsbee, L. J., Wagner, J. A., Borgia, J. F., Drinkwater, B. L., Gliner, J. A., and Bedi, J. F., Eds. Academic Press, New York, 1978, 335–350.
31. Hannon, J. P., G. J. Klain, D. M. Sudman, and F. J. Sullivan. Nutritional aspects of high altitude exposure in women. *Am. J. Clin. Nutr.* 29:604–613, 1976.
32. Hannon, J. P. Nutrition at high altitude. In: *Environmental Physiology: Aging, Heat and Altitude*. Horvath, S. M. and Yousef, M. K., Eds. Elsevier/North-Holland, New York, 1980, 309–327.
33. Hansen, J. E., L. H. Hartley, and R. P. Hogan III. Arterial oxygen increase by high-carbohydrate diet at altitude. *J. Appl. Physiol.* 33:441–445, 1972.
34. Honig, A. The diuretic effect of acute hypoxia in humans: relationship to hypoxic ventilatory responsiveness and renal hormones. Invited editorial. *J. Appl. Physiol.*, 78:375–376, 1995.
35. Honig, A. Role of the arterial chemoreceptors in the reflex control of renal function and body fluid volumes in acute arterial hypoxia. In: *Physiology of the Peripheral Arterial Chemoreceptors*, Acker, H. and O'Regan, R.G., Eds. Elsevier/North-Holland, Amsterdam, 1983, 395–429.
36. Honig, A. Peripheral arterial chemoreceptors and reflex control of sodium and water homeostasis. *Am. J. Physiol.* 257 (*Regul. Integ. Comp. Physiol.* 26):R1282–R1302, 1989.
37. Hoyt, R. W., M. J. Durkot, V. A. Forte, Jr., L. J. Hubbard, L. A. Trad, and A. Cymerman. Hypobaric hypoxia (380 torr) decreases intracellular and total body water in goats. *J. Appl. Physiol.* 71:509–513, 1991.
38. Hoyt, R. W., T. E. Jones, T. P. Stein, G. McAninch, H. R. Lieberman, E. W. Askew, and A. Cymerman. Doubly labeled water measurement of human energy expenditure during strenuous exercise. *J. Appl. Physiol.* 71:16–22, 1991.
39. Hoyt, R. W., T. E. Jones, C. J. Baker-Fulco, D. A. Schoeller, R. B. Schoene, R. S. Schwartz, E. W. Askew, and A. Cymerman. Doubly labeled water measurement of human energy expenditure during exercise at high altitude. *Am. J. Physiol.* 266 (*Regul. Integ. Comp. Physiol.* 35):R966–R971, 1994.
40. Hoyt, R. W. and A. Honig. Body fluid and energy metabolism at high altitude. In: *Handbook of Physiology: Adaptation to the Environment.*, Blatteis, C. M. and Fregley, M. J., Eds., New York: Oxford University Press for the American Physiological Society. 1995.
41. Jain, S. C., W. L. Wilke, and A. Tucker. Age-dependent effects of chronic hypoxia on renin-angiotensin and urinary excretions. *J. Appl. Physiol.* 69:141–146, 1990.
42. Jain, S. C., J. Bardhan, Y. Y. Swamy, B. Krishna, and H. S. Nayar. Body fluid compartments in humans during acute high-altitude exposure. *Aviat. Space Environ. Med.* 51:234–236, 1980.
43. Jain, S. C., J. Bardhan, Y. V. Swamy, A. Grover, and H. S. Nayar. Body water metabolism in high altitude natives during and after a stay at sea level. *Int. J. Biometeorol.* 25:47–52, 1981.

44. Johnson, T. S., and P. B. Rock. Acute mountain sickness. *N. Engl. J. Med.* 319:841–845, 1988.
45. Johnson, H. L., C. F. Consolazio, L. O. Matoush, and H. J. Krzywicki. Nitrogen and mineral metabolism at altitude. *Fed. Proc.* 28:1195–1198, 1969.
46. Jones, R. M., F. T. LaRochelle, Jr., and S. M. Tenney. Role of arginine vasopressin on fluid and electrolyte balance in rats exposed to high altitude. *Am. J. Physiol.* 240 (*Regul. Integ. Comp. Physiol.* 9):R182–R186, 1981.
47. Jones, R. M., C. Terhaard, and S. M. Tenney. Mechanism of reduced water intake in rats at high altitude. *Am. J. Physiol.* 240 (*Regul. Integ. Comp. Physiol.* 9):R187–R191, 1981.
48. Jung, R. C., D. B. Dill, R. Horton, and S. M. Horvath. Effects of age on plasma aldosterone levels and hemoconcentration at altitude. *J. Appl. Physiol.* 31:593–597, 1971.
49. Karim, F. and M. Al-Obaidi. Modification of carotic chemoreceptor-induced changes in renal haemodynamics and function by carotid baroreflex in dogs. *J. Physiol. London* 466:599–610, 1993.
50. Karim, F., S. M. Poucher, and R. A. Summerill. The effects of stimulating carotid chemoreceptors on renal haemodynamics and function in dogs. *J. Physiol. London* 392:451–462, 1987.
51. Kilburn, K. H., and A. R. Dowell. Renal function in respiratory failure. Effects of hypoxia, hyperoxia, and hypercapnia. *Arch. Intern. Med.* 127: 754–762, 1971.
52. Koller, E. A., M. Schopen, M. Keller, R. E. Lang, and M. B. Valloton. Ventilatory, circulatory, endocrine, and renal effects of almitrine infusion in man. A contribution to high altitude physiology. *Eur. J. Appl. Physiol.* 58:419–425, 1989.
53. Koller, E. A., A. Buhrer, L. Felder, M. Schopen, and M. B. Valloton. Altitude diuresis: Endocrine and renal responses to acute hypoxia of acclimatized and non-acclimatized subjects. *Eur. J. Appl. Physiol.* 62:228–234, 1991.
54. Kraning, K.K., II. A Computer Simulation for Predicting the Time Course of Thermal and Cardiovascular Responses to Various Combinations of Heat Stress, Clothing and Exercise. Technical Report T13-91. U.S. Army Research Institute of Environmental Medicine, Natick, MA, 1991.
55. Kronenberg, R. S., and C. W. Drage. Alteration of the ventilatory and heart rate responses to hypoxia and hypercapnia with aging in normal man. *J. Clin. Invest.* 52:1812–1819, 1973.
56. Krzywicki, H. J., C. F. Consolazio, H. L. Johnson, W. C. Nielsen, and R. A. Barnhart. Water metabolism in humans during acute high-altitude exposure (4300 m). *J. Appl. Physiol.* 30:806–809, 1971.
57. Lusk, G. *The Elements of the Science of Nutrition*, 4th ed. Academic Press, New York, 1928. (Reprinted in 1976 by Johnson Reprint, New York.)
58. Mathew, L., P. M. Gopinathan, S. S. Purkayastha, J. Sen Gupta, and H. S. Nayar. Chemoreceptor sensitivity and maladaptation to high altitude in man. *Eur. J. Appl. Physiol.* 51:137–144, 1983.
59. Mhyre, L. G., D. B. Dill, F. G. Hall, and D. K. Brown. Blood volume changes during three-week residence at high altitude. *Clin. Chem.* 16:7–14, 1970.
60. Milledge, J. S. Respiratory water loss at altitude. *Int. Soc. Mount. Med. Newsl.* 2(3):5–7, 1992.
61. Pauli, H. G., B. Truniger, J. Klarsen, and R. O. Mulhausen. Renal function during prolonged exposure to hypoxia and carbon monoxide. II. Electrolyte handling. *Scand. J. Clin. Lab. Invest.* 22 (Suppl.) 103:61–67, 1968.
62. Phillips, R. W., K. L. Knox, W. A. House, and H. N. Jordan. Metabolic responses in sheep chronically exposed to 6,200 m simulated altitude. *Fed. Proc.* 28:974–977, 1969.
63. Reeves, J. T., R. F. Grover, and J. E. Cohn. Regulation of ventilation during exercise at 10,200 ft in athletes born at low altitude. *J. Appl. Physiol.* 22:546–554, 1967.
64. Rennie, D., S. Bezruchka, G. Roberts, J. L. Ivy, and H. N. Hultgren. Viewpoints: Water intake at high altitude. *J. Wildern. Med.* 4:224–227 (1993).

65. Santee, W. R., and R. W. Hoyt. Recommendations for Meteorological Data Collection During Physiological Field Studies. Technical Report T94-9. U.S. Army Research Institute of Environmental Medicine, Natick, MA, 1994.
66. Schnakenberg, D. D., L. F. Krabill, and P. C. Weiser. The anorectic effect of high altitude on weight gain, nitrogen retention and body composition of rats. *J. Nutr.* 101: 787–795, 1971.
67. Schoeller, D. A. Measurement of energy expenditure in free-living humans by using doubly labeled water. *J. Nutr.* 118:1278–1289, 1988.
68. Singh, M. V., S. C. Jain, S. B. Rawal, H. M. Divekar, R. Parshad, A. K. Tyagi, and K. C. Sinha. Comparative study of acetazolamide and spironolactone on body fluid compartments on induction to high altitude. *Int. J. Biometeorol.* 30:33–41, 1986.
69. Stickney, J. C., D. W. Northup, and E. J. Van Liere. The effect of anoxic anoxia on urine secretion in anaesthetized dogs. *Am. J. Physiol.* 147: 616–621, 1946.
70. Surks, M. I., K. S. K. Chinn, and L. O. Matoush. Alterations in body composition in man after acute exposure to high altitude. *J. Appl. Physiol.* 21: 1741–1746, 1966.
71. Swenson, E. R., T. B. Duncan, S. V. Goldberg, G. Ramirez, S. Ahmad, and R. B. Schoene. The diuretic effect of acute hypoxia in humans: relationship to hypoxic ventilatory responsiveness and renal hormones. *J. Appl. Physiol.* 1995 (in press).
72. Tucker, A., Reeves, J. T., Robertshaw, D., and R. F. Grover. Cardiopulmonary response to acute altitude exposure: Water loading and denitrogenation. *Respir. Physiol.* 54:363–380 (1983).
73. Tunny, T. J., J. Van Geldern, R. D. Gordon, S. A. Klemm, S. M. Hamlet, W. L. Finn, G. M. Carney, and C. Brand-Maher. Effects of altitude on atrial natriuretic peptide: the bicentennial Mount Everest expedition. *Clin. Exp. Pharmacol. Physiol.* 16:287–291, 1989.
74. U.S. Standard Atmosphere, 1976. National Oceanic and Atmospheric Administration, National Aeronautics and Space Administration, and U.S. Air Force. 1976. U.S. Government Printing Office, Washington, DC, 1976.
75. Van Liere, E. J. The effect of anoxia on the alimentary tract. *Physiol. Rev.* 21: 307–322, 1941.
76. Whithey, W. R., J. S. Milledge, E. S. Williams, B. D. Minty, E. I. Bryson, N. P. Luff, M. W. J. Older, and J. M. Beeley. Fluid and electrolyte homeostasis during prolonged exercise at altitude. *J. Appl. Physiol.* 55: 409–412, 1983.

Chapter **10**

RENAL, ENDOCRINE, AND HEMODYNAMIC EFFECTS OF WATER IMMERSION IN HUMANS

—————————————————————————— Murray Epstein

CONTENTS

I. Introduction...198

II. Characterization of the "Afferent" Limb of the
   Immersion Model.......................................198

III. Characterization of the "Efferent" Limb of the
   Immersion Model.......................................199
   A. Renal Water Handling...............................199
      1. Mechanisms of the Diuresis......................199
   B. Renal Sodium Handling..............................200
      1. Dissociation of Natriuresis from Diuresis.......200
      2. Mechanisms of the Natriuresis...................200
      3. Nephron Sites of Decreased Sodium Reabsorption..200
      4. Mechanisms of Decreased Sodium Reabsorption....202
   C. The Renin–Angiotensin–Aldosterone System..........202
   D. Arginine Vasopressin (AVP) or Antidiuretic
      Hormone (ADH).....................................204
   E. Renal Prostaglandins...............................204
   F. Atrial Natriuretic Peptides (ANF)..................205
   G. Renal Natriuretic Peptide (Urodilatin).............205
   H. Kaliuretic Peptide.................................205
   I. Humoral Natriuretic Factor (OLF)...................206
   J. Catecholamines and Dopa-Dopamine Systems..........207

IV. State of Physical Fitness..............................207

V. Considerations for Selecting Water Immersion for Studies
of Volume Homeostasis 208

VI. Studies of Disorders Characterized by Deranged
Volume Homeostasis 208

VII. Conclusions..209

References 210

I. INTRODUCTION

Water immersion is one of the oldest therapeutic methods. Knowledge of the therapeutic qualities of water immersion dates back to the earliest days of humanity.[8,9] It is ironic that the recent widespread interest in water immersion as an investigative tool received its impetus not from centuries of hydrotherapeutic practice, but from the modern space program. Reports of orbital manned space flights indicate that astronauts undergo a striking natriuresis and diuresis, thought to be a consequence of the cephalad redistribution of body fluids that takes place in a gravity-free environment.[36,47] Because the redistribution of blood volume induced by water immersion parallels that of weightlessness, the water immersion model has been utilized as a means of investigating both normal physiology and deranged volume homeostasis on earth.[9,47]

Water immersion to the neck (NI) has long been known to produce a marked diuresis.[8,36] Several lines of evidence[1,4,8,9,36,47] suggested that this effect is mediated by a redistribution of blood volume with a relative increase in central blood volume. The past two decades have witnessed the characterization of many of the hemodynamic alterations of immersion, as well as the delineation of the myriad effects of immersion on renal function and hormonal change.[8,9,10] Studies of the "efferent" limb of the immersion model have demonstrated that NI produces a marked natriuresis, kaliuresis, and diuresis, suppression of the renin–aldosterone system, augmentation of renal vasodilatory prostanoids and atrial natriuretic peptides.

II. CHARACTERIZATION OF THE "AFFERENT" LIMB OF THE IMMERSION MODEL

Although NI has long been postulated to produce a redistribution of blood volume with a relative increase in central blood volume,[8,36] only in the past

---

Portions of this chapter are adapted from a previous review by the author in *M. Physiol. Rev.* 72:563–621, 1992 and are reprinted here with permission.

two decades have data been forthcoming in humans subjects to substantiate this postulate. After the initiation of head-out water immersion, there is an acute increase in central blood volume of 700 ml with a concomitant increase in central venous pressure from 3 to 15 mm Hg.[1,8,47] Mean cardiac output increases by 32% and mean stroke volume by 35%.[1,9,47] Both right atrial and pulmonary arterial transmural pressure gradients increase, as does central venous pressure (CVP) and transmural CVP,[34] whereas systemic vascular resistance decreases.[1,7,9,47] Begin et al.[4] determined central hemodynamics serially during a 4-h immersion period utilizing an acetylene rebreathing method. This study confirmed the 25–36% increment in cardiac index previously noted to occur acutely during immersion[1] and demonstrated that this increment was sustained throughout the period of study. Subsequently, we compared the relative central hemodynamic responses of water immersion to those of standard saline infusion.[43] With the identical noninvasive rebreathing method cited earlier,[4] the increment in cardiac output induced by head-out water immersion has been shown to be similar to that documented during the extracellular fluid (ECF) volume expansion attained by acute saline administration (2 l/120 min) equivalent to 3% body weight.[43]

III. CHARACTERIZATION OF THE "EFFERENT" LIMB OF THE IMMERSION MODEL

A. RENAL WATER HANDLING

Chronologically, the initial emphasis on characterizing the renal effects of immersion was directed to the documentation of changes in renal water handling.[3] Within the past three decades, Behn et al.[5] and Epstein et al.[16,17] succeeded in characterizing the magnitude and composition of the diuresis. Both groups of investigators observed differing diuretic responses depending on the state of hydration of the study subjects. Although the increase in urine flow (V) induced by immersion was attributable to both an increase in free-water clearance (C_{H_2O}) and osmolal clearance (C_{osm}), the major determinant of the increase in V was attributable to an increase in C_{H_2O} to 4.3 ml/min.[16,19] In contrast to studies of hydrated subjects,[16,19] the immersion-induced increase in V in the fluid-restricted subjects occurred solely as a function of an increase in C_{osm} with free-water reabsorption ($T^c_{H_2O}$) remaining constant throughout immersion.[27] These results indicate that the magnitude and composition of the diuresis occur as a function of the state of hydration of the subject.

1. Mechanisms of the Diuresis

Several mechanisms have been documented to contribute to the diuresis attending immersion. These include: (1) suppression of antidiuretic hormone (ADH), (2) increased delivery of filtrate to the diluting site, (3) increase in the release of endogenous renal prostaglandins, (4) augmentation of atrial natriuretic factors (ANF) and urodilatin and (5) decrease in sympathetic nervous system activity.

B. RENAL SODIUM HANDLING

We characterized the natriuretic response during various sodium intakes and various depths of immersion.[16,17,19,26,27,33] Our studies[33] of mildly sodium-depleted subjects (dietary intake of 10 mEq/d) disclosed that the absolute increase in sodium excretion was less than 7 mEq/6h, reflecting the constraints imposed by the sodium-depleted and volume-contracted state of the subjects. In a subsequent study[16] carried out with a sodium intake more nearly approximating that of the normal diet (150 mEq/d), sodium-replete normal subjects demonstrated an earlier (hour 1 vs. hour 4) and more profound (72 mEq/6h vs. 7 mEq/6h) natriuresis than during sodium depletion (Figure 1). Water immersion to the waist[26] did not induce a natriuresis in either sodium-depleted or sodium-replete subjects, presumably because a lessened pressure gradient induced less central hypervolemia.

1. Dissociation of Natriuresis from Diuresis

Although immersion is usually associated with both a diuresis and a natriuresis, the two events do not necessarily always occur together. Thus, overnight fluid restriction abolished the diuresis of immersion without attenuating the natriuresis.[27] Similarly, the administration of aqueous vasopressin to immersed hydrated normal subjects undergoing immersion abolished the diuresis while the natriuresis remained intact.[14] The differences in the temporal profile of the diuresis and natriuresis of immersion merit reemphasis. The diuresis of immersion is usually manifest by hour 1 or 2. In contrast, the natriuresis is progressive and usually peaks by hour 3 or 4. Together, these observations suggest the presence of separate mechanisms for the diuretic and natriuretic responses.

2. Mechanisms of the Natriuresis

The demonstration of a highly significant increase in the fractional excretion of sodium during immersion indicates that the natriuresis is attributable primarily to an increased tubular rejection of sodium rather than to alterations in the filtered sodium load.

3. Nephron Sites of Decreased Sodium Reabsorption

Several lines of evidence suggest that the decreased sodium reabsorption occurs at multiple sites in the nephron. The demonstration of a progressive kaliuresis during immersion[16,19] suggests that the natriuresis of immersion is multifactorial and is mediated in part by an increased rejection of sodium proximal to the diluting site, as well as due to an additional component secondary to a decline in circulating aldosterone. This hypothesis is supported by our data that indicate sodium excretion was enhanced when free-water

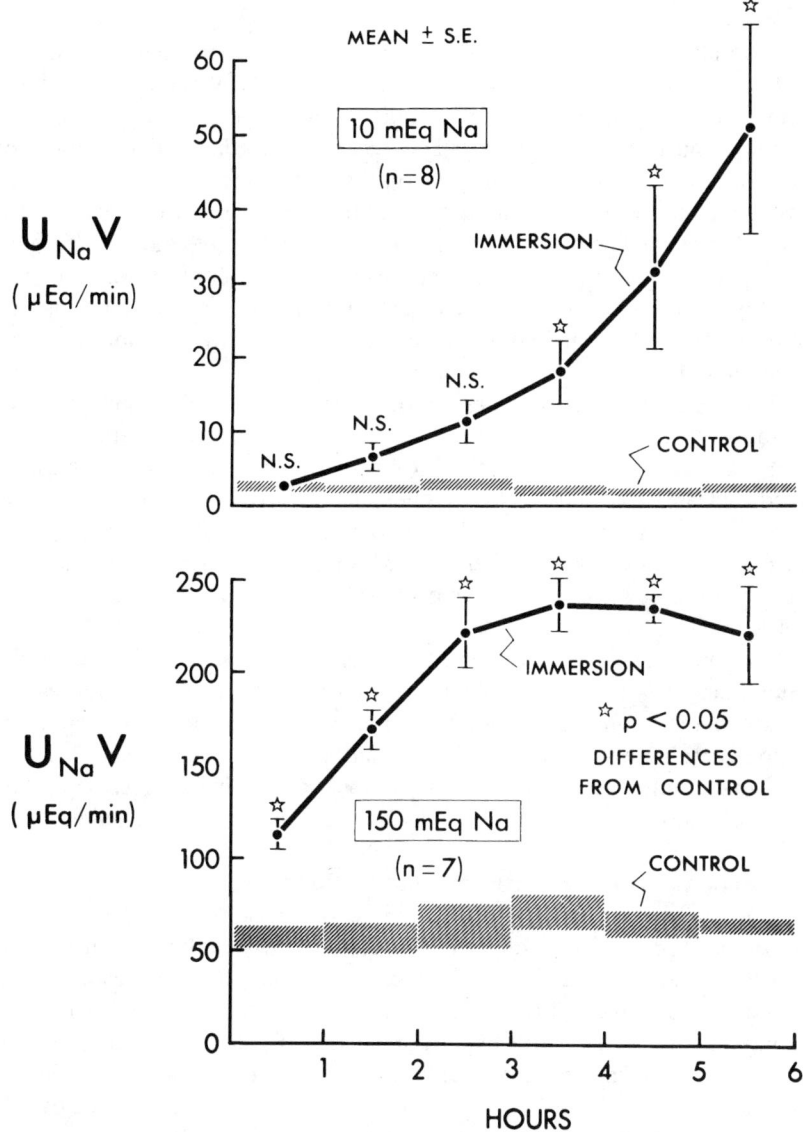

FIGURE 1 Comparison of effects of immersion on rate of sodium excretion ($U_{Na}V$) in subjects in balance on low-sodium (top) and high-sodium (bottom) diets. Shaded areas represent mean ± SE for control studies. A significant increase in $U_{Na}V$ occurs within the initial hour in sodium-replete subjects, but is delayed to the 4th hour in subjects ingesting a sodium-restricted diet. (Data from sodium-restricted subjects from Reference 33; for sodium-replete subjects from Reference 16; figure from Epstein M., *Physiol. Rev.* 72:563–621, 1992. With permission.)

clearance was augmented. This suggests an increase in sodium delivery to the diluting site.[16,19]

In an attempt to further define the sites in the nephron where increased rejection of sodium occurs, Rabelink et al.[50] examined several renal functional parameters during immersion, including lithium clearance (C_{Li}) and renal phosphate and uric acid handling. They carried out quantitative analysis of segmental tubular sodium reabsorption based on C_{Li} and demonstrated a progressive increase of C_{Li}. To the extent that this variable constitutes a quantitative index of solute delivery from the proximal tubules into the thin descending loop of Henle, these authors proposed that the lithium data suggest disruption of the glomerulotubular balance during immersion — that is, the filtered load of sodium increases, whereas absolute proximal sodium reabsorption did not change.

Additional attempts to characterize the intrarenal loci of sodium reabsorption have utilized phosphate and uric acid clearance as directional markers of sodium reabsorption in the proximal tubule. Epstein et al.[8] demonstrated that absolute and fractional phosphate excretion was not altered by 5 h of immersion compared with the corresponding values during a time control study. Rabelink et al.[50] have confirmed these observations. In addition, Rabelink et al.[50] demonstrated that uric acid clearance was not augmented during immersion.

In summary, studies carried out to quantitatively assess segmental tubular sodium reabsorption based on lithium, phosphate, and uric acid clearances and during hypotonic saline expansion have indicated that decreased sodium reabsorption at multiple sites in the nephron contributes to the natriuresis of immersion. Conceivably, these mechanisms contribute in varying degrees depending on the volume status and underlying disease state, to the ultimate natriuresis.

4. Mechanisms of Decreased Sodium Reabsorption

The mechanisms mediating the natriuresis are multifactorial and include aldosterone suppression, augmentation in ANF, a possible humoral natriuretic factor (OLF), an augmentation of renal prostaglandins, and a decrease in sympathetic nervous activity (Figure 2). Clearly, suppression of aldosterone contributes importantly to the natriuresis of immersion.[19] Enhanced release of endogenous renal prostaglandins also contributes to the natriuresis, at least in volume-contracted subjects.[22,23] Increasing evidence suggests that an atrial natriuretic factor[24] and possibly a human ouabain-like compound contribute in part to the natriuresis. Suppression of sympathetic nervous system activity also contributes to the natriuresis.[39] Finally, the roles of alterations in transcapillary Starling forces and intrarenal blood flow distribution remain to be evaluated.

C. THE RENIN–ANGIOTENSIN–ALDOSTERONE SYSTEM

Several lines of evidence have suggested the possibility that water immersion would suppress the renin–angiotensin–aldosterone system. Over 30 years ago, Bartter and Gann[2] demonstrated that constriction of the supradiaphragmatic inferior vena cava consistently increased aldosterone secretion, presumably by producing relative volume depletion above the constriction. Subsequent studies have demonstrated a parallel increase in PRA in the dog with inferior vena cava constriction. Since immersion to the neck produces an opposite hemodynamic redistribution, characterized by an increase in intrathoracic volume, one would anticipate a suppression of both PRA and aldosterone.

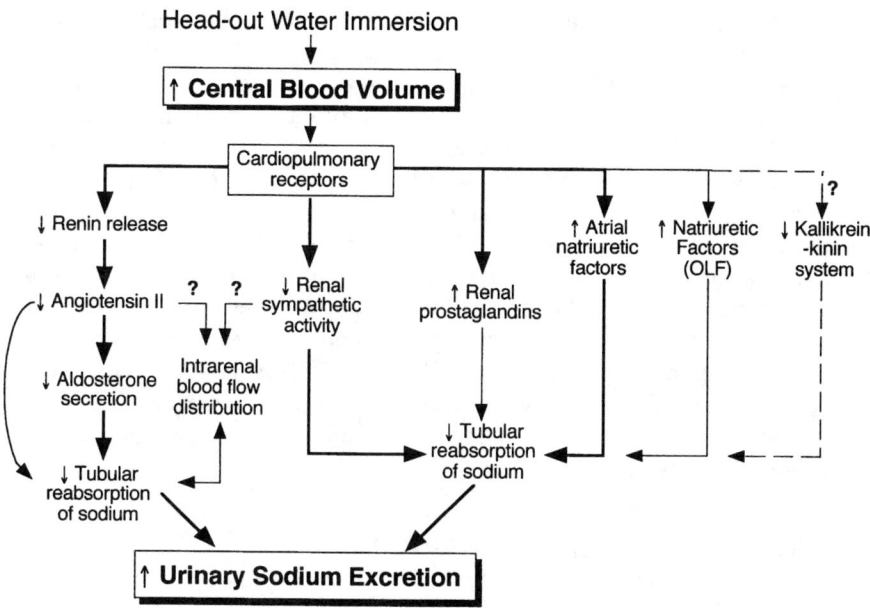

FIGURE 2 Schematic drawing of possible mechanisms whereby immersion-induced central hypervolemia induces natriuresis. Heavy arrows indicate pathways for which evidence is available. Diverse hemodynamic, renal, and hormonal effectors act in concert to promote the natriuresis. (From Epstein, M., *Physiol. Rev.* 72:563–621, 1992. With permission.)

We have systematically characterized the changes of the renin–angiotensin–aldosterone axis during water immersion and have confirmed this formulation.[28,33] Blood was collected serially at 30-min intervals to determine plasma renin activity (PRA) and plasma aldosterone (PA).[28] Immersion resulted in a progressive suppression of PRA within the first 30 min and a significant suppression of PA by 60 min of immersion.[28] By 210 min, PRA was suppressed maximally to 38% of the prestudy value. Cessation of immersion was associated with a prompt return of PRA toward prestudy values as early as 30 min of recovery.

As detailed previously,[8] activation of left atrial and cardiopulmonary receptors with a resultant decrease in sympathetic nerve traffic to the kidney contributes importantly to the suppression of renin release.

D. ARGININE VASOPRESSIN (AVP) OR ANTIDIURETIC HORMONE (ADH)

Although AVP suppression during water immersion has been documented only within the past decade, considerable evidence had suggested the possibility of such a change. Many investigators reported an increase in solute-free water clearance during head-out water immersion.[5,8,9,16,19,36] In addition, the administration of AVP abolishes the diuresis of immersion.[14,36]

Over 20 years ago, we utilized a sensitive and specific radioimmunoassay for urinary ADH to document the effects of immersion on urinary ADH excretion.[27] Immersion resulted in a progressive decrease in ADH excretion from 80 ± 7 to 37 ± 61 µU/min. Furthermore, cessation of immersion was associated with a marked rebound, with ADH excretion increasing from 37 to 177 µU/min during the recovery hour.[27]

The availability of a precise and highly reproducible radioimmunoassay for plasma AVP prompted us to characterize the effects of immersion-induced acute isoosmotic volume expansion on plasma AVP in normal human subjects.[30] Normal subjects were studied after 14 h of dehydration on two occasions: control and during 4 h of NI. Blood was obtained every 30 min for AVP. Although AVP did not change during the control period, throughout NI it showed prompt and sustained suppression ($p < 0.05$ vs. control). There were no concomitant changes in plasma osmolality. These data support the concept that acute isoosmotic central volume expansion in humans results in a suppression of plasma AVP.

E. RENAL PROSTAGLANDINS (PGE)

Additional studies demonstrated a profound effect of NI on endogenous prostaglandin synthesis. Studies in sodium-replete subjects disclosed that immersion is associated with a progressive increment in renal PGE excretion, reaching a peak by hour 2 of immersion.[22] PGE excretion returned to prestudy levels during the postimmersion hour. Subsequent studies conducted after the administration of indomethacin (50 mg q6h × 5) disclosed that this cyclooxygenase inhibitor attenuated but did not prevent the immersion-induced increment in PGE.[22] In other words, pretreatment with indomethacin decreased basal PGE excretion by more than 50% and lessened the excretion of PGE during the subsequent immersion. A similar pattern was noted when five of the subjects treated with indomethacin were restudied after dietary sodium restriction.[22]

Although indomethacin produced similar levels of PGE excretion in both the sodium-replete and sodium-depleted groups,[22] it did not significantly alter cumulative sodium excretion in the sodium-replete group. In contrast, it virtually abolished the natriuretic response in the sodium-depleted subjects. Such observations lend support to the formulation that renal prostaglandins constitute determinants of renal sodium handling under conditions of diminished effective volume.[21]

In contrast to previous reports suggesting a parallelism between renal prostaglandin levels and the renin–aldosterone axis, immersion resulted in a dissociation of these two hormonal systems, with a suppression of PRA while PGE excretion was enhanced.[23]

F. ATRIAL NATRIURETIC PEPTIDES (ANF)

ANF are found in secretory granules of the atria, and immunoreactive ANF (irANF) has been detected in animal and human plasma.[18,44,46,52] This hormone exerts potent natriuretic and renal hemodynamic effects. The available evidence indicates that augmentation of atrial volume and stretch can lead to increased plasma irANF.[9,18,44,46] Hence, it seemed possible that augmentation of ANF release may contribute to the effects of cardiopulmonary blood volume expansion on the kidney. Consequently, we studied the effect of central volume expansion induced by water immersion to the neck on the kinetics of ANF release, and the relationship of ANF to renal excretory function[24] in 13 normal, sodium-replete subjects (Figure 3). Immersion resulted in a prompt and marked increase in plasma irANF from 7.8 ± 1.8 to 19.4 ± 3.8 fmol/ml. These levels fell to 6.3 ± 1.4 fmol/ml after 60 min recovery and were associated with reversible increases in both V rate and in sodium excretion; and with decreases in both PRA ($-66 \pm 3\%$) and PA ($-57 \pm 6\%$). These findings support the postulate that ANF constitutes one of the effectors of the natriuresis of immersion, and presumably of volume homeostasis in normal humans.

G. RENAL NATRIURETIC PEPTIDE (URODILATIN)

The demonstration that the 32-amino acid peptide [ANP-(95-126)], known as urodilatin, possesses natriuretic and diuretic properties in humans has prompted studies to assess its role during immersion. Recently, Norsk et al.[48] investigated the relationship between urodilatin and renal sodium and water handling during immersion in normal subjects. Immersion induced an increase in renal urodilatin and guanosine 3',5'-cyclic monophosphate (cGMP) excretion. Because they demonstrated a correlation between renal urodilatin excretion and both urine flow and sodium excretion, these investigators concluded that urodilatin may participate as one of the mechanisms mediating the natriuresis and diuresis of immersion in humans.

H. KALIURETIC PEPTIDE

Kaliuretic peptide is a newly characterized peptide hormone consisting of amino acids 79–98 of the ANF prohormone.[10-12,45,52,54] This peptide has the strongest potassium-excreting properties in animals[45] and humans[54,55] of all the atrial natriuretic peptides (ANP). In addition to stimulating potassium excretion, kaliuretic peptide has blood pressure lowering and diuretic properties.[45,53,54,55] This peptide originates from the 98 amino acid N-terminus of ANF prohormone by proteolytic processing to a peptide consisting of amino acids

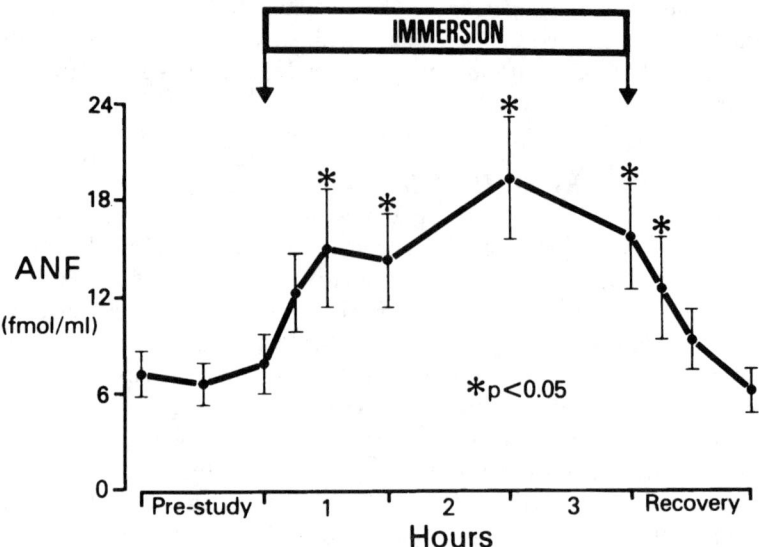

FIGURE 3 Effect of water immersion on plasma ANF levels in 13 normal subjects. Within 30 min, immersion induced a marked increase in ANF that was sustained throughout immersion. Recovery was associated with a prompt return to the prestudy level. Results are mean ± SE. *p <0.05 or more compared with the level at the end of the prestudy period. (Reproduced from Epstein, et al., *J. Clin. Invest.* 79:738–745, 1987. With permission.)

68–98, and then with further processing kaliuretic peptide is formed. We have recently demonstrated that kaliuretic peptide circulates in healthy humans and that its levels are augmented markedly and respond to water immersion.[54,55] It is likely that augmented kaliuretic peptide levels contribute to the natriuresis, diuresis, and modest kaliuresis observed in individuals undergoing water immersion.

I. HUMORAL NATRIURETIC FACTOR (OLF)

Evidence has been adduced suggesting that NI stimulates the release of a circulating natriuretic factor that may contribute to the encountered natriuresis. This bioassayable factor presumably is identified with an ouabainlike factor that cross-reacts with a digitalis receptor.[6,40] We therefore undertook to determine whether the natriuresis of NI is associated with increased activity of a natriuretic factor.[12] Urine collected during both seated control and NI studies was fractionated, and the fractions were tested in the rat assay preparation using animals with a single remnant kidney. With the control fractions, there was no significant change in sodium excretion. However, the fractions from the NI study resulted in significant increments in both $U_{Na}V$ and FE_{Na}.[12]

Recently Hamlyn et al.[40] have purified and structurally identified by mass spectroscopy an endogenous substance from human plasma that binds with high affinity to the ouabain receptor and that is indistinguishable from the cardenolide ouabain. We await studies to delineate the effects of immersion on OLF responsiveness.

J. CATECHOLAMINES AND DOPA-DOPAMINE (DA) SYSTEMS

Because stimulation of left atrial and cardiopulmonary receptors in experimental animals results in reduced autonomic nervous system activity, it might be anticipated that maneuvers such as water immersion that augment central blood volume might decrease plasma catecholamine levels. In addition, such alterations might participate in the encountered changes in renal function. Although there have been two previous attempts to examine the response of catecholamines during water immersion,[37,51] methodological considerations and divergent observations have precluded firm conclusions regarding the effect of immersion on catecholamines. We therefore designed a study utilizing more updated methodology to evaluate possible changes in the activities of the sympathetic nervous and dopa-DA systems that could contribute to the diuretic and natriuretic response of immersion. We measured plasma and urinary concentrations of norepinephrine (NE) its intraneuronal metabolite dihydroxyphenylglycol (DHPG), epinephrine (EPI), dopa, and DA in normal subjects during water immersion.[39] The urinary NE excretion was suppressed consistently during immersion. The urinary excretory rates of EPI and DHPG were also decreased. Urinary excretion of dopa, DA, and DHPG, a neuronal metabolite of NE, changed in a triphasic pattern, with decreased excretion during the first hour of immersion ($p<0.01$), small but consistent increases during the next 2 h, and decreased excretion, to below baseline, during recovery ($p < 0.01$ for dopa and DA). Our findings suggest that the neurohormonal contribution to the natriuretic response during central hypervolemia is multifactorial and includes persistent sympathoadrenal suppression and a late increase in dopa-DA activity.

IV. STATE OF PHYSICAL FITNESS

As detailed in my earlier extensive review,[9] several lines of evidence suggested that the state of physical fitness of the subjects may constitute an important determinant of the renal response during immersion. In one such study, the renal response to immersion was compared in trained and untrained subjects. Trained subjects manifested an attenuated natriuretic response to immersion compared with the untrained subjects. These preliminary observations required confirmation in rigorous studies.

V. CONSIDERATIONS FOR SELECTING WATER IMMERSION FOR STUDIES OF VOLUME HOMEOSTASIS

The delineation of the water immersion model has facilitated its application by many studies to investigations of renal function and hormonal responsiveness in both normal humans and in diverse disease states including edematous disorders.[9,11,20,25,32,41,49] Traditional attempts to assess the effects of volume alterations and hypervolemia have utilized rapid volume expansion with exogenous solutions, including saline, mannitol, and albumin. As we have detailed previously, however, several of these maneuvers have a number of drawbacks.[9,11] For example, saline infusion nonspecifically increases the volume of all fluid compartments and induces concomitant alterations in plasma composition precluding definitive statements regarding the etiological role of alterations in plasma volume.

In contrast to the more traditional attempts to achieve extracellular volume expansion, water immersion has several attributes that commend its use. As summarized in Table 1, the volume stimulus of immersion is promptly reversible after cessation of immersion in contrast to the relatively sustained hypervolemia that follows saline administration and thus constitutes an important attribute in minimizing any risk to the study patients. In contrast to saline administration, the volume stimulus of immersion occurs in the absence of changes in plasma composition.[9,19] In addition, the central hypervolemia of water immersion is caused partly by hydrostatic compression of peripheral veins and a consequent decline of venous capacitance, whereas the central hypervolemia of saline administration is due to an elevation of mean circulatory filling pressure as a consequence of the increased vascular volume.[9]

VI. STUDIES OF DISORDERS CHARACTERIZED BY DERANGED VOLUME HOMEOSTASIS

As detailed in a recent review,[9] the immersion model has been utilized successfully as an investigative tool for studying abnormal sodium and water homeostasis in patients with decompensated cirrhosis,[11,20,29] nephrotic syndrome,[41,49] and, to a lesser extent essential hypertension.[13,25]

Aside from its utility in investigating the pathogenesis of hypertension, the water immersion model has also been used successfully in studies of antihypertensive agents in this patient population. A recent example is the application of water immersion to characterize the natriuretic properties of calcium antagonists.[13]

TABLE 1 Salient Features of the Model of Head-Out Water Immersion in Humans

1. Immersion produces a *prompt* redistribution of circulating blood with a relative central hypervolemia.
2. Cardiac output is increased by 25–33% and central blood volume by approximately 700 ml.
3. The alterations in central hemodynamics are *sustained* throughout a 4-h immersion period and are promptly reversible following cessation of immersion.
4. Immersion-induced central hypervolemia is associated with a profound and progressive natriuresis and diuresis. These alterations are promptly reversible following cessation of immersion.
5. The central hemodynamic and renal effects of immersion are equal in magnitude to those induced by acute saline administration (2l saline/2h).
6. The alterations in renal sodium, potassium, and water handling in the sodium-replete state generally occur with a concomitant increase in renal plasma flow but in the absence of changes in GFR.
7. Immersion is associated with a prompt and profound (approximately two-thirds) suppression of PRA and plasma aldosterone. Cessation of immersion is associated with a prompt return of both PRA and PA to prestudy levels.
8. Immersion induces a prompt, marked, and sustained augmentation of atrial natriuretic factor (ANF). Cessation of immersion is associated with a prompt return of ANF to prestudy levels.
9. Immersion induces an augmentation of renal prostaglandins as assessed by an increase in urinary PGE and 6-keto-PGF$_{1\alpha}$ excretion.
10. The above alterations in renal function, renin-aldosterone, and ANF responsiveness occur in the absence of changes in plasma composition.

From Epstein, M., *Physiol. Rev.* 72:563–621, 1992. With permission.

VII. CONCLUSIONS

The studies reported here indicate renewed interest in the changes in physiology brought about by immersion. In the last few years, several laboratories have succeeded in delineating further the circulatory, renal, and endocrine changes induced by water immersion in humans. These studies have demonstrated that immersion in the seated posture results in a redistribution of blood volume with a relative central hypervolemia. Consequently, profound alterations in fluid and electrolyte homeostasis ensue, including a marked natriuresis, kaliuresis, and diuresis as well as a suppression of the renin-aldosterone system and ADH release. Concomitantly, release of renal PGE, ANF, and urodilatin is stimulated.

Although a delineation of the hormonal and renal responses to immersion is of importance in understanding the normal physiology of volume regulation, it must be underscored that the utility of this model transcends this immediate application. For example, characterization of the effects of immersion has facilitated studies of the pathophysiology of clinical states associated with deranged volume homeostasis, such as advanced liver disease. Thus, water immersion has been used successfully to delineate the determinants of sodium and water retention in patients with decompensated cirrhosis[11,20,29] and nephrotic syndrome.[41,49] Similarly, the immersion model has been utilized to assess the renin–aldosterone responsiveness of anephric patients[32] and patients with secondary hyperaldosteronism.[20] Finally, the numerous similarities between the effects of water immersion and those of manned space flight on the renal and cardiovascular systems commend the use of water immersion as an experimental analogue of weightlessness.[9,36,47]

REFERENCES

1. Arborelius, N., Jr., Balldin, U. I., Lilja, B., and Lundgren, C. E. G. Hemodynamic changes in man during immersion with the head above water. *Aerospace Med.* 43:592–598, 1972.
2. Bartter, F. C. and Gann, D. S. On the hemodynamic regulation of the secretion of aldosterone. *Circulation* 21:1016–1023, 1960.
3. Bazett, H. C., Thurlow, S., Corwell, C., and Stewart, W. Studies on the effects of baths on man. II. The diuresis caused by warm baths together with some observations on urinary tides. *Am. J. Physiol.* 70:430–452, 1924.
4. Begin, R., Epstein, M., Sackner, M. A., Levinson, R., Dougherty, R., and Duncan, D. Effects of water immersion to the neck on pulmonary circulation and tissue volume in man. *J. Appl. Physiol.* 40:293–299, 1976.
5. Behn, C., Gauer, O. H., Kirsch, K., and Eckert, P. Effects of sustained intrathoracic vascular distension on body fluid distribution and renal excretion in man. *Pfluegers Arch.* 313:123–135, 1969.
6. Buckalew, V. M. Natriuretic hormone. In: *The Kidney in Liver Disease,* 3rd ed., Epstein, M. Ed., Hanley & Belfus, Philadelphia, 1996, 359–372.
7. Echt, M., Lange, L., and Gauer, O.H. Changes of peripheral venous tone and central transmural venous pressure during immersion in a thermo-neutral bath. *Pfluegers Arch.* 352:211–217, 1974.
8. Epstein, M. Renal effects of head-out water immersion in man: Implications for an understanding of volume homeostasis. *Physiol. Rev.* 58:529–581, 1978.
9. Epstein, M. Renal effects of head-out water immersion in humans: A 15 year update. *Physiol. Rev.* 72:563–621, 1992.
10. Epstein, M. Studies of volume homeostasis in man utilizing the model of head-out water immersion. *Nephron* 22:9–19, 1978.
11. Epstein, M. Renal sodium handling in liver disease. In: *The Kidney in Liver Disease*, 4th ed., Epstein, M., Ed., Hanley & Belfus, Philadelphia, 1996, 3–31.
12. Epstein, M., Bricker, N. S., and Bourgoignie, J. J.. The presence of a natriuretic factor in urine of normal men undergoing water immersion. *Kidney Int.* 13:152–158, 1978.
13. Epstein, M. and De Micheli, A. G. Natriuretic effects of calcium antagonists. In: Epstein, M., *Calcium Antagonists In Clinical Medicine.* Hanley & Belfus, Philadelphia, 1992, 349–366.
14. Epstein, M., DeNunzio, A. G., and Loutzenhiser, R. D. Effects of vasopressin administration on diuresis of water immersion in normal humans. *J. Appl. Physiol.* 51:1384–1387, 1981.
15. Epstein, M., DeNunzio, A. G., and Ramachandran, M. Characterization of the renal response to prolonged immersion in normal man. Implications for an understanding of the circulatory adaptation to manned spaceflight. *J. Appl. Physiol.* 49:184–188, 1980.

16. Epstein, M., Duncan, D., and Fishman, L. M. Characterization of the natriuresis caused in normal man by immersion in water. *Clin. Sci.* 43:275–287, 1972.
17. Epstein, M., Duncan, D. C., and Meek, B. The role of posture in the natriuresis of water immersion in normal man. *Proc. Soc. Exp. Biol. Med.* 142:124–127, 1973.
18. Epstein, M. and Gerzer, R. Natriuretic peptides and the kidney. In: Massry, S. G. and Glassock, R. J., Eds., *Textbook of Nephrology.* Vol. 1, 3rd ed. Williams & Wilkins, Baltimore, 1995. 227–231.
19. Epstein, M., Katsikas, J. L., and Duncan, D.C. Role of mineralocorticoids in the natriuresis of water immersion in normal man. *Circ. Res.* 32:228–236, 1973.
20. Epstein, M., Levinson, R., Sancho, J., Haber, E., and Re, R. Characterization of the renin-aldosterone system in decompensated cirrhosis. *Circ. Res.* 41:818–829, 1977.
21. Epstein, M. and Lifschitz, M. Volume status as a determinant of the influence of renal PGE on renal function. *Nephron* 25:157–159, 1980.
22. Epstein, M., Lifschitz, M., Hoffman, D. S., and Stein, J. H. Relationship between renal prostaglandin E and renal sodium handling during water immersion in normal man. *Circ. Res.* 45:71–80, 1979.
23. Epstein, M., Lifschitz, M., Re, R., and Haber, E. Dissociation of renin-aldosterone and renal prostaglandin E during volume expansion induced by immersion in normal man. *Clin. Sci.* 59:55–62, 1980.
24. Epstein, M., Loutzenhiser, R. D., Friedland, E., Aceto, R. M., Camargo, M. J. F., and Atlas, S. A. Relationship of increased plasma ANF and renal sodium handling during immersion-induced central hypervolemia in normal humans. *J. Clin. Invest.* 79:738–745, 1987.
25. Epstein, M., Loutzenhiser, R. D., and Levinson, R. Spectrum of deranged sodium homeostasis in essential hypertension. *Hypertension,* 8:422–432, 1986.
26. Epstein, M., Miller, M., and Schneider, N. S. Depth of immersion as a determinant of the natriuresis of water immersion. *Proc. Soc. Exp. Biol. Med.* 146:562–566, 1974.
27. Epstein, M., Pins, D. S., and Miller, M. Suppression of ADH during water immersion in normal man. *J. Appl. Physiol.* 38:1038–1044, 1975.
28. Epstein, M., Pins, D. S., Sancho, J., and Haber, E. Suppression of plasma renin and plasma aldosterone during water immersion in normal man. *J. Clin. Endocrinol. Metab.* 41:618–625, 1975.
29. Epstein, M., Pins, D. S., Schneider, N., and Levinson, R. Determinants of deranged sodium and water homeostasis in decompensated cirrhosis. *J. Lab. Clin. Med.* 87:822–839, 1976.
30. Epstein, M., Preston, S., and Weitzman, R. E. Iso-osmotic central blood volume expansion suppresses plasma arginine vasopressin in normal man. *J. Clin. Endocrinol. Metab.* 52:256–262, 1981.
31. Epstein, M., Re, R., Preston, S., and Haber, E. Comparison of suppressive effects of water immersion and saline administration on renin-aldosterone in normal man. *J. Clin. Endocrinol. Metab.* 49:358–363, 1979.
32. Epstein, M., Sancho, J., Perez, G., Haber, E., Re, R., and Loutzenhiser, R. Volume as a determinant of plasma aldosterone in anephric man. *J. Clin. Endocrinol. Metab.* 46:309–316, 1978.
33. Epstein, M. and Saruta, T. Effect of water immersion on renin-aldosterone and renal sodium handling in normal man. *J. Appl. Physiol.* 31:368–374, 1971.
34. Gabrielsen, A., Johansen, L. B., and Norsk, P. Central cardiovascular pressures during graded water immersion in humans. *J. Appl. Physiol.* 75:581–585, 1993.
35. Gauer, O. H. Mechanoreceptors in the intrathoracic circulation and plasma volume control. In: *The Kidney in Liver Disease,* Epstein, M., Ed., Elsevier, New York, 1978, 3–17.
36. Gauer, O. H., Henry, J. P., and Behn, C. The regulation of extracellular fluid volume. *Ann. Rev. Physiol.* 32:547–595, 1970.
37. Goodall, M., McCally, M., and Graveline, D. E. Urinary adrenaline and noradrenaline response to simulated weightless state. *Am. J. Physiol.* 206:431–436, 1964.

38. Gower, W. R., Jr., Chiou, S., Skolnick, K., and Vesely, D. L. Molecular forms of circulating atrial natriuretic peptides in human plasma and their metabolites. *Peptides,* 15:861–867, 1994.
39. Grossman, E., Goldstein, D. S., Hoffman, A., Wacks, I. R., and Epstein, M. The effects of water immersion on the sympathoadrenal and dopa-dopamine systems in humans. *Am. J. Physiol.* 262:R993–R999, 1992.
40. Hamlyn, J. M., Blaustein, M. P., Bova, S., DuCharme, D. W., Harris, D. W., Mandel, F., Mathews, W. R., and Ludens, J. H. Identification and characterization of a ouabain-like compound from human plasma. *Proc. Natl. Acad. Sci. U.S.A.* 88:6259–6263, 1991.
41. Krishna, G. G. and Danovitch, G. M. Effects of water immersion on renal function in the nephrotic syndrome. *Kidney Int.* 21:393–401, 1982.
42. Lange, L., Lange, S., Echt, M., and Gauer, O. H. Heart volume in relation to body posture and immersion in a thermo-neutral bath. A roentgenometric study. *Pfluegers Arch.* 352:219–226, 1974.
43. Levinson, R., Epstein, M., Sackner, M. A., and Begin, R. Comparison of the effects of water immersion and saline infusion on cerebral haemodynamics in man. *Clin. Sci. Mol. Med.* 52:343–350, 1977.
44. Maack, T., Camargo, M. J. F., Kleinert, H. D., Laragh, J. N., and Atlas, S. A. Atrial natriuretic factor: Structure end function properties. *Kidney Int.* 27:607–615, 1985.
45. Martin, D. M., Peavahouse, J. B., Trigg, D. J., Vesely, D. L., and Beurkert, J. E. Three peptides from the ANF prohormone NH_2-terminus are natriuretic and/or kaliuretic. *Am. J. Physiol.* 258:F1401–F1408, 1990.
46. Needleman, P., Adams, S. P., Cole, B. R., et al. Atriopeptins as cardiac hormones. *Hypertension* 7:469–482, 1985.
47. Norsk, P. and Epstein, M. Manned space flight and the kidney. *Am. J. Nephrol.* 11:81–97, 1991.
48. Norsk, P., Drummer, C., Johansen, L. B., and Gerzer, R. Effect of water immersion on renal natriuretic peptide (urodilatin) excretion in humans. *J. Appl. Physiol.* 74:2881–2885, 1993.
49. Peterson, C., Madsen, B., Perlman, A., Chan, A. Y. M., and Myers, B. D. Atrial natriuretic peptide and the renal response to hypervolemia in nephrotic man, *Kidney Int.* 34:825–831, 1988.
50. Rabelink, T. J., Koomans, H. A., Boer, W. H., Van Rijn, H. J., and Mees, E. J. D. Lithium clearance in water immersion-induced natriuresis in humans, *J. Appl. Physiol.* 66:1744–1748, 1989.
51. Skipka, W. K., Deck, A., and Bonning, D. Effect of physical fitness on vanillylmandelic acid excretion during immersion. *Eur. J. Appl. Physiol. Occup. Physiol.* 35:271–276, 1976.
52. Vesely, D. L., Atrial natriuretic hormones. Prentice Hall, Englewood Cliffs, NJ, 1992, 1–256.
53. Vesely, D. L., Douglass, M. A., Dietz, J. R., Giordano, A. T., McCormick, M. T., Rodriguez-Paz, G., and Schocken, D. D. Negative feedback of atrial natriuretic peptides. *J. Clin. Endocrinol. Metab.* 78:1128–1134, 1994.
54. Vesely, D. L., Douglass, M. A., Dietz, J. R., Giordano, A. T., McCormick, M. T., Rodriguez-Paz, G., and Schocken, D. D. Prohormone atrial natriuretic peptide 79-98 (kaliuretic stimulator) lowers blood pressure and increases potassium excretion. *Circulation* 88:I331, 1993.
55. Vesely, D. L., Douglass, M. A., Dietz, J. R., Gower, W. R., Jr., McCormick, M. T., Rodriguez-Paz, G., and Schocken, D. D. Three peptides from the atrial natriuretic factor prohormone amino terminus lower blood pressure and produce a diuresis, natriuresis, and/or kaliuresis in humans. *Circulation* 90:1129–1140, 1994.

Part III

SPECIAL CONSIDERATIONS IN REGARD TO BODY FLUID BALANCE DURING EXERCISE

Chapter 11

AGE, GENDER, AND FLUID BALANCE

Marta D. Van Loan
Richard A. Boileau

CONTENTS

I. Introduction...215

II. Fluid Compartments......................................216

III. Fluid Volume: Infancy, Childhood, and Adolescence...........216
   A. Infancy...216
   B. Childhood and Adolescence...........................217

IV. Young, Middle-Aged, and Older Adults......................223

V. Summary...228

References..229

I. INTRODUCTION

The essential molecule of life — water. Water is the single largest component of the body, representing about 50–70% of body weight for the adult man and about 40–60% of body weight for the average adult woman. Moreover, water normally comprises about 72% of the lean body mass (LBM) or fat-free mass (FFM) for both young adult men and women. Infants, on the other hand, contain more fluid than adults relative to their body weight, consisting of about 70-85% of body weight as water.[8] The wide range of values for the proportion of total body water to body weight (TBW/WT) among individuals is primarily a function of the amount of body fat, inasmuch as fat in adipose tissue is a major contributor to an increase in WT without a corresponding increase in TBW. Maintenance of proper fluid balance is necessary for a variety of biological functions — adequate blood volume, the integrity of the cardiovascular system, providing an environment for biochemical reactions in cells, and the regulation of body temperature, to name a few. Failure to maintain a proper fluid balance can affect an individual's health such that cognitive function and physical performance are diminished or impaired; more serious health consequences such as hypertension and pulmonary edema can also occur.

To understand fluid balance, one must first recognize the various compartments through which water is distributed. In this chapter we will focus on the fluid compartments' changes with growth and development, the possible differences between genders, and the changes associated with aging.

II. FLUID COMPARTMENTS

Normally the FFM of an individual contains 72–73% water. Therefore, the larger the FFM the greater the amount of TBW, with the cells of the FFM constituting the largest reservoir of body water.

TBW is partitioned into two basic compartments, intracellular and extracellular. Intracellular fluid (ICF) is confined to the cells and comprises about 40–50% of WT. The extracellular fluid (ECF) space consists of several compartments, among which are the interstitial, plasma, intraocular, cerebrospinal, and bone fluid spaces. Water between the cells and blood vessels, or *interstitial water*, is 10–15% of adult WT; however, in an infant most of the fluid in the body is found in the interstitial space. Water found in the plasma, referred to as *intravascular fluid*, is responsible for maintaining a constant blood volume and constitutes about 4–5% body weight. The combination of interstitial fluid and intravascular fluid is ECF, which makes up approximately 17–20% of WT (Figure 1). In our discussion of TBW and its various compartments, it is important to acknowledge that these water compartments are dynamic in nature and that water flows back and forth between compartments as needed to maintain fluid homeostasis and the integrity of the organism.

III. FLUID VOLUME: INFANCY, CHILDHOOD, AND ADOLESCENCE

A. INFANCY

McCance and Widdowson[21] described the body as consisting of a watery part and fat; the watery part was subdivided into two fractions, the cell mass and the extracellular fluids. They also noted that the newborn infant contained a higher proportion of water than the adult, specifically about 82% of the FFM. Fomon and colleagues,[8,9] in an analysis of several studies, reported that at birth boys and girls did not differ in water, fat, protein, or osseous and nonosseous mineral contents. Furthermore, they found that about 61% of the TBW pool

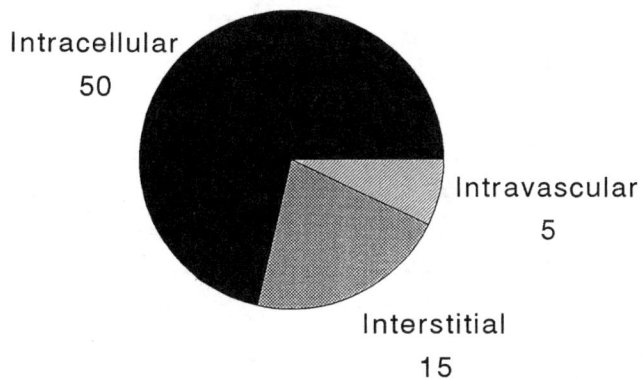

FIGURE 1 Body water compartments as a percentage of body weight.

was ECF, with about 39% ICF, giving an ECF/ICF ratio of about 1.5 for newborn boys and girls. As a percentage of FFM, however, TBW accounts for about 79–80%.

During the early months of life, WT increases progressively, with almost a threefold increase by the age of 1 year. According to Guo et al.[13] the rate of weight gain is greatest in the first 2 months of life, with an average increase of 33 g/d for boys and 28 g/d for girls. During this time the most notable change is a large shift in the distribution of water between the ECF and ICF compartments. Although there is only a slight increase in absolute amount of TBW (1–2%), it is representative of an overall decrease in %TBW. Generally, ECF decreases from about 50% of FFM to almost 42% while ICF increases from about 30 to 37% of FFM. These changes are similar for both boys and girls (Table 1). Friis-Hansen and colleagues[12] also observed a decline in %TBW from birth through the first year. Values varied from 70 to 83% of body weight in newborn babies, declining to 53–65% from 6 months to 1 year.

B. CHILDHOOD AND ADOLESCENCE

Gradual changes continue throughout childhood and by 2 years of age the proportion of ECF drops another 2%, with a corresponding increase in ICF. By the age of 5 years, however, gender differences begin to appear in the distribution of TBW. As a percentage of FFM, TBW declines slowly from the value observed at 1 year (79%) to about 77% by 5 years of age (Table 1). During this period, the decrease in ECF and the increase in ICF, proportional to TBW, is larger in boys than girls. This change most likely is indicative of a larger cell mass in the boys compared to the girls. As a percentage of WT, TBW declines from about 70% at birth for both boys and girls to about 65% for boys and 62% for girls by 10 years of age, based on the analyses of Fomon et al.[9] (Table 1; Figure 2).

TABLE 1 Body Fluids as a Percentage of Body Weight from Infancy through Adolescence by Age, Gender, and Race[a]

Author (Age)	Males			Females		
	TBW	ECF	ICF	TBW	ECF	ICF
Foman						
(birth)	69.6 (80.6)	42.5 (49.3)	27.0 (31.3)	68.6 (80.6)	42.0 (49.3)	26.7 (31.3)
(1 yr)	61.2 (79.0)	32.9 (42.5)	28.3 (36.5)	60.1 (78.8)	31.8 (41.6)	28.3 (37.1)
(2 yr)	62.9 (78.1)	31.9 (39.6)	31.0 (38.5)	62.2 (78.2)	31.5 (39.5)	30.8 (38.7)
(5 yr)	65.4 (76.6)	30.0 (35.2)	35.4 (41.4)	64.6 (77.6)	31.0 (37.3)	33.6 (40.3)
(10 yr)	64.8 (75.1)	26.7 (31.0)	38.0 (44.1)	62.0 (76.9)	28.1 (34.9)	33.9 (42.0)
Fris-Hansen						
(birth)	78.6					
(9 mo–1yr)	56–53					
(2 1/2 yr)	58.5					
(7 yr)	59.3					
(11 yr)	53.4					
Boileau et al.						
(Prepub) W	59.7 (75.1)			58.5 (76.0)		
(Prepub) B	66.2 (74.7)			59.1 (75.4)		
(Pubesc) W	60.8 (75.0)			54.7 (74.6)		
(Pubesc) B	64.5 (74.5)			58.1 (76.3)		
(Post) W	61.0 (73.2)			54.9 (73.3)		
(Post) B	64.8 (73.3)			56.7 (74.1)		
Haschke et al.						
(9 yr)	65.4 (75.5)					
(11 yr)	63.6					
(12 yr)	63.0					

Age, Gender, and Fluid Balance

(13 yr)	63.5	
(14 yr)	65.2	
(15 yr)	65.5	
Hunt & Heald		
(12 yr)	61.4	
(13 yr)	61.6 (80–89)	
(14 yr)	62.9	
(15 yr)	63.1 (70–79)	
(16 yr)	64.8	
(17 yr)	64.9	
(18 yr)	64.3	
Bruce et al.		
(6 yr) M & F	48.8	26.1
(11 yr)	51.9	25.6
(17 yr)	49.9	25.5
Schutte		
(10–11 yr)	60.9	22.8
(11–12 yr)	58.6	26.3
(12–13 yr)	59.2	24.2
(13–14 yr)	62.2	
(14–15 yr)	62.1	
(15–16 yr)	64.0	
(16–17 yr)	62.0	
(17–18 yr)	60.4	

[a] Values are percentage of WT, with percentage of FFM shown in parentheses.

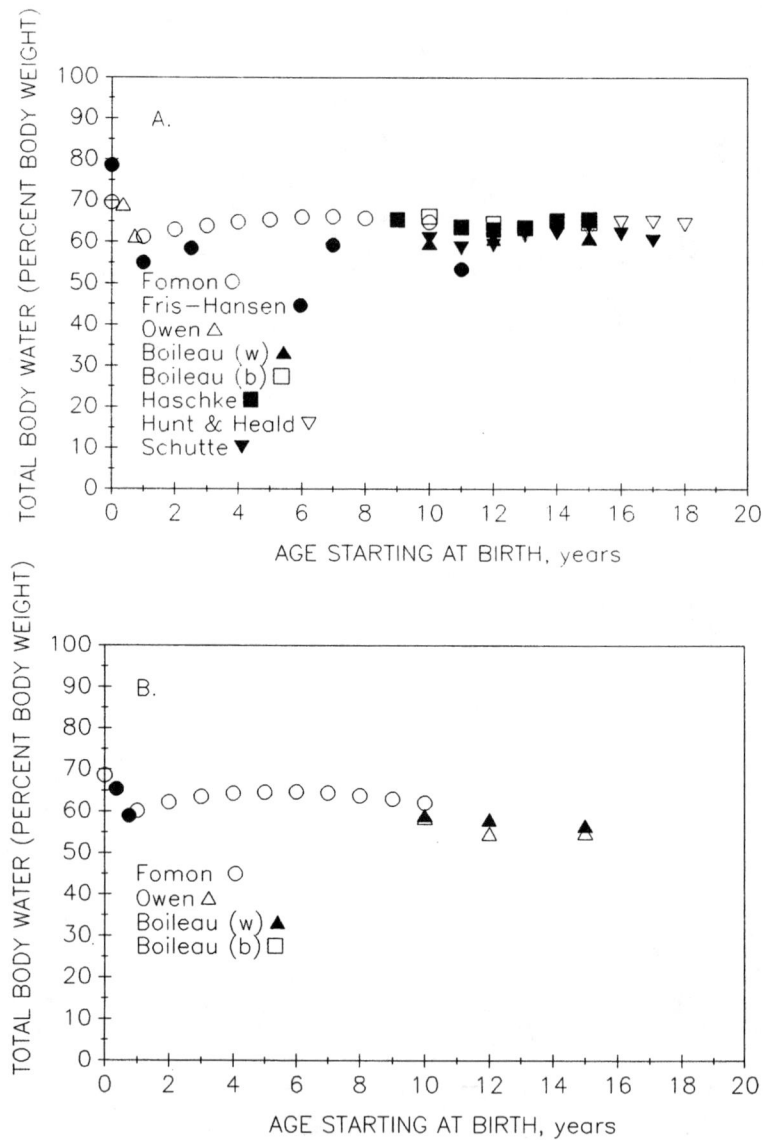

FIGURE 2 Total body water as a percentage of body weight for males (A) and females (B) from birth through adolescence.

Similar changes in the various body compartments continue over the next 5 years. By the age of 10, the water content of FFM is about 75 and 77%, respectively, for boys and girls. Boys continue to show a larger increase in ICF compared to girls.

Boileau and co-workers[3] examined racial, gender, and age differences by comparing changes among African-American and Caucasian children and adults. They found that TBW/WT was higher in males (61.6%) than in females (55.8%), with the largest differences in the pubertal, postpubertal, and adult groups. Additionally, TBW/FFM decreased from prepubescence (75% boys, 76% girls) to young adulthood (72% males, 73% females) by 0.38% annually, resulting in an overall decline of 2.8% in each gender. Additional cross-sectional data by Boileau et al. at the University of Illinois (personal communication) on 395 children and youth ages 7–17 years are represented in Figure 3. A gradual decrease in the water fraction (FW) of WT is observed for both boys and girls through the age of 12 years, with girls continuing to decrease thereafter. In boys, however, the FW increases abruptly at ages 12–13 years and remains significantly higher than in girls. This increase in the FW of boys is associated with a relative decrease in body fatness as well as an increase in the absolute FFM. Also shown in Figure 3 is the age-related change in water content of the FFM, with the FFM computation based on a four-compartment model from density, TBW, and bone mineral measurements. A decrease of 1–2% in the fraction of water in fat-free mass (FWFFM) was noted in both boys and girls in spite of an absolute increase in TBW over the age range. The decrease in FWFFM with age and maturation in children is consistent with observations in other studies.[3,9,18]

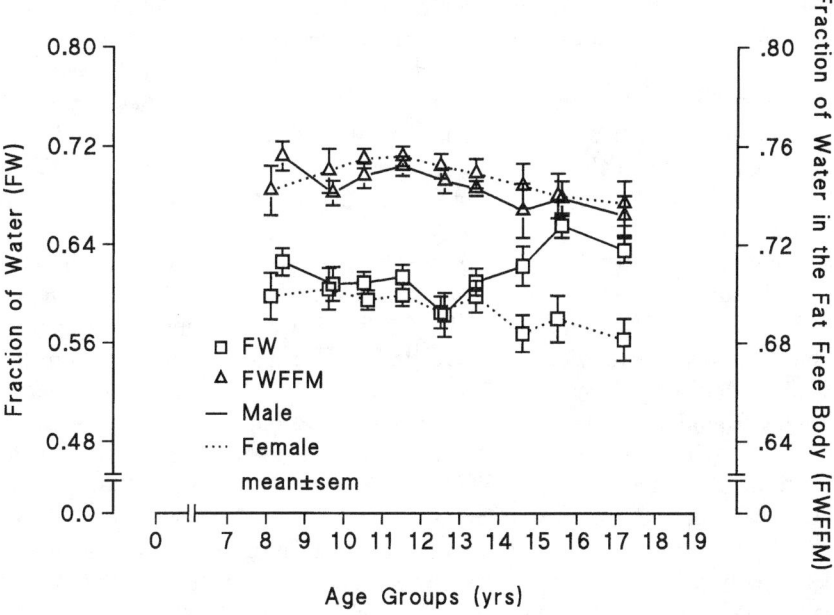

FIGURE 3 Total bodywater as a fraction of body weight (left axis) and as a fraction of fat-free mass (right axis) in boys and girls.

Haschke[14,15] found that TBW/WT decreased between 9 and 11 years of age, remained stable through 13 years of age, and increased again through the age of 14. Hunt and Heald[18] examined body constituents in adolescent boys 12–18 years of age. TBW was estimated using deuterium dilution and expressed as a percentage of WT. In addition, body composition was measured by densitometry, enabling estimation of the FWFFM. They determined that mature hydration was attained by about 11 years of age; however, this has not been generally confirmed by other investigators. Subsequent analysis by Lohman et al.[20] revealed a decline across the 12–18 age range in FWFFM of about 0.5% per year. Schutte[28] in his investigation of racial differences across age found that in African-American boys 10–18 years of age, TBW as a percentage of WT, fluctuated from 58 to 60% between 10 and 13 years of age, to a high of 64% at 16 years and was followed by a slight decline to 60% by 18 years. More recently, Hewitt et al.[16] examined the effects of hydration level on the estimation of fat mass (FM) in children (ages 5–10), young adults (ages 22-39), and older adults (ages 65-84). FFM was estimated from the four-compartment model. Comparisons were made between the traditional two-compartment model and the multicompartment model to determine the extent to which estimates of FM were influenced by variation in the TBW/FFM ratio. The water content of WT was higher in the boys and girls than either the young adults or older adults. The mean values for children ranged from 57.2% for the girls to 63.0% for the boys, whereas the adults had values of 59% or less. Using results from the multicompartment model, TBW/FFM ratios were determined and, based on the four-compartment model, found that the boys and girls had FWFFM values of 73.1 and 72.2%, respectively. The corresponding values for the adult groups were between 70.7 and 72.6%. They concluded that, when adjustments were made to the calculation of FFM for variation in body constituents such as TBW and bone mineral, the TBW/FFM ratio in children was similar to that of adults, a finding that disagrees with the data presented in Figure 4.

Studies by Schutte[28] and Slaughter[29] have focused on differences in TBW between African-American and Caucasian children. Schutte found a significant difference in TBW per unit of height (TBW/HT) when comparing the results from 172 African-American boys, 10–18 years of age, with results from the work of Mellits and Cheek[23] on Caucasian children and adolescents. However, Schutte found no differences between racial groups when expressed as TBW/WT. These results are similar to those of Slaughter et al.[30] for boys. In addition, Slaughter et al. examined the relationship between TBW/HT and TBW/WT in both African-American and Caucasian girls. Again, no differences were found between the racial groups within a given gender group; however, between the gender groups girls had lower values for both TBW and TBW/WT compared to the boys. For the boys, TBW values ranged from 60.0 to 62.7% of WT compared to 54.9 to 55.2% for the girls.

Clearly, major changes take place during this growth period. The changes include: (1) a shift or decrease in the proportion of extracellular fluid, (2) an

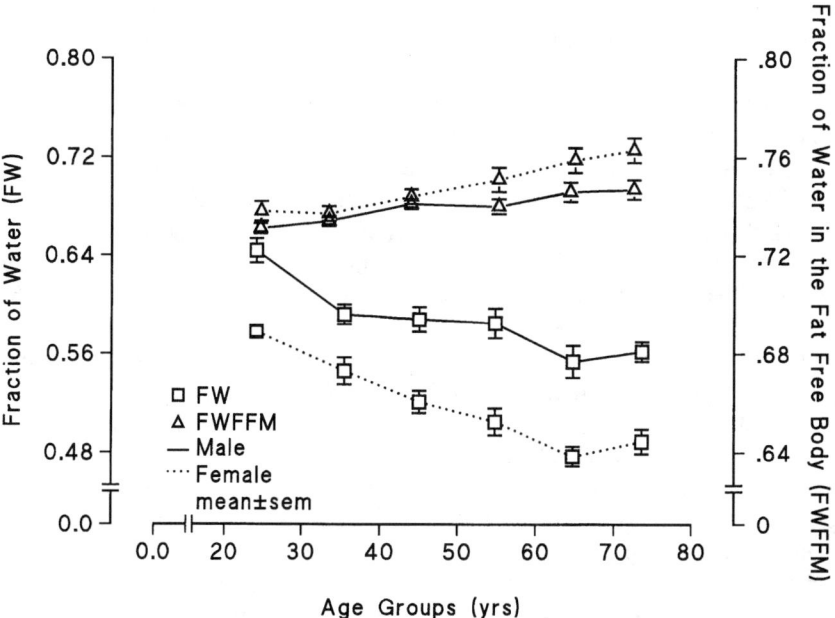

FIGURE 4 Total bodywater as a fraction of body weight (left axis) and as a fraction of fat-free mass (right axis) in adult men and women.

increase in the amount of intracellular fluid commensurate with an increase in FFM, and (3) a decrease in the water fraction of the FFM. These changes are supported by the data presented in Table 1 and are considered to be representative of the changes taking place in growing children. However, there is a noticeable lack of data documenting changes in fluid compartments for children of Asian or Hispanic ancestry.

IV. YOUNG, MIDDLE-AGED, AND OLDER ADULTS

Based primarily on results obtained from animal research, Moulton[24] suggested that chemical maturity was reached at 4.4% of the life expectancy. Using a life expectancy of 80 years for human beings and Moulton's 4.4% value, one might conclude that chemical maturation in the human is reached at about 3.5 years of age. The data discussed earlier in this chapter, relative to changes in body fluids, suggest that 3.5 years of age does not coincide with chemical stability or maturation in the human. Nonetheless, animal research can provide valuable information about the composition of mature species. For example, Pace and Rathbun,[26] using guinea pigs, determined that the water content of FFM was 72.4% and the N/FFM ratio was 3.5% with similar results observed in the rat, rabbit, cat, dog, and monkey. As for the chemical growth of male human beings, Forbes[11] observed that changes in Na, K, and water, from midfetal life to young adulthood followed a differential curve. He calculated that in young adulthood 54% of WT was water, while Allen and colleagues[1] determined that on the average there was 0.784 kg of water/kg of WT less bone mineral and fat. Allen et al. further noted in their study of body composition in a group of men ($n = 23$) and women ($n = 7$) that the water content of the body fluctuated between 0.816 kg/kg WT to 0.752 kg/kg WT (less bone and fat) depending on when the TBW determination was made relative to the last ingestion of fluid by the individual. They observed values ranging from 45 to 65% water in body weight. Research by Edelman et al.[7] using a multiple-tracer dilution technique, also found TBW/WT ratios ranging from 51.5 to 62.0% for women and men, respectively. Additional fluid measurements made by Edelman and others included the exchangeable sodium and potassium spaces, as measures of ECF and ICF compartments. Their results suggest that ECF ranges from 40.7 to 46.8%, and ICF values are 41.0–41.4% of WT for adult women and men. Edleman et al. also point out that these values may vary depending on the methods employed for estimating ECF. Furthermore, "true" ICF, when using exchangeable sodium as the tracer, is not simply the result of subtracting ECF from TBW because the resulting value includes some bone matrix sodium. Lesser et al.,[19] using inert gases and isotope tracer techniques, assessed changes in TBW, FFM, and FM in men and women aged 19 to 68 years studied cross-sectionally. These investigators noted a decrease in the TBW/FFM ratio with age; the means were 71.4, 70.7, and 70.5% for age groups that were 19–29 years, 30–41 years, and 59–68 years of age, respectively. In addition, they noted a decrease in the ICF fraction with aging and a corresponding increase in the ECF fraction.

Cohn et al.[5,6] in a study of 123 healthy adults, 20–79 years of age, showed that FFM decreased with age by about 12% and 19% for males and females, respectively. Like Bruce et al.[4] Cohn et al.[5,6] also observed a decline in TBW with age by about 6 l for each gender; this was equivalent to a decrease of 12% in women and 17% in men. Relative to WT, the largest proportion of TBW was observed in both men and women between 20 and 29 years of age with average values of 59.0 and 50.7%, respectively. Similar to Bruce et al.[4] TBW/WT declined to 50.5% for men and 44.9% for women 70–79 years of age. In relation to FFM, the fraction variation ranged from 73.9% for 30–39-year-old men to 80.7% for 50–59-year-old men followed by a decline to 80.1% at 70–79 years. For women, TBW/FFM ratio ranged from 74.9% during the 20–39 age span to 86.0% at 50–59 years, declining to 80.1% at 70–79 years. Although the work by Cohn and colleagues may be considered the most extensive work to date to examine multiple body compartments using highly sophisticated techniques, it is limited as in most other studies somewhat because of its cross-sectional approach to changes associated with aging rather than following individuals longitudinally. Boileau and co-workers (personal communication) collected TBW data on 307 men and women ages 20–80 and expressed them as FW and FWFFM. The FWFFM was based on body composition analysis employing the four-compartment model. FW was higher for males in all decades and decreased across age for both sexes. Mean differences of 7.5 l (15%) and 3.5 l (11%) were observed across the age ranges for males and females, respectively. Interestingly, the FWFFM increased by about 2% in both males and females, a result in general agreement with Cohn et al.[6] but not always observed in other samples.

Research by Baumgartner et al.[2] also demonstrated a change in TBW in elderly people. In a cross-sectional study of 98 men and women ages 65–94, the authors found that the aqueous fraction of WT was 57% for men and 51% for women. They also determined, using a four-compartment model, that the water fraction of FFM averaged 74.3% and 74.4% for men and women, respectively. These investigators noted that "it has not been established that the ECF/ICF ratio changes systematically with aging" but they offered the suggestion that the variance of the ratio increases in older individuals thus giving an impression of an overall change associated with aging. Schoeller,[27] in a review of the literature, found that TBW decreases with age and, for women, the decrease is small up to age 60 and declines rapidly after 60. For men, however, the decrease in TBW starts in middle age and continues through old age. In spite of the decrease in TBW, Schoeller found that the average hydration of FFM remained constant, indicating a general decrease in FFM with age.

Heymsfield et al.[17] using neutron activation techniques, assessed multiple body compartments from *in vivo* elemental analysis. In a group of men ($n = 8$) and women ($n = 12$) whose average ages were 65 and 55, respectively, they found that TBW/WT was 58.8% for men, 53.3% for women, and 55.8% for the total group; as a fraction of FFM, water was 72.5% for this group. In two separate studies — Osserman et al.,[25] with young men, and McMurrey et al.,[22] with young men and women — in which subjects' average ages ranged from 27 to 37, TBW/WT ranged from 61% for Osserman's young men to 54.3 and 48.6% for McMurrey's young men and women, respectively. These values are similar to those reported by Heymsfield et al.[17] in the older group of individuals, suggesting that during the middle-aged years fluid volumes remain stable. Osserman and co-workers[24] also found that water represented 71.7% of the total FFM. In one of the larger studies conducted with women, Young et al.[30] compared a group of young women, ages 16–30, with older women, 30–70. They found that in the 16–30 age group TBW represented 51.7% of WT and remained stable between ages 30–40 and 40–50 with average values of 49.3% and 48.6%, respectively. However, starting with the 50–60 age group and continuing through the 60–70 age group, TBW/WT declined to values of 44.1% and 42.2%.

Further research conducted by Pierson et al.[27] with adult men ($n = 30$; ages 20–80) and women ($n = 28$; ages 19–73) confirmed the findings of others by demonstrating that TBW/WT was higher in men than women, with values ranging from about 65% WT at age 20, and that the water content of the body declined with age, to about 58% WT for men and 52% WT for women. This is indicative of a faster rate of loss for women compared to men.

TABLE 2 Body Fluids of Young, Middle-Aged, and Older Men and Women[a]

Author (Age)	Males			Females		
	TBW	ECF	ICF	TBW	ECF	ICF
Hewitt et al.						
(31 mean age)	59.4 (71.4)		(33 mean age)	52.3 (71.1)		
(70 mean age)	51.9 (73.0)			46.0 (72.7)		
Edelman et al.	62.0	41.4	46.8	51.5	41.0	40.7
Lesser et al.						
(19–29 yr) M & F	56.2 (71.4)	14.8 (18.2)	42.6 (52.9)			
(30–41 yr) M & F	56.5 (70.7)					
(59–68 yr) M & F	45.4 (70.5)	13.6 (21.0)	31.7 (49.5)			
Bruce et al.						
(20–29 yr) M & F	52.4	25.8	26.5			
(30–39 yr) M & F	55.1	25.3	29.8			
(40–49 yr) M & F	56.3	27.6	28.7			
(50–59 yr) M & F	48.6	25.6	22.9			
Cohn et al.						
(20–29 yr)	59.0 (76.3)	24.2	31.4	53.7 (74.9)	24.3	27.0
(30–39 yr)	56.3 (75.9)	26.2	32.4	49.8 (74.9)	24.4	24.7

(40–49 yr)	55.5 (80.4)	23.5	32.0	49.0 (80.2)	24.5	23.7
(50–59 yr)	54.9 (80.7)	24.6	30.4	43.7 (86.0)	22.0	22.3
(60–69 yr)	52.1 (78.8)	25.6	28.0	45.2 (82.6)	24.0	21.7
(70–79 yr)	50.5 (85.4)	25.1	25.4	44.9 (80.1)	25.0	22.3
Baumgartner et al.						
(74–75 yr)	57.0 (74.3)			51.0 (74.4)		
Heymsfield et al.						
(55 yr)	58.8			53.3		
(65 yr)						
Osserman et al.						
(18–46 yr)	61.0 (71.8)					
McMurrey et al.						
(23–54 yr)	54.3	23.4	30.9	48.6	22.8	25.8
Young et al.						
(16–30 yr)				51.7		
(30–40 yr)				49.3		
(40–50 yr)				48.6		
(50–60 yr)				44.1		
(60–70 yr)				42.2		

[a]Values are a percentage of WT, with percentage of FFM shown in parentheses.

Researchers in Sweden[4] studied 134 males and 342 females, ages 20–70, and found that TBW/WT gradually declined from 61.4% at age 26 to 51.8% at 61. They also observed a decline in ICF/WT from a high of 29.8% in the fourth decade to a low of 22.9% in the sixth decade. Furthermore, this decline in ICF/WT could not be entirely explained by a corresponding increase in WT in older individuals, suggesting that there may be a loss of FFM occurring as part of the aging process. Forbes,[10] in a review of research with older individuals, also reported that the decline in TBW observed with aging was due to the loss of ICF volume, although ECF remained constant. As a result, the ratio of ECF/TBW rose with age, from an average of 0.42 at 30 years to 0.48 at 80 years. The ECF/ICF ratios also rose from 0.72 to 0.92, respectively. McMurrey and others[22] also measured ECF and ICF volumes for both men and women. For men, ECF/WT was 23.4% and ICF/WT was 30.9% while the same ratios for women were 22.8% and 25.8%, respectively. The larger ICF/WT fraction for men is indicative of a larger FFM compared to women. Pierson et al.[27] also observed a gradual loss in ECF relative to weight with age for men, while for women ECF did not change significantly with age. ICF was similar for both genders, relative to weight, in the young adult years but decreased markedly with age, the decline being 50% steeper in women than men. The authors suggest that the loss of skeletal muscle (approximately 80% ICF by weight) and its replacement by an increase in adipose tissue (about 3% ICF), explains the decline in ICF for both genders. The ECF/ICF ratio shows a gradual increase with age in both genders, the increase resulting from the decrease in ICF, primarily.

V. SUMMARY

Body fluid volumes change with growth and development and with the aging process; however, more similarities exist than initially are apparent. Fluid changes during infancy are the most dramatic fluid changes in the life cycle because they occur in a relatively short period of time, with an 8–9% decline in TBW/WT during the first year of life. From 1 to 10 years of age, fluid volume changes are more gradual; ECF declines and ICF increases in both genders. The TBW/WT value reported by Fomon[9] for 10-year-old boys is similar to values reported by several others [3,14,15,18] for postpubescent and adolescent boys up to age 18. A lack of data for girls makes similar comparison impossible. Data for fluid volumes in young, middle-aged, and older adults demonstrate stability from young adulthood through middle age, with values for TBW/WT ranging from 55 to 60% for men and 50 to 55% for women. Similarly, ECF and ICF values, referenced to WT, also remain stable for these same age groups with values about 25% for ECF for both genders, and ICF about 32% for men and about 25% for women. In the older age groups, (over 60 years), TBW/WT declines average about 50% for men and about 45% for women. Although ECF remains stable for older individuals,

ICF shows a decline to about 25–28% of WT for men and 21–22% for women. Finally, the fluid changes associated with age and gender can be summarized by the work of Pierson et al.,[27] who showed that: (1) TBW as a percentage of WT was slightly higher in men at all ages, primarily due to the larger FFM; (2) water content decreases with age in both genders but the rate of decline is faster in women; (3) extracellular water is similar in both men and women initially but males lose ECF/WT with age, whereas females show no significant change in ECF/WT with age; (4) ICF starts at similar levels for both men and women and demonstrates a steep decline with age; and (5) ECF/ICF ratio generally increases with age in both sexes primarily due to a decrease in ICF.

In conclusion, adults as well as children and adolescents experience changes in body fluid compartments. During the adult years, however, the changes are slower. Changes in body fluids during the adult years, particularly in middle-aged and older adults, suffer from a lack of longitudinal data; most results are from cross-sectional studies and may not be representative of changes at the individual level.

REFERENCES

1. Allen, T. H., Welch, B. E., Trujillo, T. T., and Roberts. J. E. Fat, water and tissue solids of the whole body less its bone mineral. *J. App. Physiol.* 14:1009–1012, 1959.
2. Baugartner, R. N., Heymsfield, S. B., Lichtman, S., et al. Body composition in elderly people: Effect of criterion estimates on predictive equations. *Am. J. Clin. Nutr.* 53:1345–53, 1991.
3. Boileau, R. A., Lohman, T. G., Slaughter, M. H., et al. Hydration of the fat-free body in children during maturation. *Hum. Biol.* 56:651–66, 1984.
4. Bruce, A., Andersson, M., Arvidsson B., and Isaksson, B. Body composition. Prediction of normal body potassium, body water and body fat in adults on the basis of body height, body weight, and age. *Scand. J. Clin. Lab. Invest.* 40:461–473, 1980.
5. Cohn, S. H., Vartsky, D., Yasumura, S. Sawitsky, A., Zanzi, I, Vaswani, A., and Ellis, K.J. Compartmental body composition based on total-body nitrogen, potassium, and calcium. *Am. J. Physiol.* 239:E524–E530, 1980.
6. Cohn, S. H., Vaswani, A., Yasumura, S., et al. Assessment of cellular mass and lean body mass by noninvasive nuclear techniques. *J. Lab. Clin. Med.* 105:305–11, 1985.
7. Edelman, I. S., Olney, J. M., James, A. H., Brooks, L., and Moore, F. D. Body composition: Studies in the human being by the dilution principle. *Science* 115:447–454, 1952.
8. Fomon, S. J. Body composition of the male reference infant during the first year of life. *Pediatrics* 40:863–70, 1967.
9. Fomon, S. J., Haschke, F., Ziegler, E. E., et al. Body composition of reference children from birth to age 10 years. *Am. J. Clin. Nutr.* 35:1169–75, 1982.
10. Forbes, G. B. *Human Body Composition: Growth, Aging, Nutrition, and Activity.* Springer-Verlag, New York, 1987, 182–184.
11. Forbes, G. B. Methods for determining composition of the human body: With a note on the effect of diet on body composition. *Pediatrics* 477–494, 1962.
12. Friis-Hansen, B. J., Holliday, M., Stapleton, T., et al. Total body water in children. Annual Meeting of the Society for Pediatric Research, 1950.
13. Guo, S., Roche, A. F., Fomon, S. J., et al. Reference data on gains in weight and length during the first two years of life. *J. Pediatr.* 119:355–62, 1991.

14. Haschke, F. Body composition of adolescent males. Part I. Total body water in normal adolescent males. Part II. Body composition of the male reference adolescent. *Acta Pediatr. Scand.* (Suppl. 307):1–23, 1983.
15. Haschke, F. Body composition during adolescence. In: *Body Composition Measurements in Infants and Children*. Report of the 98th Ross Conference. Ross Laboratories, Columbus, OH, 1987, 76-83.
16. Hewitt, M. J., Going, S. B., Williams, D. P., et al. Hydration of fat-free body mass in children and adults: Implications for body composition assessment. *Am. J. Physiol.* 265 (*Endocrinol. Metab.* 28) E88–95, 1993.
17. Heymsfield, S. B., Waki, M., Kehayias, J., et al. Chemical and elemental analysis of humans in vivo using improved body composition models. *Am. J. Physiol.* 261 (*Endocrinol. Metab.* 24):E190–98, 1991.
18. Hunt, E. E. and Heald, F. P. Physique, body composition, and sexual maturation in adolsecent boys. *Ann. N.Y. Acad. Sci.* 110:532–544, 1963.
19. Lesser, G. T., Kumar, I., and Steele, J. M. Changes in body composition with age. *Ann. N.Y. Acad. Sci.* 110:576–88, 1963.
20. Lohman, T. G., Boileau, R. A., and Slaughter, M. H. Body composition in children and youth. In: *Advances in Pediatric Sports Sciences,* Boileau, R. A., Ed., Human Kinetics Publisher, Champaign, IL. 1984, 29–57.
21. McCance, R. A. and Widdowson, E. M. A method of breaking down the body weights of living persons into terms of extracellular fluid, cell mass and fat, and some applications of it to physiology and medicine. *Proc. R. Soc. London* 138:115–130, 1951.
22. McMurrey, J. D., Boling, E. A., Davies, J. M., Parker, H. V., et al. Body composition: Simultaneous determination of several aspects by the dilution principle. *Metabolism* 7:651–667, 1958.
23. Mellits, E. D. and Cheek, D. B. Growth and bodywater. In: *Human Growth,* Cheek, D. B., Ed., Lea and Feibiger, Philadelphia, PA. 1968.
24. Moulton, C. R. Age and chemical development in mammals. *J. Biol.Sci.* 57:79–97, 1923.
25. Osserman, E. F., Pitts, G. C., Welham, W. C., and Behnke, A. R. In vivo measurements of body fat and body water in a group of normal men. *J. Appl. Physiol.* 2:633–639, 1950.
26. Pace, N. and Rathbun, E. N. Studies on body composition. III. The body water and chemically combined nitrogen content in relation to fat content. *J. Biol. Chem.* 158:685–91, 1945.
27. Pierson, R. N., Wang, J., Colt, E. W., and Neuman, P. Body composition measurements in normal man: The potassium, sodium, sulfate and tritium spaces in 58 adults. *J. Chronic Dis.* 35:419–428, 1982.
28. Schoeller, D. A. Changes in total body water with age. *Am. J. Clin. Nutr.* 50:1176–81, 1989.
29. Schutte, J. E. Prediction of total body water in adolescent males. *Hum. Biol.* 52:382–391, 1980.
30. Slaughter, M. H., Lohman, T. G., Boileau, R. A., et al. Differences in the subcomponents of fat-free body in relation to height between black and white children. *Am. J. Hum. Biol.* 2:209–17, 1990.
31. Young, C. M., Blondin, J., Tensuan, R., et al. Body composition studies of "older" women, thirty to seventy years of age. *Ann. N.Y. Acad. Sci.* 110:589–607, 1963.

Chapter 12

HORMONAL CONTROL OF FLUID BALANCE IN WOMEN DURING EXERCISE

Suzanne M. Fortney

CONTENTS

I. Introduction..232

II. Female Hormones and Body Fluids.........................232
   A. The Menstrual Cycle....................................232
      1. Hormonal Fluctuations............................232
      2. Observed Changes in Body Weight, Fluid Balance, and
         Blood Volume During the "Normal Menstrual Cycle"......233
      3. Premenstrual Syndrome...........................236
      4. Potential Mechanisms for Menstrually Induced Changes
         in Fluid Balance....................................237
   B. Oral Contraceptives, Body Fluids, Exercise.................241
   C. Pregnancy 241

III. Effect of Heat Exposure on Body Fluids in Women............242
   A. Acute Heat Exposure 242
      1. Effect of Estrogen–Progesterone on Temperature
         Regulation..242
      2. Women "Glow" Rather Than Sweat 243
      3. Blood Volume Regulation During Resting Heat Exposure...244
   B. Heat Acclimation......................................245
      1. Special Concern for Women in the Tropics 245
      2. Ability of Women to Heat Acclimate 245

IV. Effect of Exercise on Body Fluid Balance in Women 246
   A. Acute Exercise 246
      1. Acute Exercise and Water Balance 246

      2. Acute Exercise and Plasma Volume 247
      3. Dehydration–Rehydration Considerations 247
  B. Chronic Exercise..248
      1. Chronic Exercise and Blood Volume 248
      2. Chronic Exercise and Menstrual Function 249

V. Summary..250

Acknowledgments 251

References 251

I. INTRODUCTION

Fluid and electrolyte balance is tightly regulated in humans. Even during severe exercise, the decrease in blood volume is only about 5 to 10%, with a 15 to 20 mOsm/kg increase in plasma osmolality. Chronic aerobic exercise and to a lesser extent resistive exercise may result in an upward resetting of baseline fluid and electrolyte balance. Similarly, exposure to chronic heat or cold may produce a 5 to 10% shift in the baseline blood volume and electrolyte content. Precise neural and hormonal mechanisms integrate fluid intake, fluid absorption, and fluid excretion. Detailed discussions of the regulatory mechanisms for fluid and electrolyte balance are presented in Chapters 1 and 3.

In women, these same neural and hormonal mechanisms are in place to maintain a consistent baseline level of fluid and electrolyte balance. However, due to the cyclic fluctuations in female reproductive hormones, this baseline level is not constant, with blood volume varying by as much as ±10% during a normal menstrual cycle[46] and, incredibly, increasing as much as 40% during a normal, single-fetus pregnancy.[88]

A fascinating but often overlooked area of research is the study of what happens when conflicts arise between reproductive and exercise–thermal demands on fluid and electrolyte balance. "Athlete's amenorrhea" may be the result when exercise–thermal demands impinge on reproductive demands. Altered exercise or thermal responses and tolerances may be expected when reproductive demands impinge on exercise–thermal demands.

II. FEMALE HORMONES AND BODY FLUIDS

A. THE MENSTRUAL CYCLE
1. Hormonal Fluctuations

The menstrual cycle can be divided arbitrarily into two stages, the follicular or preovulatory phase and the luteal or postovulatory phase. Ovulation is defined as the day of luteinizing hormone peak and is a distinct characteristic that triggers the release of the ovum from the developing ovarian follicle.

Two primary gonadotropic hormones — luteinizing hormone and follicular stimulating hormone — are cyclically released from the anterior pituitary gland and regulate the ovarian secretion of two primary classes of female steroid hormones, estrogens and progesterones. Three estrogens — estrone, 17-β estradiol, and estriol — are secreted from the ovaries during the menstrual cycle and each shows a similar pattern of excretion as illustrated in Figure 1 for 17-β estradiol. In the human, 17-β estradiol is the most biologically active estrogen. Therefore, when most authors refer to the "estrogen concentration," they are referring to the activity of 17-β estradiol. During the follicular phase, all three estrogen levels are lowest during the first week and rapidly rise to a peak 1–2 d before ovulation. After ovulation, there is a rapid fall back toward the preovulatory levels, followed by a gradual buildup and plateau during the middle of the luteal phase and a sudden decline 3–5 d before menses. Preovulatory estrogen is produced primarily by the developing ovum and postovulatory estrogen is produced primarily by the corpus luteum.

Progesterone levels remain low during the follicular and early luteal phases of the cycle, with a gradual rise and peak in the middle of the luteal phase. Approximately 5 d before menses, progesterone levels rapidly fall to preovulatory levels. Progesterone is secreted from the corpus luteum and its increase during the luteal phase is used clinically as evidence of normal ovulatory function.[1]

It has long been known that estrogens and progesterones have multiple biological actions that include direct and indirect effects on fluid and electrolyte balance.[12,33,49,83,110,152] In addition, other fluid–electrolyte-altering hormones vary during the menstrual cycle (Table 1). Prolactin,[21,47] aldosterone (ALD),[32,55,76] arginine vasopressin (AVP),[145] cortisol,[52] and testosterone concentrations[58,92] have all been shown to increase during ovulation, during the luteal phase, or during both times. Atrial natriuretic factor was found to decrease during the luteal phase, possibly as a compensatory response to the natriuretic effect of increased plasma progesterone during this phase.[72]

2. Observed Changes in Body Weight, Fluid Balance, and Blood Volume During the "Normal Menstrual Cycle"

Water retention[138,140] and body weight gain[62,105,108] are frequent side effects of menstrual function. In about 25% of women these changes can lead to severe water retention, one of the clinical symptoms of premenstrual syndrome.[6,9,98] It has been estimated that approximately 50% of women experience weight gain premenstrually, although often without clinical symptoms.[104] Thorn et al.[139] studied a group of 50 normal women and found that in the week before menses, 24 gained 1 or more kilograms that could not be attributed to dietary changes. A second period of weight gain was found to occur in 38 of the 50 women near the time of ovulation.

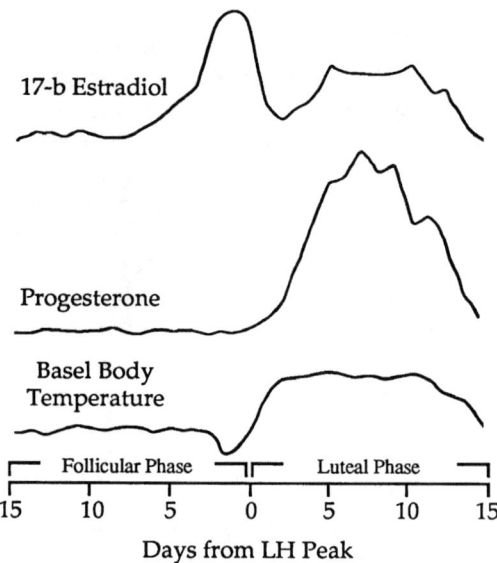

FIGURE 1 Hormonal fluctuations associated with the menstual cycle; where day 0 represents the day of ovulation. Adapted from Mishell et al., *Am. J. Obstet. Gynecol.*, 3:60–65, 1971, and Berne and Levy, in *Physiology*, 2nd ed., C.V. Mosby, St. Louis, 1988, 1012.

Table 1 Fluid/Electrolyte Regulating Hormones that Fluctuate During the Menstrual Cycle

	Peri-Ovulatory Period	Luteal Phase
Estrogen	↑ (96)	↑ (96)
Progesterone	—	↑ (96)
Prolactin	↑ (21, 47)	↑ (47)
Aldosterone (ALD)	↑ (76)	↑ (32, 55, 76, 95)
Arginine Vasopressin (AVP)[a]	↑ (44)	—
Cortisol	↑ (52)	↑ (52)
Testosterone[b]	↑ (58)	↑ (92)
Adrenocorticotropic Hormone (ACTH)	↑ (52)	—
Atrial Natriuretic Hormone (ANF)	—	↓ (72)

[a] Increased plasma AVP is not a consistent finding, however, a decreased osmotic threshold for AVP release and thirst in the luteal phase has been reported consistently.[129,145]

[b] "Percentage free" or unbound testosterone.

Edwards and Baylis[38] studied the urinary and electrolyte excretion patterns of eight normal women in response to water loading during the follicular and luteal phases of the menstrual cycle. Urine volume, excretion of sodium and potassium, and osmolar free water clearances were similar in the follicular and luteal phases when the women were supine. The normal response to moving from the supine to the upright position is to reduce urinary water and electrolyte excretion. This response was significantly potentiated in the luteal phase, leading the author to conclude that the compensatory mechanisms for water and salt retention are potentiated during the luteal phase. Changes in leg volume and distensibility,[77] accentuated stress-provoked systemic vasoconstriction,[11,90] impaired ability to vasoconstrict leg blood vessels upon standing,[62] and increased capillary permeability[74] have all been documented during the luteal phase and may contribute to a greater pooling of blood or a greater fluid filtration to the interstitium. Thus, much of the weight gain associated with the late luteal phase of the menstrual cycle may be caused by fluid retention in the interstitial compartment.

The effect of the menstrual cycle on the vascular fluid compartment is less understood. Red cell mass is assumed to remain fairly constant during a menstrual cycle, and the loss of red cells in most women during menstruation averages only about 25 ml.[125] However, estrogens are secreted in a cyclic pattern and are known to have an antierythropoetic effect.[36] Whether there is a cyclic pattern of red blood cell production in the bone marrow in response to fluctuating estrogen levels is unknown.

Plasma volume may be expected to change in a more dynamic manner than the red cell mass. Elevated estrogen levels in animals and humans have been associated with increased fluid intake, a reduced osmotic threshold for thirst,[145] increased water turnover,[24,30,138,139,140] decreased sodium excretion,[109] increased ALD secretion,[32,55] increased AVP,[10,13,145] and reduced interstitial tissue and plasma oncotic pressures.[105] These actions may be expected to cause or accompany an expansion in plasma volume. Further evidence of an increased blood volume associated with estrogens includes significant increases in hemodynamic variables such as left ventricular end diastolic volume, stroke volume, cardiac index, and skin blood flow immediately following acute estrogen administration to women.[143]

In an attempt to assess changes in plasma volume during the menstrual cycle, we obtained early-morning finger blood samples from eight normal supine women throughout at least one complete menstrual cycle.[46] Plasma volume was determined using radioisotope dilution in each woman at the beginning of the cycle and changes in hematocrit and hemoglobin concentrations were used to estimate fluctuations in plasma volume. As shown in Figure 2, significant fluctuations in plasma volume occurred for each woman during a normalized menstrual cycle. Although there was considerable variability in the overall pattern from woman to woman, for each woman a transient increase in plasma volume occurred near the day of predicted ovulation, day 14 in Figure 2, and a second, more gradual increase occurred near the end of the cycle.

One observation from our study[46] and from a cross-sectional study of hematocrit changes during the menstrual cycle[144] is that blood volume would appear to be unaltered during the menstrual cycle if hematocrit values are compared only between midfollicular and midluteal phases. Previous investigators,[105] who obtained blood samples only at these two sampling times, have

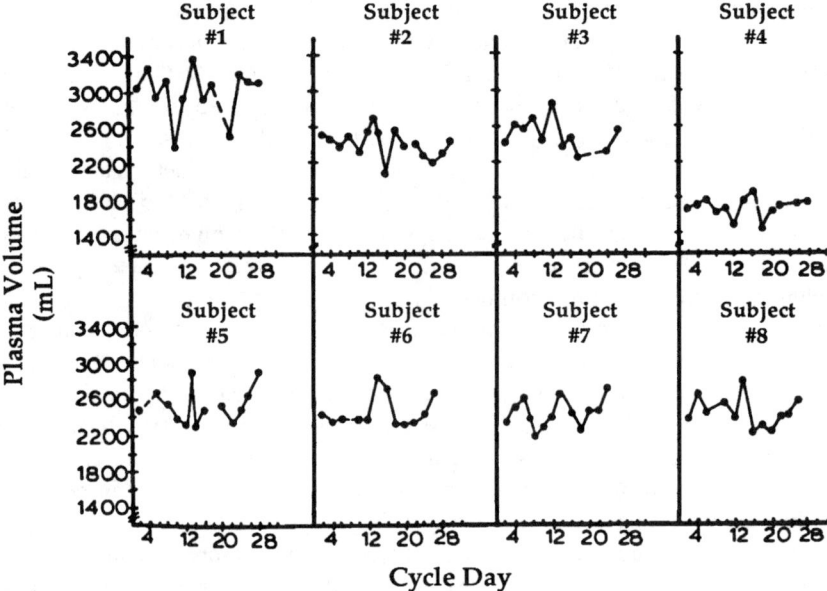

FIGURE 2 Plasma volume of eight women during normalized 28-d menstrual cycles; where ovulation is represented as day 14.[46]

made this conclusion. Other studies in which blood samples were drawn once a week[13,145] also failed to identify significant changes in hematocrit as a function of the menstrual cycle. The increases in plasma volume during a menstrual cycle are transient and easily missed if cycle stage is not verified and if samples are not drawn frequently.

3. Premenstrual Syndrome (PMS)

PMS was first described by Frank in 1931.[104] The diagnostic criteria are now well accepted and include a follicular phase free of symptoms, recurrence of symptoms in the luteal phase, and the relief of symptoms during menstruation.[141] A variety of physical and psychological symptoms—including cramps, painful breasts, a feeling of swelling, irritability, and depression—have been known to occur during the 3–5 days before menses. Water retention was first suggested as the pathological mechanism of PMS for both the somatic and mental symptoms.[136] However, recently it has been noted that the occurrence of PMS symptoms often does not correlate with premenstrual weight gains, and many women who sustain significant fluid retention remain asymptomatic.[141] However, one consistent finding in women with PMS symptoms has been an increase in capillary filtration coefficient. Tollan et al.[141] used the capillary wick technique to measure changes in tissue pressures and strain gauge plethysmography to measure capillary filtration in the legs of ten women with well-defined PMS. Measurements were compared in each woman in the follicular and luteal phases. The capillary filtration coefficient increased 30%

in the luteal phase and was accompanied by a mean 3.6 mmHg reduction in interstitial colloid osmotic pressure without significant change in body weight. The authors concluded that their results support the hypothesis that the etiology of PMS is related to an altered fluid distribution rather than fluid retention per se.

That changes in fluid volume and fluid retention associated with PMS may be related to estrogen or progesterone fluctuations is strongly supported by the fact that PMS occurs almost exclusively in ovulatory women.[99] Although the exact mechanism for PMS is still a matter of debate,[9,104] popular theories involve excess estrogen, reduced progesterone, or abnormally high estrogen–progesterone ratio.

The excess estrogen theory was supported by Bäckstrom and co-workers.[7] This very complicated theory begins with the observation that women with PMS have lower levels of both estrogen and progesterone 8–9 days before menstruation as compared to women without PMS. Estrogen is a potent inhibitor of follicular-stimulating hormone release. The reduced levels of estrogen during the midluteal phase of the cycle may allow follicular-stimulating hormone levels to rise in the PMS women, stimulating proliferation of a second set of follicles that begin producing estrogen while progesterone levels remain depressed. Thus, by the fifth day before menstruation, PMS women had significantly elevated estrogen and estrogen-progesterone ratios when compared to the control group.

What would be the consequences of an unusually high estrogen or estrogen–progesterone ratio? In another paper, Bäckstrom et al.[6] discussed evidence that estrogens have a direct excitatory effect on the central nervous system, an effect counteracted by progesterone. Symptoms such as irritability, headaches, and anxiety may result from overstimulation of the limbic system by excess estrogen. Progesterone therapy is one of the treatments of PMS. Thus, the elevated estrogen–progesterone ratio may contribute to the psychological symptoms of PMS.

4. Potential Mechanisms for Menstrually-Induced Changes in Fluid Balance

a. Estrogens and Fluid Retention

Estrogen administration to dogs has been shown to cause fluid and sodium retention and increases in body weight.[26,30,73,139] This fluid-retaining effect was independent of adrenal function[139] but dependent on the presence of an intact posterior hypophysis.[30] These results suggest that estrogens may increase body fluids by altering pituitary secretion of vasopressin and most likely do not involve increased adrenal secretion of ALD.

In sheep, Ueda et al.[142] measured the cardiovascular and hemodynamic responses during a continuous 3-week infusion of 17-β estradiol. They reported that estrogen administration resulted in a 20% increase in blood volume that was directly correlated with the change in estradiol concentration ($r = 0.72$).

This finding of water retention following exogenous estrogen administration has also been reported in humans. Estradiol monobenzoate in oil (0.14 to 0.20 mg/kg body weight) was injected intramuscularly daily for 1 week in 11 women. A slight and transient decrease in urinary output of sodium and water was accompanied by significant increases in body weight, extracellular fluid volume (thiocyanate), and plasma volume as estimated from decreases in serum protein, and venous hematocrit.[110] In another study, 16 women being treated for minor menstrual irregularities were administered two to four doses of either estrone or α–estradiol intramuscularly. In all patients, there was a consistent lowering of hematocrit and hemoglobin concentrations during the 4–10 d of treatment. On cessation of estrogen treatment, blood values returned to initial levels within 5–9 d.[152] Dignam et al.[33] studied the effects of intravenous administration of up to 50 mg estradiol to 18 postmenopausal women and 1 woman without ovaries. Although they found inconsistent changes in urine flow, sodium and chloride excretion were reduced with estrogen administration. The authors speculated that the estrogen effect may be due to a direct effect on the renal tubules. This option of a direct estrogen effect on the kidney is strengthened by the observation of specific renal estrogen receptors.[93]

b. Estrogen–Progesterone and the Kidney

Despite the previous observation of estrogen-induced fluid retention in adrenalectomized animals,[139] another possible mechanism for an enhanced sodium and water retention involves an indirect estrogen effect to increase renin substrate production by the kidneys, which would increase production of angiotensin II and ALD. ALD concentration peaks at ovulation[76,95,135] and is higher in the luteal phase than during the follicular phase.[32,55] The ovulatory peak in ALD secretion could explain the fluid retention and plasma volume expansion at this time, but what about during the luteal phase? Fluid retention occurs in the late luteal phase, a time when both estrogen and progesterone levels are falling. To answer this puzzle, the antinatriuretic effect of progesterone must be considered. Progesterone is a weak mineralocorticoid that may function as a competitive antagonist to the estrogen-stimulated increase in ALD during the luteal phase. Fluid retention would occur when progesterone levels fall near the end of the luteal phase and "unmask" the salt-retaining actions of the elevated ALD.

Other investigators have speculated that changes in kidney function during the menstrual cycle may occur through direct actions of estrogen or progesterone to alter the hypothalamic production of AVP. The observation by Dance et al.[30] that the fluid-retaining effect of exogenous estrogen is blocked by removal of the posterior pituitary in dogs supports this hypothesis. Several authors[44,112] have found increases in AVP in normal women at the time of ovulation and others[32] have found no consistent difference between early follicular and midluteal levels. Estrogen administration to postmenopausal women was accompanied by a threefold increase in AVP. This effect was blocked when progesterone was administered.[44] Therefore, in the midluteal phase when progesterone levels are elevated, the estrogen-induced increase in AVP may be blocked. Thus, here again estrogen and progesterone may have opposing actions in regulating fluid balance during the menstrual cycle.

c. Estrogen–Progesterone and the Peripheral Vasculature

Whether the fluid retention associated with the periovulatory and late luteal phases of the menstrual cycle result in a positive fluid balance and whether fluid will be retained in the vascular or the interstitial compartment depend on concurrent changes in the peripheral vasculature. An increase in vascular compliance would promote fluid retention, especially in the vascular compartment, while a decrease in vascular compliance would stimulate urine production and fluid movement to the interstitial compartment.

The specific role of estrogen–progesterone on the regulation of the peripheral circulation is not yet known. There may be direct effects of these hormones on the blood vessel walls or indirect effects through their action to alter blood volume and other hormones. The influence of natural and synthetic estrogens on different tissues, arteries, and veins has been evaluated extensively in animal studies. The results have varied depending on the species studied, tissue used, and doses applied. Natural and synthetic estrogens often exhibit completely opposite effects on the same tissue.[11]

In a recent study, estrogen (1 mg 17 β-estradiol) was administered sublingually to postmenopausal women and changes in femoral artery blood flow were measured by using a duplex ultrasound technique. Estrogen administration resulted in an immediate, 1 to 2 hours, 30% increase in femoral blood flow with no change in mean arterial pressure or heart rate. The authors suggested their results may indicate a direct action of estrogen on the vascular wall and speculated that the mechanism, which occurred too rapidly to be accounted for by the "classical steroid receptor mechanism," may have been due to a direct endothelial stimulation of nitric oxide release.[114]

The whole body systemic response to estrogen appears to be an increase in compliance, lowering of blood pressure, and increase in skin and muscle blood flow. Estrogen administration to sheep resulted in vasodilation in the uterus and skin blood vessels,[102] a decrease in mean arterial blood pressure,[142] and decreased total systemic vascular resistance.[102] In humans, blood pressure is lowest near ovulation and during the midluteal phases when estrogen levels are highest,[37,62] and increases to the highest level during menses, when estrogen levels are lowest.[37] Finger and forearm skin blood flow and finger skin temperature show cyclic changes with the menstrual cycle, with a higher resting skin blood flow in the luteal phase compared to the follicular.[11] Calf blood flow increases near ovulation and in the early luteal phase.[78] All of these changes suggest that estrogen increases vascular compliance, at least in the basal resting condition.

Upon provocation, however, vasoconstrictor responses appear to be enhanced by estrogen. The vasopressor response to immersion of the hand in cold water is enhanced in the luteal phase when compared to follicular,[11] and

Bartelink et al.[11] speculated that this was due to an effect of estrogen to upregulate α_2-adrenergic vasoconstrictor receptors. Estrogen administration to rats has been shown to potentiate the vasoconstrictor responses to norepinephrine, epinephrine, and vasopressin but to have no influence on vasoconstrictor actions of dopamine, seratonin, or angiotensin.[3] The well-known hypertensive effect of oral contraceptives may be due to the effects of estrogen that increase renin — and, therefore, angiotensin II vasoconstrictor activity — as well as blood volume.[14]

Progesterone appears to have dose-dependent effects leading to vasoconstriction or vasodilation, the latter possibly due to an influence on the vasodilating β-adrenergic receptors.[11] Therefore, the net effect of the menstrual cycle on blood vessel compliance also may depend on the estrogen–progesterone ratio, rather than the concentration of each individual hormone.

d. Estrogens–Progesterones and Capillary Permeability

Estrogens have been postulated to increase capillary permeability either through a direct vascular effect or through an indirect effect to increase renin.[74] Progesterones, on the other hand, have been shown to decrease vascular permeability.[74] Estrogen-induced changes in capillary permeability may be a mechanism contributing to the weight gain and edema seen in some women during the periovulatory and late luteal phases.

e. Thirst and Appetite During the Menstrual Cycle

Changes in fluid balance during the menstrual cycle may be influenced by estrogen-induced changes in fluid intake. Thirst has been reported to vary during the menstrual cycle, with approximately 25% of women reporting an increase in thirst premenstrually.[139] Fluid intake is regulated by the hypothalamus, an area known to contain estrogen receptors. A direct, central-neural effect of estrogens on fluid intake has been postulated but awaits confirmation.[145] It has also been postulated that estrogen may affect fluid intake indirectly through its stimulation of the renin–angiotensin system. Angiotensin II is a well-known dipsinogen.

The primary stimulus for thirst is an increase in plasma osmolality. Three separate studies[13,129,145] have assessed thirst and AVP responses to graded increases in plasma osmolality in normal women and noted marked differences during the menstrual cycle. Each study reported a slight but significant 3- to 5-mOsm reduction in baseline plasma osmolality in the luteal phase accompanied by reduction of the osmotic thresholds for thirst and AVP secretion. In two of the studies[13,129] a significant reduction in the gain of the AVP-osmolality response occurred in the luteal phase, as indicated by a reduced slope of the increase in AVP with increasing osmolality. Each study speculated that these changes in renal salt sensitivity may be related to changes in estrogen or progesterone.

Nutrient intake in women has been shown to vary during the menstrual cycle.[29,108] Near ovulation, when endogenous levels of estrogen were high, women ate less; just after ovulation, when estrogen levels declined, total nutrient intake increased. These differences were due solely to fluctuations in carbohydrate intake, with no significant change in protein or fat consumption.[29] Dalvit-McPhillips[29] speculated that estrogen's effect to reduce carbohydrate intake may involve activation of a serotonergic mechanism. In the central nervous system, serotonin receptors occur primarily in the midbrain and hypothalamus and are believed be involved in the regulation of food intake. Estrogen, like carbohydrates, may increase trytophan levels, promoting serotonin synthesis and reducing hunger.

Food intake also may be influenced during the menstrual cycle by an effect of progesterone to increase metabolism. Basal metabolic rate[128] and 24-h energy expenditure[147] were higher during the luteal phase. For example, Solomon et al.[128] found that the resting metabolic rate of six healthy women confined to a metabolic unit was lowest approximately 1 week before ovulation, when progesterone levels are very low, and increased during the luteal phase with a sudden fall at the onset of menstruation.

B. ORAL CONTRACEPTIVES, BODY FLUIDS, EXERCISE

The effects of estrogen–progesterone on body fluids and vascular responses are more pronounced in women who use oral contraceptives. This was particularly evident prior to 1973, before low-dose estrogen pills — those containing less than 50 μg of ethinyl estradiol — came on the market.[96] Oral contraceptive use in some women has been shown to be associated with enhanced fluid and sodium retention,[18,109] a decreased glomerular filtration rate,[109] body weight gain,[146] increased plasma volume,[84,146] and increased cardiac output.[84,86,146] This increase in salt and fluid retention was postulated by Prashad et al.[109] to potentially reduce maximal exercise capacity in weight-bearing modes of exercise. On the other hand, Lehtovirta et al.[84] suggested the increased cardiac output may increase short-term intense exercise capacity.

The estrogen content of the contraceptive pill is associated with increased blood pressure, even with doses as low as 35 μg.[96] This could be caused by the increased blood volume as well as by stimulation of renin-substrate production.[14,70,146] Simultaneously, however, renin production decreases and blood–renin activity has been reported to either increase[14,146] or decrease.[70] There is some indirect evidence that progesterones may contribute to the blood pressure changes with oral contraceptives; however, estrogens still contribute the primary pressor effect.[96]

C. PREGNANCY

An increase in blood volume with pregnancy is one of the "hallmarks of a successful pregnancy."[88] At full term, maternal blood volume may increase as much as 40%, because of a 45–55% increase in plasma volume and a 20–30% increase in red cell mass. Initially the greater increase in plasma volume compared to red cell mass was thought to be a nutritional deficit, but it is now recognized that even well-nourished pregnant women have this response.

During a normal pregnancy, both estrogen and progesterone levels increase by approximately 100%. This increase has been shown to be associated with a resetting of both volume and osmotic receptors that result in an increased fluid turnover, decreased plasma sodium and osmolality, and decreased osmotic threshold for thirst and AVP secretion.[31,106] The net result of such changes in the volume homeostasis system is that the "effective blood volume" does not change with pregnancy despite an absolute increase in volume.

Longo et al.[88] observed that the increase in blood volume is directly proportional to the weight of the fetus or placenta, or both. Thus, with twins or other multiple pregnancies, blood volume increases in direct proportion to the number of fetuses. As the fetus develops, the placenta produces estrogens that may exert a positive feedback for fetal growth. The increased estrogen secretion stimulates the renin–angiotensin–ALD system, resulting in increased fluid and salt retention. This results in expansion of the plasma volume. At the same time, other placental products—prolactin, growth hormone, chorionic somatotropin—stimulate erythropoietin production. The increased blood volume is accompanied by an increased blood flow in the low-resistance uteroplacental circulation that stimulates fetal growth and further estrogen production.

Exercise during pregnancy is accompanied by reductions in uterine blood flow, thus potentially compromising fetal oxygenation and heat exchange. However, unless the exercise is unusually prolonged or severe, or other complications have occurred in the pregnancy, no adverse effects from the exercise itself should ensue. The expanded blood volume of the mother not only acts to maintain fetal oxygen delivery but also functions as a "sink" for the metabolically produced heat.[94]

III. EFFECT OF HEAT EXPOSURE ON BODY FLUIDS IN WOMEN

A. ACUTE HEAT EXPOSURE
1. Effect of Estrogen–Progesterone on Temperature Regulation

The biphasic changes in body temperature associated with the menstrual cycle were first described by van de Velde in 1904.[61] Basal body temperature during the follicular phase is fairly constant until just before ovulation. A transient decrease in body temperature precedes ovulation and is followed by a progressive rise in body temperature during the luteal phase. With the onset of menses, body temperature decreases by about 0.5°C back to the follicular-phase level.

The observed rise in body temperature during the luteal phase is believed to be a direct effect of progesterone. The administration of progesterone to castrated women[71] or men[117] caused a prompt rise in body temperature, while estrogen administration had an opposing effect. Estrogen administered with progesterone, however, did not counteract the progesterone-induced thermogenesis.

The mechanism by which progesterone increases body temperature is not clear but may be through a direct, central neural action to increase the setpoint temperature. For example, the threshold core temperatures for sweating and vasodilation are elevated in the luteal phase,[57,66,67,82,132] resulting in the regulation of body temperature at a higher level and a widening of the thermal comfort zone.[28] Another possible mechanism by which progesterone may increase body temperature is through an action to increase heat production. Resting metabolic rate is approximately 10% greater in the luteal phase than in the follicular phase.[66,147]

Although progesterone acts to increase core temperature, estrogen has an opposing action. In a study with postmenopausal women, Tankersley et al.[137] reported that estrogen-replacement therapy influenced central thermoregulatory neurons to lower body-temperature set point by decreasing the sweating and vasodilatory thresholds. This effect may be responsible for the transient drop in body temperature prior to ovulation. However, during the luteal phase when estrogen levels increase, this effect is negated by an opposing action of the elevated progesterone levels. The setpoint of body temperature is, therefore, dependent on the estrogen–progesterone ratio.

2. Women "Glow" Rather Than Sweat

There is an old saying that "horses sweat, men perspire, and women glow." The physiological basis for this saying may reside in a gender-based difference in the mechanism by which body heat is dissipated. Several authors have observed that in a hot-humid environment women are as able as men to sustain changes in body core temperature, despite a lower sweat output even when fully heat acclimated.[50,107,123,124,150,153] Under such conditions, women have been shown to have a significantly higher skin blood flow, perhaps giving them a more "glowing" appearance. The enhanced skin blood flow, together with a 10% greater surface-area-to-body-mass ratio, results in a greater capacity for nonevaporative heat loss.

The mechanism for a conservation of sweat loss in women in a hot-humid environment most commonly has been attributed to an increased susceptibility to hydromeiosis, or the so-called "sweat-gland fatigue."[20,50,124,148,153] The greater density[80] and lower average flow rates per gland[22,50,113] may make women more susceptible to a mechanical obstruction of the sweat-gland pores due to swelling of cutaneous epidermal cells. Araki[4] further found that as women became more physically trained and attained a higher sweat rate, they became even more susceptible to hidromeiosis. They concluded that this ability to reduce sweat output improved a woman's capacity for "useful sweating" in this particular environment. Wyndham et al.[153] concluded that "the male in these hot-humid conditions is a prolific, wasteful sweater, whereas the female adjusts her sweat rate better to the required heat loss."

In a hot-dry environment, the gender differences in sweating rate are greatly reduced[115] or completely disappear, assuming equal levels of fitness and heat acclimation.[50,124,149] Under such conditions, most sweat evaporates off the surface of the skin, dissipating body heat. Thus, a high-sweat rate in these conditions is a distinct advantage.

3. Blood Volume Regulation During Resting Heat Exposure

If women are more efficient sweaters than men, then one might predict they would have a smaller decrease in plasma volume during prolonged exercise or heat exposure. However, studies that compare changes in plasma volume between subjects are greatly complicated by effects of fitness, acclimation, and hydration status. Therefore, it is not surprising that results comparing plasma-volume changes in men and women during heat stress are equivocal. Senay[122] reported that during 10-h passive hot-dry-heat exposures, plasma volume decreased in women at a rate 1.5 times faster than similarly stressed men. Röcker et al.[116] on the other hand reported a smaller total decrease in plasma volume in women during 4-h intermittent sauna. During cycle exercise at a mild intensity (30% $\dot{V}O_2$ max), Senay and Fortney[121] reported that women hemoconcentrated while men either maintained their plasma volume or hemodiluted. Wells[150] on the other hand, reported hemodilution during mild cycle exercise in a group of women who were possibly more fit than those of Senay and Fortney.[121] Drinkwater et al.[35] reported that for trained women, the changes in plasma volume during mild (30% $\dot{V}O_2$ max) treadmill exercise in a cool (28°C), warm (35°C), or hot environment (48°C) were similar to men. In none of the foregoing studies were potential menstrual cycle effects taken into account.

It has been shown that there is a delay in the onset of sweating in the luteal phase of the menstrual cycle when compared to the follicular phase.[66,82,132] However, once sweating is initiated, the slope of the sweating response is either the same[82,132] or greater[57,66] in the luteal phase. Therefore, based only on the sweating response it would be difficult to predict the effect of the menstrual cycle on body-fluid responses to exercise or heat stress. If estrogens increase capillary permeability,[74] one would expect a greater loss of plasma volume during the luteal phase when compared to early follicular. However, because plasma concentrations of ALD and AVP[32] are elevated in the luteal phase at rest and during exercise, these hormonal changes would be expected to conserve body fluids during the luteal phase. Senay[122] found no effect of menstrual cycle stage on the plasma volume response to passive heat exposure, and Stephenson[131] reported that the decrease in plasma volume during the luteal phase was twice that seen in the follicular phase during a 167-min passive heat exposure.

During mild cycle exercise (30% $\dot{V}O_2$ max) in a hot environment, Gabelein and Senay[51] reported a reduced resting plasma volume in the luteal phase accompanied by a smaller reduction in plasma volume during exercise. Similar findings were obtained during a severe cycle exercise bout (80% $\dot{V}O_2$ max).[131] In each of these studies exercise and heat stress obliterated the baseline menstrual cycle differences in resting plasma volume. Stephenson and Kolka[133] suggested that the lower resting plasma volume in the luteal phase stimulated greater release of fluid-retaining hormones such as ALD and AVP, which acted to conserve fluid losses during luteal phase exercise.

B. HEAT ACCLIMATION
1. Special Concern for Women in the Tropics?

Prior to the 1960s, it was commonly assumed that women were less heat tolerant than men, and there are numerous reports even in the scientific literature of the particularly harmful effects of a hot climate on the Caucasian female. For example, white women immigrants to Saba, an island in the West Indies, were described as "nervous and high-strung" and some of their problems were said to have been because of "the fact that the tropical climate is said to accentuate the usual woman's disorders".[111] These myths of the peculiarly delicate nature of women vis-a-vis heat were supported by the variety of tropical diseases and strong cultural factors that restricted a woman from partaking in the very activities that might acclimate her to the heat. It was recognized that a lack of physical exercise may contribute to an inability to tolerate a hot climate, as seen in the following quote: "Women in general stand the tropics less well than men, because, as a rule, they have no serious employment and considerably less domestic work at home. Almost every tropical settlement has its quota of lazy, bored, card-playing, spirit-drinking women, who would be far healthier and happier if financial circumstances forced them to do their own housework, if not some labor out of doors."[111]

2. Ability of Women to Heat Acclimate

Hertig and co-workers[64,65] were the first to critically evaluate the reports that women could not tolerate heat stress. Their studies and several others in this time period[27,42,153] reported that women were inherently less able to deal with heat as they exhibited more severe physiological as well as psychological reactions. Hertig et al.[64,65] reported that although repeated heat exposures resulted in the physiological responses characteristic of heat acclimatization — such as increased sweating, lower body temperatures, and increased tolerance — the time course of such changes was slower in women than in men. Even in the acclimated state, the women could not attain the same sweat capacity as the men. They concluded that women were inherently less able to deal with heat stress because of a smaller temperature gradient between the core and skin resulting from their reduced sweating response and a smaller reserve capacity to move blood to the skin.

However, it was soon recognized that temperature regulation is a function of the relative exercise intensity[118] and that many of these earlier studies were complicated by the fact that the women were compared to men exercising at easier relative exercise intensities. In studies where men and women with similar levels of $\dot{V}O_2$ max were compared, gender differences in thermoregulatory responses during heat acclimation were greatly reduced or eliminated,[5,69,126,149] with the exception of sweating, which remained lower in women in hot-wet environment conditions.[50,101] In a hot-dry environment, gender differences in sweating disappeared as well.[50,149]

Greenleaf et al.[56] found that untrained women hemodiluted to a similar extent as men after heat acclimation. Previous reports[45,69] that women did not hemodilute with heat acclimation may have been complicated by the fact that the women were already partially heat acclimated as a result of a previous training program.

IV. EFFECT OF EXERCISE ON BODY FLUID BALANCE IN WOMEN

A. ACUTE EXERCISE
1. Acute Exercise and Water Balance

During exercise, renal blood flow is reduced as blood is shunted from the splanchnic regions to the exercising muscles and skin. As a result, urinary excretion of water and salt is reduced during and for some time after exercise. Prashad and co-workers[109] examined the effect of the menstrual cycle and oral contraceptive use on the oliguria following a graded treadmill exercise protocol. After exercise, urine flow was reduced in all phases of the menstrual cycle by an average of 35%, to an absolute level of urine flow of 0.5 ml/min. The only exception was that during the luteal phase, urine flow was reduced to only 0.7 ml/min, which represented a 25% reduction in urine flow. Thus, an attenuated exercise effect on urine flow occurred during the luteal phase. It is, therefore, surprising that ALD levels are higher in the luteal phase than in the follicular phase. DeSouza and co-workers[32] found that although resting levels of AVP and plasma renin activity (PRA) were not altered during the menstrual cycle, ALD levels were higher during the luteal phase. Similarly, during 40 min of 80% $\dot{V}O_2$ max treadmill exercise, the increases in plasma AVP and PRA were not altered by menstrual phase, while the ALD response was potentiated during the luteal phase. One possible explanation for these seemingly contradictory observations of a greater urine loss, in spite of elevated ALD levels during the luteal phase, may be related to the concurrent rise in luteal phase progesterone. Progesterone is a competitive inhibitor of ALD[40] and may interfere with the ALD action to conserve sodium and water. Whether these menstrual cycle alterations in urine and electrolyte excretion result in significant changes in plasma volume, and thus exercise responses, is unclear at this time.

2. Acute Exercise and Plasma Volume

Change in plasma volume during exercise in a hot environment was reviewed in section III.A.3. The plasma-volume responses to exercise in a cool environment would be expected to have a similar pattern but smaller magnitude at any given level of exercise.[60] Some authors[51,131] have reported smaller changes in plasma volume in the luteal phase of the menstrual cycle during mild and moderate exercise in the heat. This finding may contribute to the increased time to exhaustion and lower blood-lactate levels reported by other authors during submaximal exercise in the luteal phase.[75,103]

The relatively modest fluctuations in plasma volume associated with the menstrual cycle would be expected to have little effect on a maximal exercise effort. Maximum oxygen uptake generally has been found to be unaffected by the stage of the menstrual cycle.[34,75] However, in a study by Schoene et al.,[119] a lower level of $\dot{V}O_2$ max was found during treadmill exercise in the luteal phase for nonathletes, while no significant menstrual effects were found for competitive female athletes. The authors discussed a possible mechanism by which the elevated progesterone levels in the luteal phase increase the respiratory drive during exercise. This increased respiratory drive could result in a greater sensation of dypsnea that may reduce the exercise performance of nonathletes.

3. Dehydration-Rehydration Considerations

One question that may arise during a prolonged athletic event is whether there are different fluid requirements for men and women. Clearly, since it is recommended that athletes replace fluid losses during exercise to maintain a peak-exercise performance,[54] and men often lose more fluid because of their larger size and possibly a less efficient sweating response, then a greater absolute fluid requirement may be necessary for men, especially in a hot-wet environment. It should also be considered, however, that the average woman has a 13% smaller plasma volume.[85] Therefore, any given absolute loss of volume represents a greater proportional decrease in plasma volume and it is critical that women rehydrate as frequently as men despite smaller absolute changes in body weight during a competition.

In a study by Byrd et al.,[23] men and women were moderately dehydrated by exercising in a hot environment so that each subject group had a comparable 3.7% reduction in body weight. The corresponding decreases in plasma volume for the female (5.3%) and male (4.6%) subjects were similar. These results suggest there are no marked gender differences in the overall regulation of body fluids during exercise; thus, for a given relative reduction in body weight there will be a similar relative decrease in plasma volume. However, this does not rule out the possibility of subtle changes in fluid handling during the menstrual cycle, as suggested by the findings of Gabelein and Senay[51] and Stephenson and Kolka[131] which showed greater relative changes in plasma volume in women during exercise in the follicular phase compared to the luteal phase.

Another question is whether the glucose content of rehydration drinks for men and women should differ. During prolonged exercise, a proposed factor limiting exercise endurance is a depletion of muscle glycogen in the exercising muscles.[64] Carbohydrate loading prior to exercise[17] and the addition of carbohydrate to rehydration fluids[54] have been suggested as a means to increase submaximal exercise endurance. Exercise training is accompanied by a shift in substrate utilization during exercise such that glucose is preferentially spared and free fatty acid utilization is increased.[68] Thus, menstrually induced hormonal actions that might alter carbohydrate utilization or stores could affect exercise endurance.

Animal studies have indicated that muscle and liver glycogen formation is markedly increased after elevation in estrogen–progesterone levels.[2] However, little is known about the effect of the human menstrual cycle on muscle glycogen dynamics. Muscle biopsy results from six women during follicular and luteal phases of their menstrual cycles suggest that resting muscle glycogen content and glycogen turnover rates after exercise were greater during the midluteal phase compared to midfollicular phase.[59,103] Such results suggest that women, especially in the luteal phase, may require less carbohydrates in a rehydration solution to increase their endurance during prolonged submaximal exertion.

It has been suggested that oral contraceptives may spare carbohydrate utilization during exercise by stimulating the release of growth hormone.[15,19] Growth hormone has a well-known antiinsulin action that results in a preferential sparing of carbohydrates and a shift to lipids as an energy substrate during exercise. Growth hormone is elevated in women who take oral contraceptives and in eumenorrheic women during the luteal phase of the menstrual cycle.[48] Also, the growth-hormone response to exercise is potentiated in women compared to men.[25]

Women in the luteal phase of the menstrual cycle have been reported to have higher levels of resting muscle glycogen and lower blood-lactate levels during prolonged submaximal exercise.[34] These changes may contribute to the increased endurance times reported in women during the luteal phase of the menstrual cycle compared to the follicular phase.[75,103] This finding of an enhanced exercise endurance during the luteal phase, however, is not a consistent finding and may be dependent upon the intensity, mode, and duration of the exercise performed.

B. CHRONIC EXERCISE
1. Chronic Exercise and Blood Volume

The effects of chronic exercise on aerobic capacity and blood volume are reported to be similar in men and women. When women undergo an intense period of aerobic training, they have relative increases in $\dot{V}O_2$ max comparable to men's,[79] and when the $\dot{V}O_2$ max is expressed relative to the lean body mass, the female value is nearly identical to or only slightly lower than the male value.[151] As with findings in men, this increase in $\dot{V}O_2$ max is accompanied by significant increases in both plasma and erythrocyte volumes.[134]

The improvements in submaximal-training responses, such as lowered heart rate, core temperature, and blood-lactate levels for a given absolute level of exercise, are of similar magnitude in women and men.[43,54] Although sweat rate increases during training in women, the maximal rate of sweating and the sensitivity of the sweating response remain less than that of trained men, at least in a hot-wet environment.[4,81,101]

As with men, the changes in plasma volume during exercise are determined by the relative exercise intensity of the activity, independent of the aerobic capacity of the individual.[91] Therefore, after training there is a smaller decrease in plasma volume at a given oxygen uptake. During prolonged intense exercise with ad lib fluid replacement, trained women are as capable as men in maintaining their hydration status. For example, after a marathon run in a mild climate (17.5–20.4°C), trained men and women had the same relative deficits in body weight (approximately 3%) without significant change in plasma volume.[100]

2. Chronic Exercise and Menstrual Function

Chronic intense exercise in some women may result in a disruption of the menstrual cycle and thus alter body-fluid regulation. When menstrual cycles fail to begin by age 16, the disorder is classified as "primary amenorrhea." If the menstrual cycles suddenly become irregular or stop in a previously cycling woman, the disorder is classified as "secondary amenorrhea." Inconsistent menstrual cycles occurring at an interval of 39–90 d are termed "oligomenorrhea." Lack of cycles or cycles occurring at intervals greater than 90 d is termed "amenorrhea".[89] "Athlete's amenorrhea" is the term used to indicate the cessation of menstrual cycles that sometimes accompanies severe exercise training and is therefore a form of secondary amenorrhea.

The reported incidence of athlete's amenorrhea varies greatly and is confounded by the lack of consistent criteria for the disorder. Most studies refer vaguely to a menstrual irregularity in athletes. A summary of studies reporting the incidence of athlete's amenorrhea can be found in an excellent review article by Loucks and Horvath.[89] Overall, the reported incidence in female athletes ranges from the same as the general population to 20 times greater. Athlete's amenorrhea is reported most frequently in younger women, who have not had children, who had a late onset of menarche, and who have a relative level of body fat less than 22%.[127] Its occurrence is also related to the frequency or duration of training sessions, the percentage of protein in the diet, the mode of training (weight bearing), and the degree of psychological stress associated with the exercise.

The exact mechanism or mechanisms by which chronic exercise alters menstrual function is a matter of extensive debate. Again, the review article by Loucks and Horvath[89] summarizes various theories that attempt to relate exercise training to mechanisms involving changes in body composition; hormonal, body fluid, thermal, or stress responses to exercise; reproductive maturity; changes in diet or energy balance; and neurotransmitters associated with psychological stress. Of the proposed mechanisms, it cannot be determined whether the primary cause is related to hypothalamic dysfunction, inappropriate hormonal feedback, or to other endocrine or metabolic dysfunctions.

The consequences of athlete's amenorrhea on fertility and osteoporosis are critical issues associated with this disorder. Consequences for fluid balance and exercise responses would be expected to be short-acting and to be associated with specific changes in estrogen–progesterone concentrations. Amenorrheic athletes have depressed levels of circulating estrogen–progesterone[8] and even "normally cycling" athletes may have a shortened luteal phase with a smaller rise in serum progesterone levels.[8] The body fluid responses of such women may, therefore, be expected to be similar to those occurring during the early follicular phase of a normal menstrual cycle. A positive effect reported in amenorrheic athletes is an increased hematocrit and total body hemoglobin that could result in an increased aerobic capacity.[41]

V. SUMMARY

Distinct cyclic fluctuations in fluid and electrolyte balance occur in women as a result of fluctuations in estrogen and progesterone during the menstrual cycle. Estrogen promotes fluid retention, while progesterone has an opposite effect through its competitive interaction with ALD. Therefore, the baseline fluid balance of a woman fluctuates as a function of the estrogen–progesterone ratio. Fluid retention occurs near ovulation during the peak estrogen surge and just before menses as progesterone levels decline. Many studies that have reported a lack of effect of the menstrual cycle on body fluids or submaximal exercise responses may have failed to detect differences due to inappropriate sampling times; most studies have compared midfollicular to midluteal phases of the menstrual cycle.

The fluctuations in plasma volume during the menstrual cycle or with oral contraceptive usage are physiologically significant and of similar magnitude to that seen after programs of physical training or heat acclimation. They would be expected to have some influence on exercise and heat responses. Menstrual cycle effects on the control of sweating and skin blood flow have been reported. Estrogen, progesterone, or both hormones may directly affect hypothalamic temperature-sensitive neurons, resulting in a central resetting of heat-loss responses. Heat-loss responses would then be affected by these central neural effects and by the fluctuations in blood volume.

Exercise endurance also has been suggested to be affected by the menstrual cycle, with greater endurance during the luteal phase. This effect may be mediated through the estrogen–progesterone actions to alter blood volume and through estrogen's effects to spare carbohydrates and preferentially utilize fats for energy.

ACKNOWLEDGMENTS

I gratefully acknowledge the technical assistance of Martha Munies (Hernandez Engineering) and Jacqueline Reeves (KRUG Life Sciences Inc.).

REFERENCES

1. Abraham, G. E., Maroulis, G. B., and Marshall, J. R., Evaluation of ovulation and corpus luteum function using measurements of plasma progesterone, *Obstet. Gynecol.*, 44:522–525, 1974.
2. Ahmed-Sorour, H. and Bailey, C. J., Role of ovarian hormones in the long-term control of glucose homeostasis glycogen formation and gluconeogenesis, *Ann. Nutr. Metab.*, 25:208–212, 1981.
3. Altura, B. M., Sex and estrogens and responsiveness of terminal arterioles to neurohypophyseal hormones and catecholamines, *J. Pharmacol. Exp. Ther.*, 193:403–412, 1975.
4. Araki, T., Matsushita, K., Umeno, K., Tsujino, A., and Toda, Y., Effect of physical training on exercise-induced sweating in women, *J. Appl. Physiol.: Respir. Environ. Exer. Physiol.*, 51(6):1526–1532, 1981.
5. Avellini, B. A., Kamon, E., and Krajewski, J. T., Physiological responses of physically fit men and women to acclimation to humid heat, *J. Appl. Physiol.: Respir. Environ. Exer. Physiol.*, 49(2):254–261, 1980.
6. Bäckström, T. and Carstensen, H., Estrogen and progesterone in plasma in relation to premenstrual tension, *J. Steroid Biochem.*, 4:257–260, 1974.
7. Bäckström, T., Wide, L. Södergärd, R., and Carstensen, H., FSH, LH, TeBG-capacity, estrogen and progesterone in women with premenstrual tension during the luteal phase, *J. Steroid Biochem.*, 7:473–476, 1976.
8. Baker, E. R., Menstrual dysfunction and hormonal status in athletic women: A review, *Fertil. Steril.*, 36(6):691–696, 1981.
9. Bancroft, J. and Bäckström, T., Premenstrual syndrome, *Clin. Endocrinol.*, 22:313–336, 1985.
10. Barron, W. M., Schrieber, J., and Lindheimer, M. D., Effect of ovarian sex steroids on osmoregulation and vasopressin secretion in the rat, *Am. J. Physiol.*, 250 (*Endocrinol. Metab.* 13):E352–E361, 1986.
11. Bartelink, M. L., Wollersheim, H., Theeuwes, A., van Duren, D., and Thien, Th., Changes in skin blood flow during the menstrual cycle: The influence of the menstrual cycle on the peripheral circulation in healthy female volunteers, *Clin. Sci.*, 78:527–532, 1990.
12. Bateman, J. C., A study of blood volume and anemia in cancer patients, *Blood*, 6:639–651, 1951.
13. Baylis, P. H., Spruce, B. A., and Burd, J., Osmoregulation of vasopressin secretion during the menstrual cycle, in *Vasopressin*, Schrier, R. W., Ed., Raven Press, New York, 1985, 241–247.
14. Beckerhoff, R., Luetscher, J. A., Beckerhoff, I., and Nokes, G. W., Effects of oral contraceptives on the renin-angiotensin system and on blood pressure of normal young women, *Hopkins Med. J.*, 132:80–87, 1973.

15. Bemben, D. A., Boileau, R. A., Bahr, J. M., Nelson, R. A., and Misner, J. E., Effects of oral contraceptives on hormonal and metabolic responses during exercise, *Med. Sci. Sports Exer.*, 24(2):434–441, 1992.
16. Berne, R. M. and Levy, M. N., The reproductive glands, in *Physiology*, 2nd Ed., C.V. Mosby, St. Louis, 1988, chap. 55.
17. Bergstrom, J., Hermansen, L., Hultman, E., and Saltin, B., Diet, muscle glycogen and physical performance, *Acta Physiol. Scand.* 71:140–150, 1967.
18. Blahd, W. H., Lederer, M. A., and Tyler, E. T., Effect of oral contraceptives on body water and electrolytes, *J. Reprod. Med.*, 13:223–225, 1974.
19. Bonen, A., Haynes, F. W., and Graham, T. E., Substrate and hormonal responses to exercise in women using oral contraceptives, *J. Appl. Physiol.*, 70(5):1917–1927, 1991.
20. Brown, W. K. and Sargent, F., II, Hidromeiosis, *Arch. Environ. Health*, 11:442–452, 1965.
21. Buckman, M. T., Peake, G. T., and Srivastava, L. S., Periovulatory enhancement of spontaneous prolactin secretion in normal women, *Metabolism*, 29(8):753–757, 1980.
22. Buono, M. J. and Sjoholm, N. T., Effect of physical training on peripheral sweat production, *J. Appl. Physiol.*, 65(2):811–814, 1988.
23. Byrd, R., Steward, L., Torranin, C., and Berringer, O. M., Sex differences in response to hypohydration, *J. Sports Med.*, 17:65–86, 1977.
24. Carlberg, K. A., Fregly, M. J., and Fahey, M., Effects of chronic estrogen treatment on water exchange in rats, *Am. J. Physiol.*, 247 (*Endocrinol. Metab.* 10):E101–E110, 1984.
25. Chakmakjian, Z. H. and Bethune, J. E., Study of human growth hormone response to insulin, vasopressin, exercise, and estrogen administration, *J. Lab. Clin. Med.*, 72:429–437, 1968.
26. Christy, N. P. and Shaver, J. C., Estrogens and the kidney, *Kidney Int.*, 6:366–376, 1974.
27. Cleland, T. S., Horvath, S. M., and Phillips, M., Acclimatization of women to heat after training, *Int. Z. Angew. Physiol., Einschl. Arbeitsphysiol.*, 27:15–24, 1969.
28. Cunningham, D. J. and Cabanac, M., Evidence from behavioral thermoregulatory responses of a shift in setpoint temperature related to the menstrual cycle, *J. Physiol.*, 63(3):236–238, 1971.
29. Dalvit-McPhillips, S. P., The effect of the menstrual cycle on nutrient intake, *Psychol. Behav.*, 31:209–212, 1983.
30. Dance, P., Lloyd, S., and Pickford, M., The effects of stilbestrol on the renal activity of conscious dogs, *J. Physiol.*, 145:225–240, 1959.
31. Davison, J. M., Shiells, E. A., Philips, P. R., and Lindheimer, M. D., Serial evaluation of vasopressin release and thirst in human pregnancy, *J. Clin. Invest.*, 81:798–806, 1988.
32. DeSouza, M. J., Maresh, C. M., Macguire, M. D., Kraemer, W. J., Flora-Ginter, G., and Goetz, K. L., Menstrual status and plasma vasopressin, renin activity, and aldosterone exercise responses, *J. Appl. Physiol.*, 67:736–743, 1989.
33. Dignam, W. S., Voskian, J., and Assali, N. S., Effects of estrogens on renal hemodynamics and excretion of electrolytes in human subjects, *J. Clin. Endocrinol. Metab.*, 16:1032–1042, 1956.
34. Dombovy, M. L., Bonekat, H. W., Williams, T. J., and Staats, B. A., Exercise performance and ventilatory response in the menstrual cycle, *Med. Sci. Sports Exer.*, 19(2):111–117, 1987.
35. Drinkwater, B. L., Denton, J. E., Kupprat, I. C., Talag, T. S., and Horvath, S. M., Aerobic power as a factor in women's response to work in hot environments, *J. Appl. Physiol.*, 41(6):815–821, 1976.
36. Dukes, P. P. and Goldwasser, E., Inhibition of erythropoiesis by estrogens, *Endocrinology*, 69:21–29, 1961.
37. Dunne, F. P., Barry, D. G., Ferriss, J. B., Grealy, G., and Murphy, D., Changes in blood pressure during the normal menstrual cycle, *Clin. Sci.*, 81:515–518, 1991.
38. Edwards, O. M. and Bayliss, R. I. S., Urinary excretion of water and electrolytes in normal females during the follicular and luteal phases of the menstrual cycle: The effect of posture, *Clin. Sci. Mol. Med.*, 45:495–504, 1973.

39. Evans, J. K., Naish, P. F., and Aber, G. M., Estrogen-induced changes in renal hemodynamics in the rat: Influence of plasma and intrarenal renin, *Clin. Sci.*, 71:613–619, 1986.
40. Fanestil, D. D. and Park, C. S., Steroid hormones and the kidney, *Ann. Rev. Physiol.*, 43:637–649, 1981.
41. Feicht, C. B., Johnson, T. S., Martin, B. J., Sparkes, K. E., and Wagner, W. W., Secondary amenorrhea in athletes, *Lancet*, 2:1145–1146, 1978.
42. Fein, J. T., Haymes, E. M., and Buskirk, E. R., Effects of daily and intermittent exposure on heat acclimation of women, *Int. J. Biometeorol.*, 10(1):41–52, 1975.
43. Flint, M. M., Drinkwater, B. L., and Horvath, S. M., Effects of training on women's response to submaximal exercise, *Med. Sci. Sports*, 6(2):89–94, 1974.
44. Forsling, M. L., Åkerlund, M., and Strömberg, P., Variations in plasma concentrations of vasopressin during the menstrual cycle, *J. Endocrinol.*, 89:263–266, 1981.
45. Fortney, S. M. and Senay, L. C., Jr., Effect of training and heat acclimation on exercise responses of sedentary females, *J. Appl. Physiol.: Respir. Environ. Exer. Physiol.*, 47(5):978–984, 1979.
46. Fortney, S. M., Turner, C., Steinmann, L., Driscoll, T., and Alfrey, C., Blood volume responses of men and women to bed rest, *J. Clin. Pharmacol.*, 34:434–439, 1994.
47. Franchimont, P., Dourcy, C., Legros, J. J., Reuter, A., Vrindts-Gervaert, Y., Van Cauwenberge, J. R., and Gaspard, U., Prolactin levels during the menstrual cycle, *Clin. Endocrinol.*, 5:643–650, 1976.
48. Frantz, A. G. and Rabkin, M. T., Effects of estrogen and sex difference on secretion of human growth hormone, *J. Clin. Endocrinol.*, 25:1470-1480, 1965.
49. Friedlander, M., Laskey, N., and Silbert, S., Effect of estrogenic substance on blood volume, *Endocrinol*ogy, 20:329–333, 1936.
50. Frye, A. J. and Kamon, E., Sweating efficiency in acclimated men and women exercising in humid and dry heat, *J. Appl. Physiol.: Respir. Environ. Exer. Physiol.*, 54(4):972–977, 1983.
51. Gaebelein, C. J. and Senay, L. C., Jr., Vascular volume dynamics during ergometer exercise at different menstrual phases, *Eur. J. Appl. Physiol.*, 50:1–11, 1982.
52. Genazzani, A. R., LeMarchand-Béraud, Th., Aubert, M. L., and Felber, J. P., Pattern of plasma ACTH, hGH, and cortisol during menstrual cycle, *J. Clin. Endocrinol. Metab.*, 41:431–437, 1975.
53. Gisolfi, C. V. and Cohen, J. S., Relationship among training, heat acclimation, and heat tolerance in men and women: The controversy revisited, *Med. Sci. Sports*, 11(1):56–59, 1979.
54. Gisolfi, C. V. and Duchman, S. M., Guidelines for optimal replacement beverages for different athletic events, *Med. Sci. Sports Exer.*, 24:679–687, 1992.
55. Gray, M. J., Strausfeld, K. S., Watanabe, M., Sims, E. A., and Solomon, S., Aldosterone secretory rates in the normal menstrual cycle, *J. Clin. Endocrinol. Metab.*, 28:1269–1275, 1968.
56. Greenleaf, J. E., Brock, P. J., Sciaraffa, D., Polese, A., and Elizondo, R., Effects of exercise-heat acclimation on fluid, electrolyte, and endocrine responses during tilt and +Gz acceleration in women and men, *Aviat. Space Environ. Med.*, 56:683–689, 1985.
57. Grucza, R., Pekkarinen, H., Titov, E-K., Kononoff, A., and Hänninen, O., Influence of the menstrual cycle and oral contraceptives on thermoregulatory responses to exercise in young women, *Eur. J. Appl. Physiol.*, 67:279–285, 1993.
58. Guerrero, R., Aso, T., Brenner, P. F., Cekan, Z., Landgren, B.-M., Hagenfeldt, K., and Diczfalusy, E., Studies on the pattern of circulating steroid in the normal menstrual cycle, *Acta Endocrinologica*, 81:133–149, 1976.
59. Hackney, A. C., Effects of the menstrual cycle on resting muscle glycogen content, *Horm. Metab. Res.*, 22:647, 1990.
60. Harrison, M. H., Effects of thermal stress and exercise on blood volume in humans, *Physiol. Rev.*, 65:149–209, 1985.

61. Harvey, O. L. and Crockett, H. E., Individual differences in temperature changes of women during the course of the menstrual cycle, *Hum. Biol.*, 4(4):453–468, 1932.
62. Hassan, A. A. K., Carter, G., and Tooke, J. E., Postural vasoconstriction in women during the normal menstrual cycle, *Clin. Sci.*, 78:39–47, 1990.
63. Hermansen, L., Hultman, E., and Saltin, B., Muscle glycogen during prolonged severe exercise, *Acta Physiol. Scand.*, 71:129–139, 1967.
64. Hertig, B. A. and Sargent, F., II, Acclimatization of women during work in hot environments, *Fed. Proc.*, 22:810–813, 1963.
65. Hertig, B. A., Belding, H. S., Kraning, K. K., Batterton, D. L., Smith, C. R., and Sargent, F., II, Artificial acclimatization of women to heat, *J. Appl. Physiol.*, 18(2):383–386, 1963.
66. Hessemer, V. and Brück, K., Influence of menstrual cycle on thermoregulatory, metabolic, and heart rate responses to exercise at night, *J. Appl. Physiol.*, 59(6):1911–1917, 1985.
67. Hirata, K., Nagasaka, T., Hirai, A., Hirashita, M., Takahata, T., and Nunomura, T., Effects of human menstrual cycle on thermoregulatory vasodilation during exercise, *Eur. J. Appl. Physiol.*, 54:559–565, 1986.
68. Holloszy, J. O., Biochemical adaptations to exercise: Aerobic metabolism, in *Exercise and Sports Science Reviews*, Wilmore, J. H., Ed., Academic Press, New York, 1973, 45–71.
69. Horstman, D. H. and Christensen, E., Acclimatization to dry heat: Active men vs. active women, *J. Appl. Physiol.: Respir. Environ. Exerc. Physiol.*, 52(4):825–831, 1982.
70. Huisveld, I. A., Derkx, F. M. H., Bouma, B. N., Erich, W. B. M., and Schalekamp, M. A. D. H., Renin-angiotensin system: Oral contraception and exercise in healthy female subjects, *J. Appl. Physiol.*, 59(6):1690–1697, 1985.
71. Israel, S. L. and Schneller, O., The thermogenic property of progesterone, *Fertil. Steril.*, 1:53–64, 1950.
72. Jensen, L.K., Svanegaard, J., and Husby, H., Atrial natriuretic peptide during the menstrual cycle. *Am. J. Obstet. Gynecol.* 161: 951–952, 1989.
73. Johnson, J. A., Davis, J. O., Baumber, J. S., and Schneider, E. G., Effects of estrogens and progesterone on electrolyte balances in normal dogs, *Am. J. Physiol.*, 219(6):1691–1697, 1970.
74. Jones, E. M., Fox, R. H., Verow, P. W., and Asscher, A. W., Variations in capillary permeability to plasma proteins during the menstrual cycle, *J. Obstet. Gynaekol.*, 73:666–669, 1966.
75. Jurkowski, J. E. H., Jones, N. L., Toews, C. J., and Sutton, J. R., Effects of menstrual cycle on blood lactate, O_2 delivery, and performance during exercise, *J. Appl. Physiol.: Respir. Environ. Exer. Physiol.*, 51(6):1493–1499, 1981.
76. Kaulhausen, H., Leyendecker, G., Benker, G., and Breuer, H., The relationship of the renin-angiotensin-aldosterone system to plasma gonadotropin, prolactin, and ovarian steroid patterns during the menstrual cycle, *Arch. Gynäkol.*, 225:179–200, 1978.
77. Keates, J. S. and Fitzgerald, D. E., Limb volume and blood flow changes during the menstrual cycle. I. Limb volume changes during the menstrual cycle, *Angiology* 20:618–623, 1969.
78. Keates, J. S. and Fitzgerald, D. E., Limb volume and blood flow changes during the menstrual cycle. II. Changes in blood flow and venous distensibility during the menstrual cycle, *Angiology* 20:624-627, 1969.
79. Kilbom, A., Physical training in women, *Scand. J. Clin. Lab. Invest.*, 28(S119):7–34, 1971.
80. Knip, A. S., Measurement and regional distribution of functioning eccrine sweat glands in male and female Caucasians, *Hum. Biol.*, 41:380–387, 1969.
81. Kobayashi, Y., Ando, Y, Okuda, N., Takaba, S., and Ohara, K., Effects of endurance training on thermoregulation in females, *Med. Sci. Sports Exer.*, 12(5):361–364, 1980.
82. Kolka, M. A. and Stephenson, L. A., Control of sweating during the human menstrual cycle, *Eur. J. Appl. Physiol.*, 58:890–895, 1989.
83. Laidlaw, J. C., Ruse, J. L., and Gornall, A. G., The influence of estrogen and progesterone on aldosterone excretion, *J. Clin. Endocrinol. Metab.*, 22:161–171, 1962.

84. Lehtovirta, P., Kuikka, J., and Pyörälä, T., Hemodynamic effects of oral contraceptives during exercise, *Int. J. Gynaecol. Obstet.*, 15:35–37, 1977.
85. Lenter, C., *Geigy Scientific Tables*, Ciba-Geigy, Basel, Switzerland, 1984, 65.
86. Littler, W. A., Bojorges-Bueno, R., and Banks, J., Cardiovascular dynamics in women during the menstrual cycle and oral contraceptive therapy, *Thorax*, 29:567–570, 1974.
87. Lloyd, P. D. and Pickford, M., The effects of stilbestrol on the renal activity of conscious dogs, *J. Physiol.*, 145:225–240, 1959.
88. Longo, L. D., Maternal blood volume and cardiac output during pregnancy: A hypothesis of endocrinologic control, *Am. J. Physiol.*, 245 (*Reg. Integ. Comp. Physiol.* 14):R720–R729, 1983.
89. Loucks, A. B. and Horvath, S. M., Athletic amenorrhea: A review, *Med. Sci. Sports Exer.*, 17(1):56–72, 1985.
90. Manhem, K., Jern, C., Pilhall, M., Shanks, G., and Jern, S., Haemodynamic responses to psychosocial stress during the menstrual cycle, *Clin. Sci.*, 81:17–22, 1991.
91. Martin, D. G., Ferguson, E. W., Wigutoff, S., Gawne, T., and Schoomaker, E. B., Blood viscosity responses to maximal exercise in endurance-trained and sedentary female subjects, *J. Appl. Physiol.*, 59(2):348–353, 1985.
92. Mathor, M. B., Achado, S. S., Wajchenberg, B. L., and Germek, O. A., Free plasma testosterone levels during the normal menstrual cycle, *J. Endocrinol. Invest.*, 8:437–441, 1985.
93. McCaffrey, T. A. and Czaja, J. A., Diverse effects of estradiol-17β: Concurrent suppression of appetite, blood pressure and vascular reactivity in conscious, unrestrained animals, *Physiol. Behav.*, 45(3):649–657, 1989.
94. McMurray, R. G. and Katz, V. L., Thermoregulation in pregnancy, implications for exercise, *Sports Med.*, 10(3):146–158, 1990.
95. Michelakis, A. M., Yoshida, H., and Dormois, J. C., Plasma renin activity and plasma aldosterone during the normal menstrual cycle, *Am. J. Obstet. Gynecol.*, 123(7):724–726, 1975.
96. Mishell, D. E., Contraception (medical progress), *N. Engl. J. Med.*, 320(12):777–787, 1989.
97. Mishell, D. R., Nakamura, R. M., Crosignani, P. G., Stone, S., Kharma, K., Nagata, Y., and Thorneycroft, I. H., Serum gonadotropin and steriod patterns during the normal menstrual cycle, *Am J. Obstet. Gynecol.*, 3:60–65, 1971.
98. Munday, M. R., Brush, M. G., and Taylor, R. W., Correlations between progesterone, oestradiol and aldosterone levels in the premenstrual syndrome, *Clin. Endocrinol.*, 14:1–9, 1981.
99. Muse, K. N., Cetel, N. S., Futterman, L. A., and Yen, S. S. C., The premenstrual syndrome, *N. Engl. J. Med.*, 311:1345–1349, 1984.
100. Myhre, L. G., Hartung, G. H., Nunneley, S. A., and Tucker, D. M., Plasma volume changes in middle-aged male and female subjects during marathon running, *J. Appl. Physiol.*, 59(2):559–563, 1985.
101. Nadel, E. R., Roberts, M. F., and Wenger, C. B., Thermoregulatory adaptations to heat and exercise: Comparative responses of men and women, in *Environmental Stress*, Folinsbee, L. J., Wagner, J. A., Borgia, J. F., Drinkwater, B. L., Gliner, J. A., and Bedi, J. F., Eds., Academic Press, New York, 1978, 29–38.
102. Naden, R. P. and Rosenfeld, C. R., Role of α-receptors in estrogen-induced vasodilatation in nonpregnant sheep, *Am. J. Physiol.*, 248 (*Heart Circ. Physiol.* 17):H339–344, 1985.
103. Nicklas, B. J., Hackney, A. C., and Sharp, R. L., The menstrual cycle and exercise: Performance, muscle glycogen, and substrate responses, *Int. J. Sports Med.*, 10(4):264–269, 1989.
104. O'Brien, P. M. S., The premenstrual syndrome, *J. Reprod. Med.*, 30(2):113–126, 1985.
105. Øian, P., Tollan, A., Fadnes, H. O., Noddeland, H., and Maltau, J. M., Transcapillary fluid dynamics during the menstrual cycle, *Am. J. Obstet. Gynecol.*, 156:952–955, 1987.

106. Olsson, K., Pregnancy — A challenge to water balance, *NIPS*, (Int. Union Physiol. Sci./Am. Physiol. Soc.) 1:131–133, 1986.
107. Paolone, A. M., Wells, C. L., and Kelly, G. T., Sexual variations in thermoregulation during heat stress, *Aviat. Space Environ. Med.*, 49(5):715–719, 1978.
108. Pliner, P. and Fleming, A. E., Food intake, body weight, and sweetness preferences over the menstrual cycle in humans, *Physiol. Behav.*, 30:663-666, 1983.
109. Prashad, D. N., Fletcher, P. A., and Cooper, M., Exercise-induced changes in urinary water and mineral output during the menstrual cycle, *Br. J. Sports Med.*, 21(1):9-12, 1987.
110. Preedy, J. R. K. and Aitken, E. H., The effect of estrogen on water and electrolyte metabolism, I. The Normal, *J. Clin. Invest.*, 35:423-429, 1956.
111. Price, A. G., *White Settlers in the Tropics*, Publ. No. 23, Stone, R. C., Ed., American Geographical Society, New York, 1939.
112. Punnonen, R., Viinamäki, O., and Multamäki, S., Plasma vasopressin during normal menstrual cycle, *Hormone Res.*, 17:90-92, 1983.
113. Rees, J. and Shuster, S., Pubertal induction of sweat gland activity, *Clin. Sci.*, 60:689-692, 1981.
114. Riedel, M., Oeltermann, A., Mugge, A., Creutzig, A., Rafflenbeul, W., Lichtlen, P., Vascular responses to 17β-oestradiol in postmenopausal women. *Eur. J. Clin. Invest.*, 25:44-47, 1995.
115. Roberts, M. F., Wenger, C. B., Stolwijk, J. A. J., and Nadel, E. R., Skin blood flow and sweating changes following exercise training and heat acclimation, *J. Appl. Physiol.*, 43:133-137, 1977.
116. Röcker, L., Kirsch, K., and Stoboy, H., The influence of heat stress on plasma volume and intravascular proteins in sedentary females, *Eur. J. Appl. Physiol.*, 36:187-192, 1977.
117. Rothchild, I. and Barnes, A. C., The effects of dosage, and of estrogen, androgen or salicylate administration on the degree of body temperature elevation induced by progesterone, *Endocrinology*, 50:485-496, 1952.
118. Saltin, B. and Hermansen, L., Esophageal, rectal, and muscle temperature during exercise, *J. Appl. Physiol.*, 21:1757–1762, 1966.
119. Schoene, R. B., Robertson, H. T., Pierson, D. J., and Peterson, A. P., Respiratory drives and exercise in menstrual cycles of athletic and nonathletic women, *J. Appl. Physiol.: Respir. Environ. Exer. Physiol.*, 50:1300–1305, 1981.
120. Schwartz, B., Cumming, D. C., Riordan, E., Selye, M., Yen, S. S. C., and Rebar, R. W., Exercise-associated amenorrhea: A distinct entity?, *Am. J. Obstet. Gynecol.*, 141:662–670, 1981.
121. Senay, L. C. Jr. and Fortney, S., Untrained females: Effects of submaximal exercise and heat on body fluids, *J. Appl. Physiol.*, 39(4):643–647, 1975.
122. Senay, L. C., Jr., Body fluids and temperature responses of heat-exposed women before and after ovulation with and without rehydration, *J. Physiol.*, 232:209–219, 1973.
123. Shapiro, Y., Pandolf, K. B., Avellini, B. A., Pimental, N. A., and Goldman, R. F., Heat balance and transfer in men and women exercising in hot-dry and hot-wet conditions, *Ergonomics*, 24(5):375–386, 1981.
124. Shapiro, Y., Pandolf, K. B., Avellini, B. A., Pimental, N. A., and Goldman, R. F., Physiological responses of men and women to humid and dry heat, *J. Appl. Physiol.: Respir. Environ. Exer. Physiol.*, 49(1):1–8, 1980.
125. Short, R. V., Oestrous and menstrual cycle, in *Reproduction in Mammals: Vol. 3, Hormonal Control of Reproduction*, Austin, C. R. and Short, R. V., Eds., Cambridge University Press, Cambridge, 1984, 124.
126. Shvartz, E. and Meyerstein, N., Effect of heat and natural acclimatization to heat on tilt tolerance of men and women, *J. Appl. Physiol.*, 28(4):428–432, 1970.
127. Sinning, W. E. and Little, K. D., Body composition and menstrual function in athletes, *Sports Med.*, 4:34–45, 1987.
128. Solomon, S. J., Kurzer, M. S., and Calloway, D. H., Menstrual cycle and basal metabolic rate in women, *Am. J. Clin. Nutr.*, 36:611–616, 1982.

129. Spruce, B. A., Baylis, P. H., Burd, J., and Watson, M. J., Variation in osmoregulation of arginine vasopressin during the human menstrual cycle, *Clin. Endocrinol.*, 22:37–42, 1985.
130. St-Louis, J., Parent, A., Larivière, R., and Schiffrin, E. L., Vasopressin responses and receptors in the mesenteric vasculature of estrogen-treated rats, *Am. J. Physiol.*, 251 (*Heart Circ. Physiol.* 20):H885–H889, 1986.
131. Stephenson, L. A. and Kolka, M. A., Plasma volume during heat stress and exercise in women, *Eur. J. Appl. Physiol.*, 57:373–381, 1988.
132. Stephenson, L. A. and Kolka, M. A., Menstrual cycle phase and time of day alter reference signal controlling arm blood flow and sweating, *Am. J. Physiol.*, 249 (*Regu. Integr. Comp. Physiol.* 18):R186–191, 1985.
133. Stephenson, L. A. and Kolka, M. A., Thermoregulation in women, in *Exercise and Sport Sciences Reviews*, Vol. 21, Holloszy, J. O., Ed., Williams & Wilkens, Baltimore, 1993, 231–262.
134. Stevenson, E. T., Davy, K. P., and Seals, D. R., Maximal aerobic capacity and total blood volume in highly trained middle-aged and older female endurance athletes, *J. Appl. Physiol.*, 77(4):1691–1696, 1994.
135. Sundsfjord, J. A. and Aakvaag, A., Plasma renin activity, plasma renin substrate and urinary aldosterone excretion in the menstrual cycle in relation to the concentration of progesterone and oestrogens in the plasma, *Acta Endocrinol.*, 71:519–529, 1972.
136. Sweeney, J. S., Menstrual edema, *J. Am. Med. Assoc.*, 103:234–236, 1934.
137. Tankersley, C. G., Nicholas, W. C., Deaver, D. R., Mikita, D., and Kenney, W. L., Estrogen replacement in middle-aged women: Thermoregulatory responses to exercise in the heat, *J. Appl. Physiol.*, 73(4):1238–1245, 1992.
138. Thorn, G. W. and Emerson, K., The role of gonadal and adrenal cortical hormones in the production of adema, *Ann. Intern. Med.*, 14(5):757–769, 1940.
139. Thorn, G. W. and Engel, L. L., The effect of sex hormones on the renal excretion of electrolytes, *J. Exp. Med.*, 68:299–312, 1938.
140. Thorn, G. W., Nelson, K. R., and Thorn, D. W., A study of the mechanism of edema associated with menstruation, *Endocrinology*, 22(2):155-163, 1938.
141. Tollan, A., Øian, P., Fadnes, H. O., and Maltau, J. M., Evidence for altered transcapillary fluid balance in women with premenstrual syndrome, *Acta Obstet. Gynecol. Scand.*, 72:238-242, 1993.
142. Ueda, S., Fortune, V., Bull, B. S., Valenzuela, G. J., and Longo, L. D., Estrogen effects on plasma volume, arterial blood pressure, interstitial space, plasma proteins, and blood viscosity in sheep, *Am. J. Obstet. Gynecol.*, 155(1):195-201, 1986.
143. Veille, J. C., Morton, M. J., Burry, K., Nemeth, M., and Speroff, L., Estradiol and hemodynamics during ovulation induction, *J. Clin. Endocrinol. Metab.*, 63:721–724, 1986.
144. Vellar, O. D., Changes in hemoglobin concentration and hematocrit during the menstrual cycle, *Acta Obstet. Gynecol. Scand.*, 53:243–246, 1974.
145. Vokes, T. J., Weiss, N. M., Schreiber, J., Gaskill, M. B., and Robertson, G. L., Osmoregulation of thirst and vasopressin during normal menstrual cycle, *Am. J. Physiol.*, 254 (*Regul. Integr. Comp. Physiol.* 23):R641–647, 1988.
146. Walters, W. A. W. and Lim, Y. L., Haemodynamic changes in women taking oral contraceptives, *J. Obstet. Gynaecol.*, 77:1007–1012, 1970.
147. Webb, P., 24-hour energy expenditure and the menstrual cycle, *Am. J. Clin. Nutr.*, 44:614–619, 1986.
148. Weinman, K. P., Slabochova, Z., Bernauer, E. M., Morimoto, T., and Sargent, F., II, Reactions of men and women to repeated exposure to humid heat, *J. Appl. Physiol.*, 22(3):533–538, 1967.
149. Wells, C. L., Responses of physically active and acclimatized men and women to exercise in a desert environment, *Med. Sci. Sports Exer.*, 12(1):9–13, 1980.
150. Wells, C. L., Sexual differences in heat stress response, *Physician Sports Med.*, 5(7):79–90, 1977.
151. Wilmore, J. H., The female athlete, *J. School Health*, 227–233, 1977.

152. Witten, C. L. and Bradbury, J. T., Hemodilution as a result of estrogen therapy. Estrogenic effects in the human female, *Proc. Soc. Exp. Biol. Med.*, 78:626–629, 1951.
153. Wyndham, C. H., Morrison, J. F., and Williams, C. G., Heat reactions of male and female Caucasians, *J. Appl. Physiol.*, 20(3):357–364, 1965.

Chapter **13**

FLUID REPLACEMENT DURING EXERCISE AND RECOVERY FROM EXERCISE

Lawrence E. Armstrong
Carl M. Maresh

CONTENTS

I. Introduction... .259

II. Environmental and Host Factors .... .260

III. Fluid Replacement During Exercise .... .262
    A. Water vs. No Fluid Replacement .... .263
    B. Water vs. [Water + NaCl] Replacement.................. .264
    C. Water vs. [Water + CHO] Replacement.................. .267

IV. CHO and NaCl Effects During Recovery from Exercise .... .270

V. Fluid Replacement: Other Influences of Exercise.............. .272

VI. Summary.. .274

References .... .275

I. INTRODUCTION

Despite the important contributions of early pioneers,[53] and the fact that the principal physiological basis for thirst (i.e., cellular dehydration) had been discovered in the late 1940s, relatively little is known about exercise-related thirst, drinking behavior, and fluid replacement.[111] From 80 to 90% of our knowledge about these topics has accumulated since the early 1960s.[68] Thus, this chapter integrates a few investigations from the World War II years with many other studies conducted during the last three decades. Its purpose is to describe factors that influence the efficacy of fluid replacement on exercise performance and recovery from exercise.

We will use the following definition of terms throughout this chapter. **Thirst**: a disturbing drive that arouses and maintains the search for and ingestion of water or other fluid.[53] **Drinking behavior**: fluid consumption that is either driven by an attempt to relieve an annoying stimulation (i.e., thirst), or motivated by learned behavior that seeks to renew or prolong an agreeable stimulation (e.g., fluid intake).[25] Therefore, thirst and the physiological need for water may not be the only causes of drinking behavior; habit, a hedonic search for pleasure, and many other factors may influence drinking behavior. **Fluid replacement**: orally restoring sweat, urine, and respiratory water losses, during or subsequent to exercise or thermal dehydration. Fluid replacement modifies the deleterious effects of dehydration on physiological, psychological, and exercise performance variables. This term is used synonymously with **fluid intake** and **fluid consumption**, which also are measurable behaviors.

II. ENVIRONMENTAL AND HOST FACTORS

Drinking behavior and fluid replacement, as described in Chapters 1 and 6 of this book, are multifaceted processes that are difficult to ascribe solely to thirst. Several environmental and host factors that influence fluid replacement during exercise and recovery are summarized below.

1. Environmental stressors (i.e., temperature, humidity, wind speed, solar radiation) result in physiological perturbations (i.e., hyperosmolality, hypovolemia) that tend to either increase or decrease fluid consumption, depending on the integration of effects exerted by these stressors.[20,63,89]
2. Environmental conditions may modify pleasure-related preferences (e.g., alliesthesia).[48] For example, a cold fluid is pleasurable during hyperthermia but unpleasant during hypothermia.[79] *Ad libitum* fluid consumption during mild-to-moderately strenuous exercise increases markedly when the ambient temperature exceeds 25°C.[123] Figure 1 illustrates this phenomenon.
3. Individual differences in learned behaviors influence fluid replacement, in that humans can be instructed to drink when thirst is absent,[78] or may learn through experience that physical and mental performance are enhanced by drinking.[10]
4. Societal customs and mores may influence fluid consumption, as evidenced by the differences in beer-drinking preferences between American and British citizens.[20,30,63] Even social rituals (i.e., consuming a beverage during a break from work, accepting the friendly offer of a

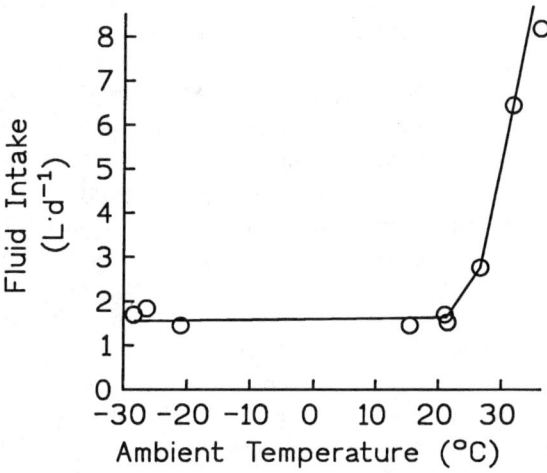

FIGURE 1 The relationship of daily fluid intake to mean ambient temperature during outdoor military maneuvers requiring moderate-to-strenuous exercise. (Redrawn from Welch, B. E., et al., *Metabolism*, 7:141, 1958. With permission.)

beverage) may enhance fluid intake in excess of drinking that is driven by sensory or somatic gratification.[20]

5. Fluid palatability affects consumption[22,79,112] and consists of beverage characteristics such as salinity, temperature, sweetness, flavor, color, viscosity, and carbonation.[11,48,62,63,112,117,120] The palatability of a fluid also may be affected by the temperature of the tongue,[61] the novelty of the fluid, the time of day, and the physiological state of the individual.[110]

6. Personal opinions regarding the effect of a fluid on one's health (i.e., nutrient, alcohol, caffeine or caloric content), body weight,[20] cost,[63] or exercise performance[8] affect beverage choice and the volume consumed. Product advertising and packaging also may influence the purchase and subsequent consumption of beverages.[20,63] Similarly, one's expectations regarding a beverage, prior to drinking, can influence palatability.[48]

7. Thirst increases during eating.[47] Between 69 and 78% of fluid replacement during normal daily activities occurs at meals.[1,48]

8. Dehydration does not result in thirst until a water deficit of 1–2% has been reached.[1,113] This water deficit may occur (a) as the daily unavoidable water loss in a mild environment, without water intake,[86] or (b) as the sweat loss incurred during 0.3–2.0 h of strenuous exercise in a hot environment.[10,78,89,113] Dehydration, due to water deprivation and increased fluid losses, is characterized by thirst and is completely relieved by administration of pure water. Dehydration due to sodium depletion does not result in thirst and is not relieved by administration

of salt-free fluids.[46,96] In contrast, the addition of high concentrations of solutes (e.g., sodium chloride) to drinking water inhibits fluid consumption partially.[2] Similarly, it has been shown that intravenous infusion of hypertonic saline (0.45 M), but not isotonic saline (0.15 M), increases plasma sodium, osmolality, subjective ratings of thirst, and water intake in humans.[106]

9. Fluid restriction for 24 h increases subjective ratings of thirst, mouth dryness, and the unpleasantness of the taste in the mouth.[107] This suggests that specific sensations are associated with dehydration and may enhance fluid replacement. Other evidence suggests that humans become thirsty before body fluid deficits occur; this thirst may arise in response to subtle oropharyngeal cues.[47]
10. Extreme gastrointestinal distension places increasingly strong inhibition on fluid consumption, before tissue repletion of lost fluid occurs.[20] Reduced sensations of mouth dryness have a similar effect.[111]
11. Humans tend to drink less when they are preoccupied or are performing physical or mental tasks.[1] Frequent rest periods, in the midst of labor or exercise, will enhance fluid consumption[45] and extend fluid replacement time.[79,120] If a fluid is readily available, it is more likely to be consumed than if it is difficult to obtain.[1,48]
12. Humans consume a greater quantity of fluid when they are calm than when they are excited.[63] Cholinergic stimulation, which tends to calm the body, facilitates drinking. Adrenergic stimulation, which tends to excite the body and call it into action (i.e., before or during exercise), inhibits drinking.[69]

The following sections of this chapter will describe ways that exercise and recovery from exercise interact with the above factors to influence fluid replacement. This complexity raises three important research design issues for physiologists. First, investigators must be aware that these influences exist and must attempt to control their effects on measurements of thirst sensations and fluid consumption. Second, because humans drink when there is no apparent physiological stimulus, psychological components should always be measured concurrently with the volume and rate of fluid intake.[62] Third, test subjects should enter each test in a state of similar hydration. This can be evaluated by simply measuring the sodium, osmolality, or color of urine,[13] and requiring rehydration when necessary.

III. FLUID REPLACEMENT DURING EXERCISE

For exercising humans, the key ingredients in replacement fluids are water, carbohydrate (CHO), and sodium chloride (NaCl). The debate regarding the efficacies of pure water vs. [water + CHO], [water + NaCl], or [water + CHO + NaCl] has continued for more than three decades and has been stimulated by three factors: (1) the desire of athletes to optimize exercise performance, (2) the profit potential of marketing sport drinks, and (3) scientific curiosity and conflicting research results. Some authorities[66,72,99] have stated that athletes require only pure water during strenuous exercise because the circulation becomes hypertonic and hypovolemic, and because a balanced diet generally provides ample water, CHO, and electrolytes for most athletic events. Others have concluded that beverages containing CHO and NaCl are equivalent[26,33,51] or superior to[40,71,84] pure water, because such beverages are more palatable (thereby increasing fluid intake) and they may provide an exogenous fuel (the CHO) when muscle and liver glycogen stores are depleted. In fact, under different circumstances all positions in this debate may be correct because there is no single replacement fluid that meets the demands of all athletes and all forms of exercise.[4] Thus, nutritional recommendations for athletes must consider the event, previous hydration status of the athlete, the need for exogenous CHO, and environmental stressors.

A. WATER VS. NO FLUID REPLACEMENT

In addition to the well-known deleterious effects of dehydration on endurance exercise performance,[4,6,10,40,77,116] heat exhaustion is the most common form of heat illness experienced by athletes.[12] Because heat exhaustion (both the water loss and salt loss varieties) is primarily a volume depletion problem,[1,5,12,77] the importance of water in health and physical performance cannot be denied. These effects were partially appreciated at the beginning of the 20th century,[81] were not conceptually integrated until 1943–1947,[1,15,108] and were not reflected in the rules of international athletic competition until the 1970s, largely as a result of the research of Pugh et al.,[109] Wyndham and Strydom,[125] and Costill et al.[33] But since 1966, few studies have compared exercise trials involving water replacement vs. no fluid intake.[100] The current fluid replacement guidelines of the American College of Sports Medicine[3] recommend that (1) approximately 500 ml of fluid be consumed about 2 hr before exercise, (2) the largest tolerable volume (e.g., 400–600 ml) be maintained in the stomach during exercise, and (3) athletes attempt to consume fluids at a rate that replaces all water lost in sweat.

Inadequate fluid replacement during endurance exercise may alter physiological function when only 1% of body weight has been lost.[66] For a 70-kg individual this amounts to only 0.7 l of sweat loss. Although it is possible that an individual could lose this amount of sweat in approximately 12 min,[10] most people would require 45–60 min of mild exercise to dehydrate to this level.[78,113] Human research has shown that the following physiological responses are potentiated during exercise by concurrent hypohydration and hyperthermia: increased rectal temperature, heart rate, plasma osmolality, and rating of perceived exertion; as well as decreased maximal aerobic power, sweat rate, exercise endurance time, plasma volume, cardiac output, stroke volume, and skin blood flow.[24,113] These responses indicate that the primary effects of body water loss are realized in thermoregulatory and cardiovascular function. Perhaps no research illustrates the potentiation of these responses better than that of Sawka and colleagues,[114] which exposed test subjects to 100 min of intermittent exercise in a 49°C environment, while either euhydrated or hypohydrated (i.e., by −3, −5, or −7% of body weight). Companion publications by Francesconi et al.[56] and Engell et al.[49] demonstrated that (1) plasma levels of renin, aldosterone, and cortisol (indicating electrolyte conservation and increased stress)[56] and (2) sensations of thirst[49] were incrementally elevated by hypohydration through 7% of body weight loss. Thirst and hormonal responses similar to these have been observed during endurance exercise in a hot environment, subsequent to a 3.8% exercise-induced hypohydration and fluid deprivation.[58,75]

In light of the multiple organ responses to restricted fluid intake, it is not surprising that endurance performance is negatively affected.[6] However, muscular strength is not altered by mild-to-moderate dehydration. Thus, inadequate fluid replacement that results in sweat losses of 1–5% of body weight can be tolerated without a loss of strength.[39,73,113] However, power during sustained or repeated bouts of exercise for longer than 30 s apparently deteriorates when moderate-to-severe dehydration (i.e., −6% or more) exists.[76] This probably results from reduced muscle blood flow, waste removal, or heat dissipation.

B. WATER VS. [WATER + NaCL] REPLACEMENT

The majority of humans perceive low concentrations of NaCl favorably. For this reason, most sport drinks contain small amounts of electrolytes because they enhance the palatability of relatively dilute carbohydrate solutions[93] and increase fluid consumption.[32,48,85,117] However, little is known about the alliesthesia-related interactions of fluid salinity with exercise and environmental conditions. For example, it has been reported that (1) alliesthesia decreases as dehydration and core body temperature increase during exercise,[11,110] and (2) adding too much of an ingredient (i.e., 12% glucose) to a fluid can reduce the appeal of that beverage during exercise.[44]

Several early observations presented conflicting findings regarding NaCl needs during residence or labor in hot environments,[78] with dietary recommendations ranging from 13 to 48 g NaCl per day.[9] Unfortunately, those human studies involved research design flaws and did not separate the effects of water depletion from salt depletion;[9,78] this is critical because pure water and pure salt depletion result in very different fluid shifts and symptoms of heat exhaustion.[122] The reported dietary intake of salt in the United States ranges from 5 to 13 g NaCl per day.[98] Empirical studies have shown that this intake is greater than the levels consumed by the inhabitants of tropical countries and that the resting human biological requirement for salt is small, ranging from only 0.1 to 0.2 g NaCl per day.[43] Other recent investigations have shown that electrolyte supplementation, including NaCl, is generally unwarranted when active individuals and athletes consume a normal Western diet and *ad libitum* water.[5,7,11,12,77] This has been verified during 4 h of physical activity in a 35°C environment;[85] during 8 h of heat exposure (41°C), including 4 h of treadmill walking on 10 consecutive days while consuming low (4 g) and moderate (8 g) quantities of NaCl;[9] and during 3 d of simulated tennis match play (4.5 h/d, 32°C).[17]

During exercise, the majority of athletes neither require nor measurably benefit from consuming electrolytes,[32] although a dilute electrolyte solution can be consumed without risk of inducing a fluid–electrolyte imbalance.[93] Inclusion of NaCl in fluid replacement drinks (< 50 meq/l) usually does not result in the expansion or retention of fluid in the vascular compartment.[42,87] However, the work of Candas and colleagues[24] demonstrates that this may occur during intermittent cycling exercise spanning 4 h (34°C). They compared the effects of five treatments (i.e., no fluid replacement, water, hypotonic, isotonic, and hypertonic sugar solutions) on cardiovascular and thermoregulatory function. Figure 2 illustrates the results of their tests. All four fluid replacement solutions were physiologically superior to the no-fluid trial, but only the isotonic fluid expanded plasma volume. More recently,[21] research from this same laboratory concluded that efficient rehydration should avoid plasma volume expansion at the expense of interstitial and intracellular rehydration. Isotonic and hypertonic beverages may act to restore plasma volume in this way.[99]

This is not meant to imply that athletes never require NaCl supplementation. Occasionally, such great emphasis has been placed on drinking requirements that the ingestion of excessive volumes of pure water or hypotonic fluid during exercise has led to hyponatremia in ultraendurance athletes.[102] This illness (defined as a plasma sodium concentration < 130 meq/l) may involve disorientation, grand mal seizure, coma, increased intracranial pressure, pulmonary edema, respiratory arrest, or death. Although four theoretical etiologies have been advanced,[8] recent evidence suggests that hyponatremia most commonly occurs when a large volume (i.e., 10 l) of hypotonic fluid is retained in the body.[8,101] The incidence of this fluid–electrolyte disorder is low in most circumstances, and usually occurs only during ultraendurance events lasting 5–20 h or more.[102] The exception is a recent case of exercise-related hyponatremia that developed in only 4 h.[8] Three interesting findings were reported in this case study, suggesting a complex etiology: (1) a "low normal" plasma sodium (134 meq/l) existed prior to exercise that may have predisposed this individual to hyponatremia; (2) an inappropriately large release of vasopressin, promoting renal water reabsorption sufficient to enhance plasma dilution, coincided with a decrease of urine volume to 0 ml/h; and (3) a large volume of fluid may have been sequestered in the gastrointestinal tract, where it acted to induce sodium movement into the intestinal lumen.[8,100] This latter phenomenon also has been proposed as part of the etiology of heat exhaustion.[5,78] Nutritional recommendations for athletes who compete in ultraendurance events should include the consumption of NaCl in fluids or solid food.[93] Consuming ample fluid is usually not a problem because a relatively slow

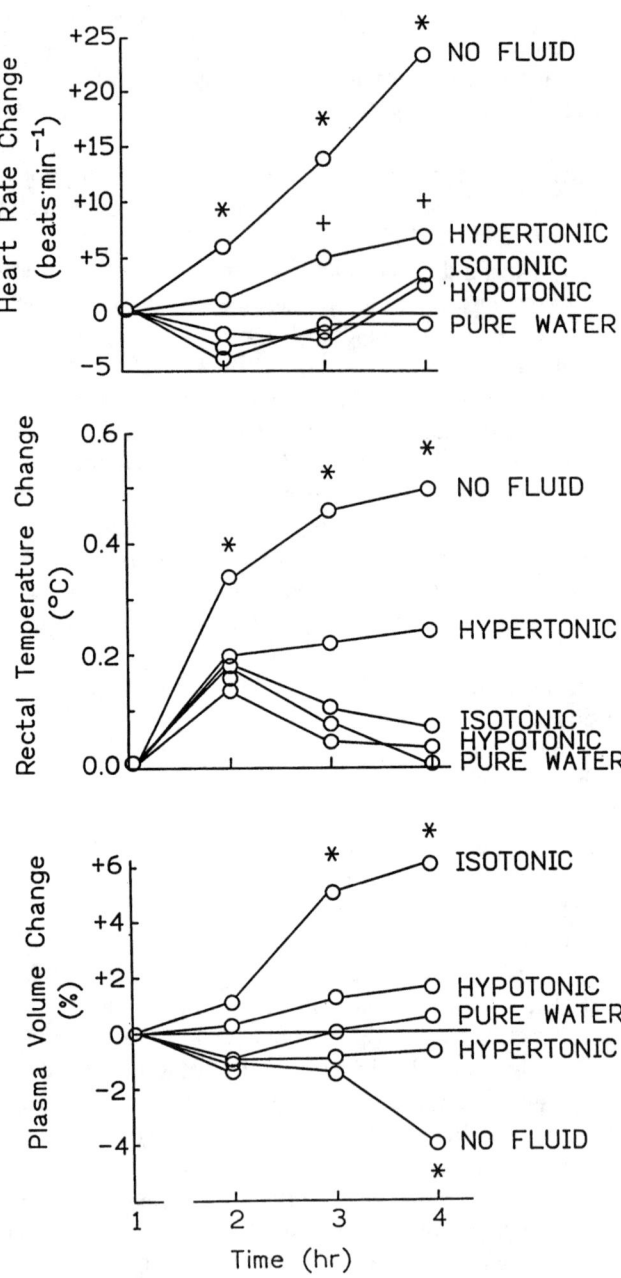

FIGURE 2 Mean changes in heart rate, rectal temperature, and plasma volume, during 4 h of intermittent cycling exercise. During five trials, subjects consumed either no fluid or rehydrated with one of four fluids. (*) Significantly different from all other treatments; (+) significantly different from the hypotonic and pure water treatments. (Redrawn from Candas, V., et al., *Eur. J. Appl. Physiol.*, 55:113, 1986. With permission.)

pace is maintained in races that are longer than the standard marathon distance (i.e., > 42 km).

A recent report considered the need for fluid replacement in soldiers who labor in the heat.[5] It concluded that salt-containing beverages are not required by all soldiers in all situations, because (1) sweat contains only 1–4 g NaCl/l, depending on one's state of heat acclimatization; (2) daily garrison meals contain 6–24 g NaCl; and (3) daily field rations contain 13 g NaCl. The greatest need for beverages containing NaCl and CHO was experienced by soldiers who lost more than 8 l of sweat per day, were not heat acclimatized, performed continuous exercise of > 60 min, did not eat a balanced diet, or were ill with diarrheal disease.

Heat cramps involve a very painful heat illness that probably is caused by a NaCl imbalance. Although the exact mechanism is unknown and few systematic scientific observations have been made, heat cramps usually occur after several hours of strenuous exercise in individuals who have lost a large volume of sweat, have drunk a large volume of unsalted water, and have excreted a small volume of urine.[77,118] The etiological similarities to hyponatremia are obvious (see above). Virtually all authors agree that NaCl depletion is involved in heat cramps. It is possible that intracellular water expansion alters the muscle membrane potential, thereby disrupting normal muscle contraction and relaxation. Heat cramps can be resolved within minutes by the administration of intravenous saline. Lightly salted beverages also bring resolution, suggesting that either fluids containing NaCl or supplemental NaCl in solid foods is warranted. As with hyponatremia, it is unlikely that NaCl will be necessary for individuals who consume a normal U.S. diet (i.e., 5–13 g NaCl/d).

Most sport drinks contain 1.2–1.8 g NaCl/l (20–30 meq sodium/l). Intestinal studies utilizing the segmental perfusion technique with a triple-lumen tube[60] have shown that doubling the sodium content of a fluid (i.e., from 25 to 50 meq/l) did not enhance water or sodium absorption. Similarly, the bioavailability of glucose in plasma, measured with a ^{3}H-glucose tracer, was not altered by increasing the content of sodium from 0 to 25–50 meq/l.[70] Therefore, if sodium is available in the gut from a previous meal, there appears to be no rationale for the presence of sodium in an oral rehydration solution.[3,114]

C. WATER VS. [WATER + CHO] REPLACEMENT

Since the mid-1980s, several authorities[28,40,74,93,116] have concluded that [water + CHO] ingestion during exercise results in prolonged endurance performance, when compared to pure water ingestion. A few of these authorities, citing previous animal[27] and human[18,27,35,37,83,84] research, have published unequivocal statements such as, "carbohydrate ingestion clearly improves performance lasting longer than 90 minutes and in which fatigue is associated with reduced bodily stores of carbohydrate."[36] We believe that unequivocal statements such as this require clarification, such as Murray's use of the phrase, "under the proper circumstances".[93] Table 1 shows that many studies found no difference between [water + CHO] supplementation versus water or placebo, in terms of endurance performance.

Our interpretation of Table 1 provides the following nine conclusions. First, because 62% of these CHO trials resulted in no significant differences between CHO-containing fluids and water, it is unlikely that CHO consumption will improve exercise performance in all recreational and athletic situations. When [water + CHO] improves endurance performance, it may be due to the maintenance of a normal blood glucose level and avoidance of hypoglycemia.[27,38,82] Indeed, some individuals are especially sensitive to a lowering of blood glucose and exhibit subjective symptoms of central nervous system fatigue that can be prevented by the consumption of glucose during endurance exercise.[14,116] These individuals comprise about one fourth of a normal athletic population.[38] In contrast, there are other individuals who exhibit none of these symptoms during exercise-induced hypoglycemia.[38,51] Therefore, it is likely that a fraction of the subjects in Table 1 were sensitive to hypoglycemia, and that this was not controlled. It appears that CHO should be consumed at least 30 min prior to the time when fatigue would normally occur, if no CHO were ingested, although there is a great variability between subjects in this regard.[40] Different authors state that the optimal rate of CHO consumption is either 0.5–1.0 g/min,[40] 1 g/min,[82] or 0.2 g/kg body weight/h.[116]

Second, there is little evidence (Table 1) that CHO supplementation in fluids affects performance when exercise lasts less than 60 min, regardless of its intensity. Third, the mean (± SD) amount of total CHO consumed was 123 ± 94 g CHO (range: 39–432) for the 23 solutions that found no significant differences between CHO-containing fluids and water or placebo, and 107 ± 99 g CHO (range: 28–432) for the 14 solutions that were significantly different from water or placebo; these total CHO values are not significantly different ($p > .05$) and their ranges are similar. Fourth, neither the exercise mode nor the experimental protocol appears to be exclusively responsible for enhanced endurance performance. However, sprint finishes at the end of prolonged exercise accounted for significant differences in four studies (Table 1). Fifth, several of these studies utilized experienced cyclists who treated exercise tests as competitive efforts. These cyclists participated in both significant[16,37,38,88,90,92] and nonsignificant[29,44,54,95] findings regarding endurance performance. Thus, it is unlikely that their training or competitive experiences biased these findings, which involved a repeated measure design in virtually all cases. None of the studies directly compared moderately fit or unfit test subjects to highly trained athletes.

Sixth, several of the CHO replacement fluids in these tests included electrolytes. The advantages of NaCl intake during exercise were described above, and the presence of NaCl affected performance to an unknown degree in these studies. The effects of carbohydrate and NaCl intake during recovery from exercise will be reviewed below. Seventh, although none of the 20 investigations in Table 1 utilized solid CHO feedings, enhanced performance

TABLE 1 The Effects of Fluid Replacement (with CHO) on Exercise Performance

Exercise Mode and Protocol	Exercise Duration (h)	Total CHO[a] Consumed (g)	Effect on Performance	Year (Ref.)
Cycling, N	2.0	90	b	1979 (83)
Cycling, N	0.5	113	NS	1981 (19)
Cycling, N	2.9	120	NS	1982 (51)
	2.7	200	NS	
Cycling, N	3.0	124	b	1983 (38)
Walk, N	5.0	120	b	1983 (84)
Run, I	2.4	160[c]	NS	1983 (57)
	2.7	180	NS	
Cycling, N	2.3	105	b	1984 (18)
Cycling, I	4.0	432	b	1986 (37)
Cycling, N	2.0	45[c]	NS	1987 (54)
		90	NS	
		90	NS	
Cycling, I	2.3	39[c]	NS	1987 (94)
	2.3	47	d	
	2.3	55	d	
Cycling, I	1.6	63[c]	b	1988 (92)
		77	b	
		96	b	
Cycling, I	2.0	116[c]	NS	1988 (44)
		231	NS	
Cycling, I	1.25	42[c]	d	1989 (95)
		55	NS	
		69	NS	
Cycling, N	0.8–1.9	28[c]	b	1989 (88)
		252	NS	
		216	NS	
		432	NS	
Run, N	2.1	50[c]	NS	1990 (124)
	2.1	50	NS	
Triathlon, N	2.3	92	NS	1990 (91)
Run, I	0.1[e]	71	NS	1991 (41)
Run, N	2.9	139	f	1992 (90)
Cycling, N	2.0	42[c]	NS	1993 (29)
		58	NS	
		58	NS	
Cycling, N	1.0	79[c]	d	1995 (16)

Note: CHO = carbohydrate; I = intermittent exercise; N = continuous exercise; NS = not significantly altered

[a] CHO type varied between studies; [b] performance was significantly improved, vs. water or placebo; [c] different types of CHO were compared; [d] high intensity performance test at end of exercise was significantly improved; [e] anaerobic power test only; [f] after a 35-km run, a 5-km time trial was significantly improved.

Modified from Murray, R., *Sports Med.*, 4:322, 1987. With permission.

may be gained by foods that are not liquid. In two studies,[52,71] blood glucose was maintained during intermittent, prolonged exercise by consumption of a chocolate bar (e.g., sucrose). Eighth, the types of carbohydrate solutions that enhanced performance included: 4% glucose, 6% glucose, 40% maltodextrin, 50% glucose polymer, [5% glucose polymer + 2% fructose], [2.3% glucose + 2.7% maltrin], [1.9% fructose + 2.1% maltrin + 2.0% sucrose], and [5.5% maltrin + 2.0% fructose]. At present, there is little evidence (Table 1) that any CHO type is superior to another.[3,88,95,116] It should be noted, however, that all subjects in one study[57] experienced gastrointestinal distress when consuming a concentrated fructose solution (0.55 N) during exercise at the rate of 600 ml/min. Ninth, one study[54] reported that a performance improvement was not observed (2.0 h of cycling) when preexercise muscle glycogen levels were elevated by consuming a high-CHO diet (i.e., $\approx$ 500 g/d).

To our knowledge, the scientific literature reveals only four situations in which CHO–electrolyte beverages may be superior to water: (1) a CHO deficiency exists in blood, liver, or muscle tissue;[116] (2) exercise is strenuous (i.e., > 70% $\dot{V}O_2$ max) and prolonged (i.e., > 50 min);[40,93,116] (3) either a NaCl deficiency,[12,77,122] hyponatremia,[8,101,102] or salt-depletion heat exhaustion[77] exists; and (4) an enhanced plasma volume expansion is desired during recovery. Other than these scenarios, there is no definitive evidence that CHO–electrolyte beverages enhance exercise performance or health, in excess of the effects derived from consuming an equal volume of water and a balanced diet.

IV. CHO AND NaCl EFFECTS DURING RECOVERY FROM EXERCISE

Relatively little is known about the physiological responses to fluid consumption subsequent to exercise. The two most relevant effects of CHO–electrolyte beverages (vs. pure water) during recovery involve the restoration of muscle glycogen and the expansion of plasma volume. These effects actually should be viewed in terms of the rate at which they occur because they both can be duplicated, albeit at a slower rate, by consuming appropriate quantities of CHO, water, and NaCl in one's daily diet.

Regarding postexercise muscle glycogen repletion, Ivy's recent review[82] provides the following recommendations: (1) ingestion of a glucose supplement in excess of 1 g/kg body weight/h optimizes muscle glycogen storage; this corresponds to the maximum rate of glucose absorption from the small bowel;[100] (2) this storage (5–8 µmol/g wet muscle mass/h) can be maintained up to 6 h after exercise if blood glucose and insulin levels are maintained; (3) glucose or glucose polymers are believed to be the most effective CHO supplements for muscle glycogen synthesis; and (4) fructose appears to be the best supplement to restore liver glycogen. The ease and rate of CHO consumption, plus new advances in nutrition products (i.e., CHO in the form of a liquid meal), are the primary reasons that supplements are recommended. Eating this amount of CHO in 6 h would be unpleasant and time-consuming for athletes who must compete more than once a day or on successive days. An excellent example of these scenarios has been published by Fallowfield and Williams.[50] They monitored two groups of subjects after they ate a controlled diet containing 6 g CHO/kg body weight and ran on a motorized treadmill for 90 min (or to exhaustion). There was no performance difference between groups for the initial 90-min run. During recovery, the CHO intake of the control group remained constant, but the high-CHO group supplemented CHO intake (to ≈ 9 g CHO/kg body weight) with a 16.5% glucose polymer solution. Subsequent to dietary treatments (i.e., consuming a control or high-CHO diet for 22.5 h), both groups repeated the exercise test. The high-CHO diet increased mean run time by 9.2 min, and the control diet decreased mean run time by 15.6 min ($\Delta = 24.8$ min, $p < .05$).

Regarding changes in plasma volume, many investigators have documented fluid movement from the intra- to extravascular space during exercise;[115] the volume of plasma water loss is linearly related to relative exercise intensity.[31] During recovery, rehydration with a glucose–electrolyte solution results in a more rapid recovery of the plasma volume deficit than when the same subjects rehydrate with water.[34] But osmotic factors may not be of supreme importance. For example, the human studies of Nose et al.[103,104,105] observed 6 test subjects during a 3-h period of recovery from mild dehydration (–2.3% of body weight), during which they consumed water and capsules containing either 0.2 g sucrose (i.e., placebo) or 0.45 g NaCl (i.e., a 1/2 normal saline solution without the taste of salt). Figure 3 illustrates the cumulative fluid intake, urine volume, net fluid gain, and change in plasma volume during their recovery. Plasma volume was restored at 30 min of the saline test, and at 120 min of the water test. Plasma sodium concentration returned to baseline in the water test at 30 min, but had not recovered in the saline test at 120 min. Cumulative fluid intake was significantly greater at 180 min of the saline test. These data were interpreted to mean that the 2.3% dehydration prompted both an osmotic (e.g., hypertonic) and a volume-dependent (e.g., hypovolemic) drive to drink. The volume-dependent drive was diminished by both fluid treatments, although the saline treatment resulted in a greater net fluid gain. This net fluid gain was affected by the greater fluid intake during the saline test, secondary to a greater plasma sodium concentration.[97] Therefore, restoration of body fluids during recovery was better in the saline test because of enhanced plasma water retention and an increased drive to drink.

Evidence also indicates that different electrolyte species induce expansion of different fluid spaces, during recovery from a body water loss of 2%.[99] A high-sodium solution favors extracellular compartment filling, whereas both high-potassium and high-CHO [9% sucrose + glucose] solutions favor intracellular rehydration.[99] The practical value of the above differences,[99,103,104] however, depends on the duration of recovery and the fluid–electrolyte contents of one's diet. A balanced diet, over 12–48 h, will provide ample fluid and electrolytes to restore plasma volume to pre-dehydration levels.[4,5,9,17,43,66,98]

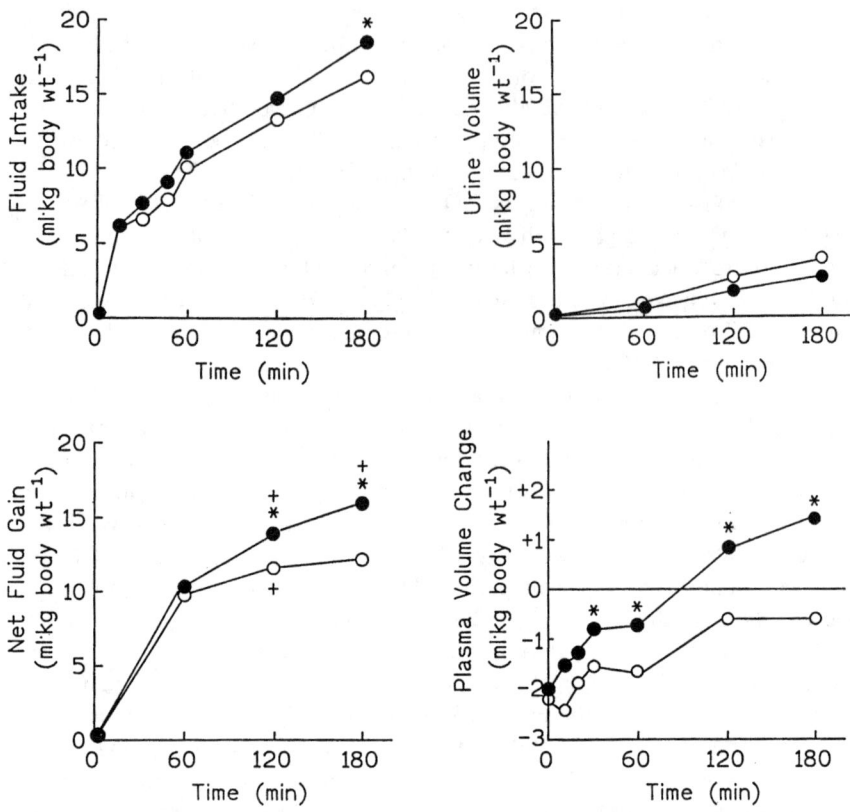

FIGURE 3 Cumulative changes of fluid intake, urine volume, net fluid gain, and plasma volume during recovery from a whole body fluid loss of 2.3%. Subjects rehydrated for 180 min, drinking either a 0.45% NaCl solution (• symbol) or water (° symbol). *significantly different from water ($p < .05$). +within-treatment difference ($p < .05$) from the 60-min point. (Redrawn from Nose, H., et al., *Fluid Replacement and Heat Stress*, National Academy Press, Washington, DC, 1994. With permission.)

V. FLUID REPLACEMENT: OTHER INFLUENCES OF EXERCISE

Exercise results in perturbations that are not present at rest. These disturbances (e.g., mental distractions, internal fluid shifts, mouth dryness, coordination) suggest that exercise per se may change drinking behavior.[80] The literature regarding drinking behavior during exercise is difficult to interpret, partly because of the many interactions of the factors described above. Chapter 14 focuses on the interactions of exercise type, duration, and intensity. With regard to fluid replacement, the following six generalizations currently may be drawn from previous publications: (1) most test subjects voluntarily choose to drink approximately 500 ml/h during exercise[100] but lose sweat at an average rate of 400–2500 ml/h;[113] (2) runners and cyclists develop symptoms of gastric "fullness" when consuming fluid at rates ≥ 800 ml/h,[100] corresponding to the maximal rate of water absorption (800–900 ml/h) by the intestines;[59,100] (3) running reduces fluid consumption more than cycling, possibly because of distractions or the difficulty of obtaining fluid;[23] (4) during exercise, idiosyncratic drinking behavior has been observed, and humans have been classified as either avid drinkers or reluctant drinkers;[80,119,121] (5) exercise and related factors (i.e., increased metabolism) inhibit drinking relatively more than heat exposure or prior dehydration;[67] and (6) fluid palatability may become a less important stimulus to drink as prolonged exercise progresses. This latter concept is depicted in Figure 4, which illustrates the cumulative fluid intake (ml) of test subjects who walked for 30 min/hr on a treadmill for 6 h (40.6°C ambient temperature). They consumed pure water at temperatures of 6, 22, and 46°C. These data[11] were interpreted to mean that the temperature of drinking water (a behavioral component) had a significant ($p < .05$) impact on fluid consumption early in these 6-h trials (i.e., alliesthesia for 6°C water was greatest). But after 2.5 h, physiological inputs (e.g., thirst, sweating, increased body temperature) overrode behavioral inputs and stimulated similar consumption of water at all temperatures. Interestingly, all groups consumed more water during exercise than during rest periods. This finding disagrees with previous studies because more water is typically consumed during rest periods[80] and meals[1] than during exercise. Evidently, some factor altered usual drinking patterns as dehydration and hyperthermia increased (from hour 0 to hour 6).

Although plasma volume can be altered by many factors (i.e., heat acclimation, exercise mode, posture, skin temperature, physical training, environmental temperature), fluid replacement may or may not influence plasma volume and subsequent physiological responses or exercise performance. The difference lies in the timing of fluid replacement.[39] When body water is lost *before* prolonged exercise, large deficits in plasma volume occur during exercise. When large amounts of body water are lost by sweating *during* exercise, very minor losses of plasma volume usually occur. This means that fluid replacement during exercise, begun in the euhydrated state, has little influence on plasma volume because only minor dehydration is experienced. Thus, the major benefit of fluid replacement during exercise appears to be the prevention of hyperthermia.[39] This may occur by preventing either plasma hyperosmolality, which decreases the rate of sweating for a given increase in core temperature,[55] or by preventing cellular dehydration.

Because plasma volume expansion results from repeated days of exercise–heat exposure,[9,12] it is reasonable that heat acclimation (see Chapter 7) also influences thirst and drinking behavior. A few investigations have evaluated the effects of heat acclimation on fluid replacement in humans, reporting increased fluid intake after 8–10 d of controlled heat-acclimation trials. This increase is due to an increased number of drinks and an increased volume per

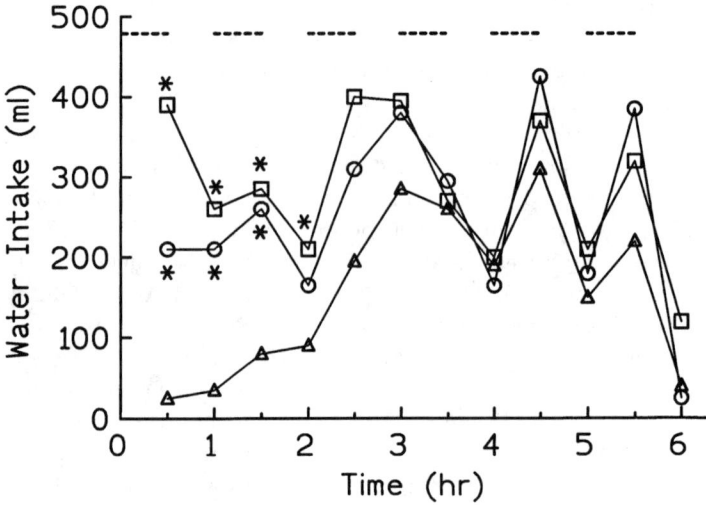

FIGURE 4 Water intake (ml/30 min) during intermittent, moderate intensity treadmill exercise (--- line) in a 40.6°C environment. Subjects consumed 6°C (O), 22°C (□), and 46°C (Δ) water *ad libitum*. *significantly different from 46°C water. (From Armstrong, L. E., Hubbard, R. W., Szlyk, P. C., Matthew, W. T., and Sils, I. V., *Aviat. Space Environ. Med.*, 56:765, 1985. With permission.)

drink.[64,65,80] The theoretical mechanism involves an elevated serum osmotic pressure caused by the loss of large volumes of hypotonic sweat,[65] and NaCl retention via the renin-angiotensin II hormonal pathway.[64] Additionally, the exercise protocol probably is of minor importance because this phenomenon has been observed during continuous cycling,[64] continuous treadmill walking,[65] and intermittent, intense treadmill running for 100 min/d.[80]

VI. SUMMARY

Elements that influence thirst and fluid replacement during and following exercise are numerous and include environmental, physiological, behavioral, social, and perceptual factors. It is important that these factors be carefully considered in the design of research projects and the interpretation of research results. Presently, it is accurate to assume that no single replacement fluid (i.e., water, [water + NaCl], or [water + CHO]) will satisfy the demands of all athletes and all forms of exercise. Regardless of the fluid consumed, the benefits derived from its ingestion depend on the time course of ingestion. Nevertheless, the importance of adequate water in maintaining health (preventing hyperthermia) and physical performance cannot be denied. Under most circumstances, athletes do not need to ingest electrolyte beverages unless their diet is deficient. Sodium in an oral rehydration solution is efficacious, however, in cases of exercise-related hyponatremia and heat cramps. Similarly, there are specific conditions in which CHO–electrolyte beverages may be superior to water, but for the vast majority of individuals who exercise (i.e., ranging from recreational sports enthusiasts to elite athletes), CHO–electrolyte beverages will not enhance exercise performance or health, in excess of the effects derived from consuming an equal volume of water and a balanced diet. During recovery from exercise, CHO–electrolyte beverages may be superior to pure water in restoring muscle glycogen levels and expanding plasma volume, but this depends on the amount of CHO and NaCl in one's daily diet and the time over which these results are desired.

REFERENCES

1. Adolph, E. F., *Physiology of Man in the Desert*, Interscience Publishers, New York, 1947, 208.
2. Adolph, E. F., Barker, J. P., and Hoy, P. A., Multiple factors in thirst, *Am. J. Physiol.*, 178:538, 1954.
3. *Exercise and Fluid Replacement*, ACSM Position Stand, *Med. Sci. Sports Exerc.*, 28:i–vii, 1996.
4. Armstrong, L. E., *Keeping Your Cool in Barcelona. The Effects of Heat, Humidity, and Dehydration on Athletic Performance, Strength, and Endurance*, U.S. Olympic Committee, Colorado Springs, CO, 1992, 1.
5. Armstrong, L. E., Considerations for replacement beverages: Fluid electrolyte balance and heat illness, in *Fluid Replacement and Heat Stress*, Marriott, B. M., Ed., National Academy Press, Washington, DC, 1994, 37.
6. Armstrong L. E., Costill, D. L., and Fink, W. J., Influence of diuretic-induced dehydration on competitive running performance, *Med. Sci. Sports Exer.*, 17:456, 1985.
7. Armstrong, L. E., Costill, D. L., Fink, W. J., Bassett, D., Hargreaves, M., Nishibata, I., and King, D. S., Effects of dietary sodium on body and muscle potassium content during heat acclimation, *Eur. J. Appl. Physiol.*, 54:391, 1985.
8. Armstrong, L. E., Curtis, W. C., Hubbard, R. W., Francesconi, R. P., Moore, R., and Askew, E. W., Symptomatic hyponatremia during prolonged exercise in heat, *Med. Sci. Sports Exer.*, 25:543, 1993.
9. Armstrong, L. E., Hubbard, R. W., Askew, E. W., De Luca, J. P., O'Brien, C., Pasqualicchio, A., and Francesconi, R. P., Responses to moderate and low sodium diets during exercise-heat acclimation, *Int. J. Sport Nutr.*, 3:207, 1993.
10. Armstrong, L. E., Hubbard, R. W., Jones, B. H., and Daniels, J. T., Preparing Alberto Salazar for the heat of the 1984 Olympic marathon, *Physician Sportsmed.*, 14:73, 1986.
11. Armstrong, L. E., Hubbard, R. W., Szlyk P. C., Matthew, W. T., and Sils, I. V., Voluntary dehydration and electrolyte losses during prolonged exercise in the heat, *Aviat. Space Environ. Med.*, 56:765, 1985.
12. Armstrong, L. E. and Maresh, C. M., The exertional heat illnesses: A risk of athletic participation, *Med. Exer. Nutr. Health*, 2:125, 1993.
13. Armstrong, L. E., Maresh, C. M., Castellani, J. W., Bergeron, M. F., Kenefick, R. W., LaGasse, K. E., and Riebe, D., Urinary indices of hydration status, *Int. J. Sport Nutr.*, 4:265, 1994.
14. Astrand, P. O. and Rodahl, K., *Textbook of Work Physiology*, McGraw-Hill, New York, 1986.
15. Bean, W. B. and Eichna, L. W., Performance in relation to environmental temperature. Reactions of normal young men to simulated desert environment, *Fed. Proc.*, 2:144, 1943.

16. Below, P. R., Mora-Rodriguez, R., Gonzalez-Alonso, J., and Coyle, E. F., Fluid and carbohydrate ingestion independently improve performance during one hour of intense exercise, *Med. Sci. Sports Exer.*, 27:200, 1995.
17. Bergeron, M. F., Maresh, C. M., Armstrong, L. E., Signorile, J. F., Castellani, J. W., Kenefick, R. W., LaGasse, K. E., Riebe, D. A., Fluid-electrolyte balance associated with tennis match play in a hot environment, *Int. J. Sport Nutrition*, 5:180, 1995.
18. Bjorkman, O., Sahlin, K., Hagenfeldt, L., and Wahren, J., Influence of glucose and fructose ingestion on the capacity for long-term exercise in well-trained men, *Clin. Physiol.*, 4:483, 1984.
19. Bonen, A., Malcolm, S. A., Kilgour, R. D., MacIntyre, K. P., and Belcastro, A. N., Glucose ingestion before and during intense exercise, *J. Appl. Physiol.* 50:766, 1981.
20. Booth, D. A., Influences on human fluid consumption, in *Thirst: Physiological and Psychological Aspects*, Ramsay, D. J. and Booth, D. A., Eds., Springer-Verlag, London, 1991, 53.
21. Bothorel, B., Follenius, M., Gissinger, R., and Candas, V., Physiological effects of dehydration and rehydration with water and acidic or neutral carbohydrate electrolyte solution, *Eur. J. Appl. Physiol.*, 60:209, 1990.
22. Boulze, D., Montastruc, P., and Cabanac, M., Water intake, pleasure, and water temperature in humans, *Physiol. Behav.*, 30:97, 1983.
23. Browns, F. E., Beckers, E., Knopfli, B., Villiger, B., and Saris, W., Rehydration during exercise: Effect of electrolyte supplementation in selective blood parameters, *Med. Sci. Sports Exer.*, 23:584, 1991.
24. Candas, V., Libert, J. P., Brandenberger, G., Sagot, J. C., Amoros, C., and Kahn, J. M., Hydration during exercise. Effects on thermal and cardiovascular adjustments, *Eur. J. Appl. Physiol.*, 55:113, 1986.
25. Cannon, W. B., *The Wisdom of the Body*, Kegan Paul, Trench, Trubner, London, 1932, 75.
26. Carter, J. E. and Gisolfi, C. V., Fluid replacement during and after exercise in the heat, *Med. Sci. Sports Exer.*, 21:532, 1989.
27. Christensen, E. H. and Hansen, O., Hypoglhamie, Arbeitsfahigkert und Ernahrung, *Skand. Arch. Physiol.*, 81:172, 1939.
28. Coggan, A. R. and Coyle, E. F., Carbohydrate ingestion during prolonged exercise: Effects on metabolism and performance, in *Exercise and Sports Science Reviews*, Vol. 19, Holloszy, J. O., Ed., Williams & Wilkins, Baltimore, 1991, 1.
29. Cole, K. J., Grandjean, P. W., Sobszak, R. J., and Mitchell, J. B., Effect of carbohydrate composition on fluid balance, gastric emptying, and exercise performance, *Int. J. Sport Nutr.*, 3:408, 1993.
30. Conner, M. T., Haddon, A. V., Pickering, E. S., and Booth, D. A., Sweet tooth demonstrated: Individual differences in preferences for both sweet foods and foods highly sweetened, *J. Appl. Psychol.*, 73:275, 1988.
31. Convertino, V. A., Keit, L. C., and Greenleaf, J. E., Plasma volume, renin, and vasopressin responses to graded exercise after training, *J. Appl. Physiol.*, 54:508, 1983.
32. Costill, D. L., Cote, R., Miller, E., Miller, T., and Wynder, S., Water and electrolyte replacement during repeated days of work in the heat, *Aviat. Space Environ. Med.*, 46:795, 1975.
33. Costill, D. L., Kammer, W. F., and Fisher, A., Fluid ingestion during distance running, *Arch. Environ. Health*, 21:520, 1970.
34. Costill, D. L. and Sparks, K. E., Rapid fluid replacement following thermal dehydration, *J. Appl. Physiol.*, 34:299, 1973.
35. Coyle, E. F., Effects of glucose polymer feedings on fatiguability and the metabolic response to prolonged strenuous exercise, in *Nutrient Utilization During Exercise*, Fox, E., Ed., Ross Laboratories, Columbus, OH, 1983, 43.
36. Coyle, E. F., Fluid and carbohydrate replacement during exercise: How much and why?, in *Sports Science Exchange*, Vol. 7, Gatorade Sport Science Institute, Chicago, 1994, 1.

37. Coyle, E. F., Coggan, A. R., and Ivy, J. L., Muscle glycogen utilization during prolonged strenuous exercise when fed carbohydrates, *J. Appl. Physiol*, 61:165, 1986.
38. Coyle, E. F., Hagberg, J. M., Hurley, B. F., Martin, W. H., Ehsani, A. A., and Holloszy, J. O., Carbohydrate feeding during prolonged strenuous exercise can delay fatigue, *J. Appl. Physiol*., 55:230, 1983.
39. Coyle, E. F. and Hamilton, M. A., Fluid replacement during exercise: Effects on physiological homeostasis and performance, in *Perspectives in Exercise Science and Sports Medicine. Vol. 3. Fluid Homeostasis During Exercise*, Gisolfi, C. V. and Lamb, D. R., Eds., Benchmark Press, Carmel, IN, 1990, 281.
40. Coyle, E. F. and Montain, S. J., Carbohydrate and fluid ingestion during exercise: Are there trade-offs?, *Med. Sci. Sports Exer.*, 24:671, 1992.
41. Criswell, D., Powers, S., Lawler, J., Tew, J., Dodd, S., Iryiboz, Y., Tulley, R., and Wheeler, K., Influence of a carbohydrate-electrolyte beverage on performance and blood homeostasis during recovery from football, *Int. J. Sport Nutr.*, 1:178, 1991.
42. Criswell, D., Renshler, S. K., Powers, S. K., Tulley, R., Cicale, M., and Wheeler, K., Fluid replacement beverages and maintenance of plasma volume during exercise: Role of aldosterone and vasopressin, *Eur. J. Appl. Physiol.*, 65:445, 1992.
43. Dahl, L. K., Salt intake and salt need, *New Engl. J. Med.*, 258:1152, 1958.
44. Davis, J. M., Burgess, W. A., Slentz, C. A., Bartoli, W. P., and Pate, R. R., Effects of ingesting 6% and 12% glucose/electrolyte beverages during prolonged intermittent cycling in the heat, *Eur. J. Appl. Physiol.*, 57:563, 1988.
45. Department of the Army, *Prevention, Treatment, and Control of heat injury*, Technical Bulletin MED 507, Washington, DC, 1980, 1.
46. Elkinton, J. R., Danowski, T. S., and Winkler, A. W., Hemodynamic changes in salt depletion and dehydration, *J. Clin. Invest.*, 25:120, 1946.
47. Engell, D., Interdependency of food and water intake in humans, *Appetite*, 10:133, 1988.
48. Engell, D. and Hirsch, E., Environmental and sensory modulation of fluid intake in humans, in *Thirst: Psychological and Physiological Aspects*, Booth, D. A. and Ramsay, D. J., Eds., Springer-Verlag, London, 1991, 382.
49. Engell, D. B., Maller, O., Sawka, M. N., Francesconi, R. P., Drolet, L., and Young, A. J., Thirst and fluid intake following graded hypohydration levels in humans, *Physiol. Behav.*, 40:229, 1987.
50. Fallowfield, J. L. and Williams, C., Carbohydrate intake and recovery from prolonged exercise, *Int. J. Sport Nutr.*, 3:150, 1993.
51. Felig, P., Cherh, A., Minigawa, A., and Wahren, J., Hypoglycemia during prolonged exercise in normal men, *New Engl. J. Med.*, 302:895, 1982.
52. Fielding, R. A., Costill, D. L., Fink, W. J., King, D. S., Hangreaves, M., and Kovaleski, J., Effect of carbohydrate feeding, frequencies and dosage on muscle glycogen use during exercise, *Med. Sci. Sports Exer.*, 17:472, 1985.
53. Fitzsimons, J. T., *The Physiology of Thirst and Sodium Appetite*, Cambridge University Press, London, 1979, 1.
54. Flynn, M. G., Costill, D. L., Hawley, J. A., Fink, W. J., and Neufer, P. D., Influence of selected carbohydrate drinks on cycling performance and glycogen use, *Med. Sci. Sports Exer.*, 19:37, 1987.
55. Fortney, S. M., Nadel, E. R., Wenger, C. B., and Bove, J. R., Effect of acute alteration of blood volume on circulatory performance in humans, *J. Appl. Physiol.*, 50:292, 1981.
56. Francesconi, R. P., Sawka, M. N., Pandolf, K. B., Hubbard, R. W., Young, A. J., and Muza, S., Plasma hormonal responses at graded hypohydration levels during exercise-heat stress, *J. Appl. Physiol.*, 59:1855, 1985.
57. Fruth, J. M. and Gisolfi, C. V., Effects of carbohydrate consumption on endurance performance: Fructose and glucose, in *Nutrient Utilization During Exercise*, Fox, E. L., Ed., Ross Laboratories, Columbus, OH, 1983, 68.

58. Gabaree, C. L. V., Thirst, plasma volume, and hormonal responses of hypohydrated males during exercise in the heat, Doctoral dissertation, University of Connecticut, Storrs, CT, 1993.
59. Gisolfi, C. V., Spranger, K. J., Summers, R. W., Schedl, H. P., and Bleiler, T. L., Effects of cycle exercise on intestinal absorption in humans, *J. Appl. Physiol.*, 71:2518, 1991.
60. Gisolfi, C. V., Summers, R., and Schedl, H., Intestinal absorption of fluids during rest and exercise, in *Perspectives in Exercise Science and Sports Medicine. Vol. 3. Fluid Homeostasis During Exercise*, Gisolfi, C. V. and Lamb, D. R., Eds., Benchmark Press, Carmel, IN, 1990, 129.
61. Green, B. G. and Frankmann, S. P., The effect of cooling the tongue on the perceived intensity of taste, *Chem. Senses Flavor*, 12:609, 1987.
62. Greenleaf, J. E., Problem: Thirst, drinking behavior, and involuntary dehydration, *Med. Sci. Sports Exer.*, 24:645, 1992.
63. Greenleaf, J. E., Environmental issues that influence intake of replacement beverages, in *Fluid Replacement and Heat Stress*, Marriott, B. M., Ed., National Academy Press, Washington, DC, 1994, 195.
64. Greenleaf, J. E., Brock, P. J., Keil, L. C., and Morse, J. T., Drinking and water balance during exercise and heat acclimation, *J. Appl. Physiol.*, 54:414, 1983.
65. Greenleaf, J. E., Douglas, L. G., Bosco, J. S., Matter, M., and Blackaby, J. R., Thirst and artificial heat acclimatization in man, *Int. J. Biometeorol.*, 11:311, 1967.
66. Greenleaf, J. E. and Harrison, M. H., Water and electrolytes, in *Nutrition and Aerobic Exercise. ACS Symposium No. 294*, Layman, D. K., Ed., American Chemical Society, Washington, DC, 1986, 107.
67. Greenleaf, J. E. and Sargent, F., Voluntary dehydration in man, *J. Appl. Physiol.*, 20:719, 1965.
68. Grossman, S. P., *Thirst and Sodium Appetite. Psychological Basis*, Academic Press, San Diego, 1990, 203.
69. Grossman, S. P., Neuropharmacology of central mechanisms contributing to control of food and water intake, in *Handbook of Physiology, Section 6. Alimentary Canal, Vol. 1. Control of Food and Water Intake*, American Physiological Society, Washington, DC, 1967, 287.
70. Hargreaves, M., Costill, D., Burke, L., McConell, G., and Febbraio, M., Influence of sodium on glucose bioavailability during exercise, *Med. Sci. Sports Exer.*, 26:365, 1994.
71. Hargreaves, M., Costill, D. L., Coggan, A., Fink, W. J., and Nishibata, I., Effect of carbohydrate feedings on muscle glycogen utilization and exercise performance, *Med. Sci. Sports Exer.*, 16:219, 1984.
72. Harrison, M. H., Heat and exercise: Effects on blood volume, *Sports Med.*, 3:214, 1986.
73. Herbert, W. G., Water and electrolytes, in *Ergogenic Aids in Sport*, Williams, M. H., Ed., Human Kinetics Publishers, Champaign, IL, 1983, 56.
74. Hickson, R. C., Carbohydrate metabolism in exercise, in *Nutrient Utilization During Exercise*, Fox, E. L., Ed., Ross Laboratories, Columbus, OH, 1983, 1.
75. Hoffman, J. R., Maresh, C. M., Armstrong, L. E., Gabaree, C. L., Bergeron, M., Kenefick, R., Castellani, J., Ahlquist, L. E., and Ward, A., Effect of hydration state on plasma testosterone, cortisol and catecholamine concentration before and during mild exercise at elevated temperature, *Eur. J. Appl. Physiol.*, 69:294, 1994.
76. Horswell, C. A., Does rapid weight loss by dehydration adversely affect high-power performance?, in *Sport Science Exchange, Vol. 3.*, Gatorade Sport Science Institute, Chicago, 1991, 1.
77. Hubbard, R. W. and Armstrong, L. E., The heat illnesses: Biochemical, ultrastructural, and fluid-electrolyte considerations, in *Human Performance Physiology and Environmental Medicine at Terrestrial Extremes*, Pandolf, K. B., Sawka, M. N., and Gonzalez, R. R., Eds., Benchmark Press, Indianapolis, 1988, 305.

78. Hubbard, R. W., Armstrong, L. E., Evans, P. K., and De Luca, J. P., Long-term water and salt deficits—A military perspective, in *Predicting Decrements in Military Performance Due to Inadequate Nutrition*, National Academy Press, Washington DC, 1986, 29.
79. Hubbard, R. W., Sandick, B. L., Matthew, W. T., Francesconi, R. P., Sampson, J. B., Durkot, M. J., Maller, O., and Engell, D. B., Voluntary dehydration and alliesthesia for water, *J. Appl. Physiol.*, 57:868, 1984.
80. Hubbard, R. W., Szlyk, P. C., and Armstrong, L. E., Influence of thirst and fluid palatability on fluid ingestion during exercise, in *Perspectives in Exercise Science and Sports Medicine. Vol. 3. Fluid Homeostasis During Exercise*, Gisolfi, C. V. and Lamb, D. R., Eds., Benchmark Press, Carmel, IN, 1990, 39.
81. Hunt, E. H., The regulation of body temperature in extremes of dry heat, *J. Hyg.*, 12:479, 1912.
82. Ivy, J. L., Carbohydrate supplements during and immediately post exercise, in *Fluid Replacement and Heat Stress*, Marriott, B. M., Ed., National Academy Press, Washington, DC, 1994, 55.
83. Ivy, J. L., Costill, D. L., Fink, W. J., and Lower, R. W., Influence of carbohydrate feedings on endurance performance, *Med. Sci. Sports Exer.*, 11:6, 1979.
84. Ivy, J. L., Miller, W., Dover, V., Goodyear, L. G., Sherman, W. M., Farrell, S., and Williams, H., Endurance improved by ingestion of a glucose polymer supplement, *Med. Sci. Sports Exer.*, 15:466, 1983.
85. Johnson, H. L., Nelson, R. A., and Consolazio, C. F., Effects of electrolyte and nutrient solutions on performance and metabolic balance, *Med. Sci. Sports Exer.*, 20:26, 1988.
86. Marriott, H. L., *Water and Salt Depletion*, Charles C Thomas, Springfield, IL, 1950, 1.
87. Maughan, R. J., Fenn, C. E., Gleeson, M., and Leiper, J. B., Metabolic and circulatory responses during exercise in man, *Eur. J. Appl. Physiol.*, 56:356, 1987.
88. Maughan, R. J., Fenn, C. E., and Leiper, J. B., Effects of fluid, electrolyte, and substrate ingestion on endurance capacity, *Eur. J. Appl. Physiol.*, 58:481, 1989.
89. Meyer, F., Bar-Or, O., Salsberg, A., and Passe, D. Hypohydration during exercise in children: Effect on thirst, drink preferences, and rehydration, *Int. J. Sport Nutr.*, 4:22, 1994.
90. Millard-Stafford, M., Starling, P. B., Rosskopf, L. B., and DiCarlo, L. J., Carbohydrate-electrolyte replacement improves distance running performance in the heat, *Med. Sci. Sports Exer.*, 24:934, 1992.
91. Millard-Stafford, M., Starling, P. B., Rosskopf, L. B., Hinson, B. T., and DiCarlo, L. J., Carbohydrate-electrolyte replacement during a simulated triathlon in the heat, *Med. Sci. Sports Exer.*, 22:621, 1990.
92. Mitchell, J. B., Costill, D. L., Houmard, J. A., Flynn, M. G., Fink, W. J., and Beltz, J. D., Effects of carbohydrate ingestion on gastric emptying and exercise performance, *Med. Sci. Sports Exer.*, 20:110, 1988.
93. Murray, R., The effects of consuming carbohydrate-electrolyte beverages on gastric emptying and fluid absorption during and following exercise, *Sports Med.*, 4:322, 1987.
94. Murray, R., Eddy, D. E., Wakasugi-Murray, T., Seifert, J. G., Paul, G. L., and Halaby, G. A., The effect of fluid and carbohydrate feedings during cycling exercise in the heat, *Med. Sci. Sports Exer.*, 19:597, 1987.
95. Murray, R., Seifert, J. G., Eddy, D. E., Paul, G. L., and Halaby, G. A., Carbohydrate feeding and exercise: Effect of beverage carbohydrate content, *Eur. J. Appl. Physiol.*, 59:152, 1989.
96. Nadal, J. W., Pedersen, S., and Maddock, W. G., A comparison between dehydration from salt loss and from water deprivation, *Am. J. Physiol.*, 134:691, 1941.
97. Nadel, E. R., Mack, G. W., and Nose H., Influence of fluid-electrolyte beverages on body fluid homeostasis during exercise and recovery, in *Perspectives in Exercise Science and Sports Medicine. Vol. 3. Fluid Homeostasis During Exercise*, Gisolfi, C. V. and Lamb, D. R., Eds., Benchmark Press, Carmel, IN, 1990, 181.

98. National Research Council, *Recommended Dietary Allowances*, 10th ed., National Academy Press, Washington, DC, 1989, 1.
99. Nielsen, B., Sjogaard, G., Ugelvig, J., Knudsen, B., and Dohlmann, B., Fluid balance in exercise dehydration and rehydration with different glucose-electrolyte drinks, *Eur. J. Appl. Physiol.*, 55:318, 1986.
100. Noakes, T. D., Fluid replacement during exercise, in *Exercise and Sport Science Reviews*, Vol. 21, Holloszy, J. O., Ed., Williams & Wilkins, Baltimore, 1993, 297.
101. Noakes, T. D., Goodwin, N., Rayner, B. L., Branken, T., and Taylor, R. K. N., Water intoxication: A possible complication during endurance exercise, *Med. Sci. Sports Exer.*, 17:370, 1985.
102. Noakes, T. D., Norman, R. J., Buck, R. H., Godlonton, J., Stevenson, K., and Pittaway, D., The incidence of hyponatremia during prolonged endurance exercise, *Med. Sci. Sports Exer.*, 22:165, 1990.
103. Nose, H., Mack, G. W., Shi, X., and Nadel, E. R., Shift in body fluid compartments after dehydration in man, *J. Appl. Physiol.*, 65:318, 1988.
104. Nose, H., Mack, G. W., Shi, X., and Nadel, E. R., Role of osmolality and plasma volume during rehydration in humans, *J. Appl. Physiol.*, 65:325, 1988.
105. Nose, H. R., Mack, G. W, Xiangrong, S., and Nadel, E. R., Role of osmolality and plasma volume during rehydration in humans, in *Fluid Replacement and Heat Stress*, Marriott, B. M., Ed., National Academy Press, Washington, DC, 1994, 143.
106. Phillips, P. A., Rolls, B. J., Ledingham, J. G. G., Forsling, M. L., and Morton, J. J. Osmotic thirst and vasopressin release in humans: A double-blind crossover study, *Am. J. Physiol.*, 248:R645, 1985.
107. Phillips, P. A., Rolls, B. J., Ledingham, J. G. G., and Morton, J. J. Body fluid changes, thirst, and drinking in man during free access to water, *Physiol. Behav.*, 33:357, 1984.
108. Pitts, G. C., Johnson, R. E., and Consolazio, F. C., Work in heat as affected by intake of water, salt, and glucose, *Am. J. Physiol.*, 142:253, 1944.
109. Pugh, L. G. C. E., Corbett, J. L., and Johnson, R. H., Rectal temperatures, weight losses, and sweat rates in marathon running, *J. Appl. Physiol.*, 23:347, 1967.
110. Rolls, B. J., Palatability and fluid intake, in *Fluid Replacement and Heat Stress*, Marriott, B. M., Ed., National Academy Press, Washington, DC, 1994, 161.
111. Rolls, B. J., Wood, R. J., Rolls, E. T., Lind, H., Lind, W., and Ledingham, J. G. G., Thirst following water deprivation in humans, *Am. J. Physiol.*, 239:R476, 1980.
112. Sandick, B. L., Engell, D. B., and Maller, O., Perception of drinking water temperature and effects for humans after exercise, *Physiol. Behav.*, 32:851, 1984.
113. Sawka, M. N. and Pandolf, K. B., Effects of body water loss on physiological function and exercise performance, in *Perspectives in Exercise Science and Sports Medicine. Vol. 3. Fluid Homeostasis During Exercise*, Gisolfi, C. V. and Lamb, D. R., Eds., Benchmark Press, Carmel, IN, 1990, 1.
114. Sawka, M. N., Young, A. J., Francesconi, R. P., Muza, S. R., and Pandolf, K. B., Thermoregulatory and blood responses during exercise at graded hypohydration levels, *J. Appl. Physiol.*, 59:1394, 1985.
115. Senay, L. C. and Pivarnik, J. M., Fluid shifts during exercise, in *Exercise and Sport Science Reviews*, Vol. 13, Terjung, R. L., Ed., Macmillan, New York, 1985, 335.
116. Sherman, W. M. and Lamb, D. R., Nutrition and prolonged exercise, in *Perspectives in Exercise Science and Sports Medicine. Volume 1. Prolonged Exercise*, Lamb, D. R. and Murray, R., Eds., Benchmark Press, Indianapolis, 1988, 213.
117. Sohar, E., Kaly, J., and Adar, R., The prevention of voluntary dehydration, in *UNESCO/India Symposium on Environmental Physiology and Psychology*, UNESCO, Paris, 1962, 129.
118. Stine, R. J., Heat illness, *J.A.C.E.P.*, 8:154, 1979.
119. Szlyk, P. C., Sils, I. V., Francesconi, R. P., and Hubbard, R. W., Patterns of human drinking: Effects of exercise, water temperature, and food consumption, *Aviat. Space Environ. Med.*, 61:43, 1990.

120. Szlyk, P. C., Sils, I. V., Francesconi, R. P., Hubbard, R. W., and Armstrong, L. E., Effects of water temperature and flavoring on voluntary dehydration in man, *Physiol. Behav.*, 45:639, 1989.
121. Szlyk, P. C., Sils, I. V., Francesconi, R. P., Hubbard, R. W., and Matthew, W. T., Variability in intake and dehydration in young men during a simulated desert walk, *Aviat. Space Environ. Med.*, 60:422, 1989.
122. Vaamonde, C. A., Sodium depletion, in *Sodium: Its Biologic Significance*, Vaamonde, C. A., Ed., CRC Press, Boca Raton, FL, 1982, 208.
123. Welch, B. E., Buskirk, E. R., and Iampietro, P. F., Relation of climate and temperature to food and water intake, *Metabolism*, 7:141, 1958.
124. Williams, C., Nute, M. G., Broadbank, L., and Vinall, S., Influence of fluid intake on endurance running performance. A comparison between water, glucose and fructose solutions, *Eur. J. Appl. Physiol.*, 60:112, 1990.
125. Wyndham, C. H. and Strydom, N. B., The danger of an inadequate water intake during marathon running, *S. Afr. Med. J.*, 43:893, 1969.

Chapter 14

EFFECTS OF ACUTE BODY WEIGHT LOSS IN WEIGHT-CONTROLLING ATHLETES

Elsworth R. Buskirk
Susan M. Puhl

CONTENTS

I. Introduction..283

II. Early Investigations 284

III. Wrestling..285

IV. Power Athletes 287

V. Lightweight Rowing.......................................288

VI. Other Related Studies.....................................289

VII. Interpretations..291

VIII. Summary...293

References 294

I. INTRODUCTION

There are a variety of reasons for athletes to reduce body weight acutely: to improve competitive performance, to enhance the possibility of competitive advantage, and to seek improvement in physical appearance. Although some dietary restrictions may be employed, acute reductions in body weight (i.e., body water) are heavily dependent on utilization of dehydration procedures. A spectrum of such procedures has been employed: extra exercise, exercise in the heat, use of hot baths or hot rooms (sauna), exercise or exposure in hot rooms while wearing water vapor-impermeable clothing, fluid intake restriction, use of diuretics and laxatives, and use of sweat-enhancing agents. Additional efforts such as forced vomiting, spitting, and bloodletting have been utilized.[15] One or more of these techniques are utilized primarily by athletes engaged in weight-class events, although gymnasts, dancers, and other athletes also employ them. Examples of weight-class sports include: wrestling, weight-lifting, boxing, karate, judo and lightweight rowing. Examples of sports or activities that involve an aesthetic component include: gymnastics, dancing, figure skating, swimming (particularly synchronized), diving, track and field, and body building. Jockeys also must meet weight limits when competing. Athletes and others who engage in acute weight reduction are usually not overfat or obese, nor are they all young people; moreover, they comprise a wide spectrum of both genders. In this brief review we will attempt to concentrate on the limited data that deal with the effects of dehydration in the weight-controlling athlete as well as related data on endurance and other relatively unique testing procedures.

It is common for athletes engaged in sports with specific weight classifications to compete in a class that is 5 to 10% below their usual weight. To achieve the competitive weight at the time of the specified weigh-in rapid or relatively acute weight-loss procedures are commonly employed. For purposes of this discussion, rapid or acute weight loss means engaging in dehydration and other procedures for a period of 72 h or less. For reviews on rapid body weight reduction and the physiological and performance consequences, see Horswill[15] and Fogelholm et al.[10] as well as portions of other chapters in this book, particularly Chapter 7, which presents summary tables of the literature relating hypohydration effects on strength, endurance, and aerobic capacity.

II. EARLY INVESTIGATIONS

Early work on the effects of hypohydration among young men has provided mixed results with respect to the effects on strength, endurance and other aspects of physical performance. Tuttle,[34] Bosco et al.,[5] and Singer and Weiss[31] concluded that weight losses up to 7% had little effect on strength and endurance. In contrast, Adolph[1] and his group's classic World War II studies in the desert found significant physiological deterioration in those walking long distances in the heat. Adolph's observations have been supported by others, namely Buskirk et al.,[7] Saltin,[28] Craig and Cummings,[9] Palmer,[25] Ribisl and Herbert,[26] and Herbert and Ribisl.[13] Although these studies exposed subjects to different regimens, evidence was provided that some aspects of performance deteriorated with rapid body weight losses (dehydration) of 4% or more.

Saltin[28] undertook dehydrating 10 young men by exposing them to thermal (sauna), metabolic (exercise), or combined thermal and metabolic procedures. Although maximal oxygen uptake ($\dot{V}O_2$ max) and cardiac output were not significantly affected (however, the sauna exposure produced a $\dot{V}O_2$ max nearly significantly different at a $p>0.05$; similarly, $\dot{V}O_2$ max with exercise in a 17 to 20°C environment yielded a $p>0.1$), maximal work time significantly decreased with all three procedures. This was true for the maximal work time on a cycle ergometer and with arm cranking. With respect to isometric muscular strength for the elbow flexors and knee extensors, neither was degraded with the 1.7 to 4.6 kg body weight losses brought about by the dehydration procedures. Interestingly, although interindividual differences were large, Saltin felt that one well-trained subject showed a smaller decrement in work time than the less well-trained subjects, an observation that Buskirk et al.[7] had also reported. Saltin concluded that hypohydration does have an impact on endurance, or the ability to sustain repeated dynamic contractions, but that the mechanism should be sought at the cellular level. Because maximal isometric force was unaffected, it implied to Saltin that the impulse traffic to the muscles and their contraction capability were both preserved.

In a subsequent study, Saltin[29] also found a significant difference in work time when hypohydrated (body weight reduction up to 5.2% with exposure to heat in a sauna). In this study of three young men, plasma volume was reduced up to 25% but there was no decrease in stroke volume with maximal cycling in the seated position on a cycle ergometer, nor was cardiac output compromised.

III. WRESTLING

The methods of acutely achieving body weight loss (hypohydration) may well vary depending on the sport and level of competition. Steen and Brownell[32] found that college wrestlers utilized sauna, rubber suits, and fluid restriction as means of losing weight to a greater extent than wrestlers in high school. International competitors can presumably use any method they wish to induce body weight loss other than the prohibited procedures involving laxatives and diuretics. No data are currently available regarding weight-loss practices of international competitors. Horswill[15] has pointed out that the virtual lack of regulation at the international level plus the 12- to 18-h period between weigh-in and competition could well permit extensive weight losses. In fact, the NCAA has instituted an extended weigh-in prior to competition interval of 20 h — a dramatic increase in the 5-h period formerly allowed — thus increasing the probability of extensive weight losses and regains.

Much of the maneuvering about rehydration could be avoided by following the simple expedient of weigh-in immediately before competition, but the organizers and sponsors of athletic competition view the logistics of handling such weigh-ins as too complicated and bow to the desires of coaches and athletes to preserve the current systems with which they have become familiar while seeking that competitive advantage. Despite such maneuvering, it appears to produce little competitive consequence because Horswill et al.[17] have found that, at least in wrestlers competing in the NCAA championships, neither acute weight gain after the weigh-in nor the weight discrepancy between opponents influenced success in the first round of the tournament. Thus, the wrestlers simply competed relatively equally at body weights that exceeded the limits of the weight class. It appears that all the maneuvering is for naught.

The strength and endurance of the handgripping muscles of college wrestlers who dehydrated to 5% body weight loss was assessed by Serfass et al.[30] A 6-min fatigue test was employed in which a hand dynamometer was squeezed maximally for a total of 180 contractions. The contraction–relaxation cycle proceeded at 1-s intervals. Performance was unaffected by the hypohydration. These results, although in agreement with those of Tuttle,[34] Saltin,[28] and Singer and Weiss,[31] contrast with those of Bosco et al.[5] The latter investigators reported a strength and endurance decrease with hypohydration. Torranin et al.[33] found similar results. Serfass et al.[30] point out that such effects seem muscle group-dependent and are demonstrable to a greater extent in subjects unaccustomed to rapid weight loss whereas wrestlers who repeatedly engage in rapid weight reduction demonstrate few if any adverse effects of hypohydration on strength and endurance.

Webster et al.[37] dehydrated college wrestlers to the average level of 4.9% body weight loss and evaluated their anaerobic power and capacity as well as their muscular strength. A 40-s protocol on a cycle ergometer was utilized to determine anaerobic power and capacity. Both were significantly reduced when the wrestlers were hypohydrated. Similarly, a graduated treadmill test to volitional exhaustion demonstrated reduced time to exhaustion. Only minimal impact was observed regarding effects of hypohydration on strength, and then only for upper-body musculature. Dehydration involved exercising in a rubberized sweatsuit (vapor barrier) during a 12-h period prior to testing session in the laboratory. The investigators concluded that such a dehydration regimen, one that many wrestlers have followed, results in a lessened capability for developing short-term power and anaerobic capacity. These results contrast with those of Jacobs,[19] who used a 30- to 60-s cycle ergometer test (Wingate test) to assess anaerobic power and found no effect on subjects who had been thermally dehydrated.

Klinzing and Karpowicz[22] developed a 2-min wrestling performance test that consisted of walking, running, jumps, and rolls. Following a dehydration regimen performance on the test was adversely affected and the anaerobic performance involved did not return to euhydration values with rehydration during a period of 1.0–3.5 h. Prolonging the rehydration period for 5 h or more returned the test results to euhydration values, which demonstrated recuperative power in relation to restoration of fluid balance.

Fogelholm et al.[11] exposed seven wrestlers and three judo athletes to 2.4 d of fluid and diet restriction as well as exercise while wearing a water vapor-impermeable suit. An average 6% weight loss was achieved with this regimen.

A 5-h loading period was allowed prior to testing so that the athletes were only 2.7 kg lighter than when the dehydration/weight-loss phase began. Performance assessments included a 30-m sprint; vertical jumps with no, 50%, and 100% extra weight; and 0–30- and 0–60-s Wingate tests (cycle ergometer) performed twice. No deterioration in performance was observed in the relatively moderate hypohydrated state. In analyzing their results in relation to other rapid-weight-loss studies, they point out that other investigators have found decreased strength (i.e., low muscle torque[18] and anaerobic performance[37]) following rapid dehydration. They also cite possible mitigating factors in that Houston et al.[18] achieved a larger weight loss in their subjects and Webster et al.[37] utilized a shorter dehydration period. Webster et al. allowed no rehydration nor were performance assessments identical in the respective studies.

Zambraski et al.[38] conducted a longitudinal study of members of the 1975 University of Iowa NCAA championship wrestling team to determine whether signs of hypohydration occurred at the time of competition. Based on urinalysis prior to weigh-in, specific gravity was elevated 0.003, osmolarity increased 160 mOsm/l, Na^+ concentration decreased 45.3 meq/l and K^+ concentration increased 71.3 meq/l. These values suggested that the wrestlers were hypohydrated prior to competition. Calculations of urinary electrolyte losses indicated a 2-d loss of 3.7% of total body Na^+ stores and 3.0% of K^+ stores. Previous studies on Iowa high school wrestling finalists were similar.[39,40] It should be noted that at the time these studies were conducted the NCAA only allowed a 5-h period for rehydration.

In a trial with four collegiate wrestlers who were national qualifiers, the wrestlers were asked to simulate the energetic requirements of a wrestling match by running to exhaustion on a treadmill 5 h after a conventional weigh-in for their weight class.[21] Rehydration was permitted during the 5-h period postweigh-in. The wrestlers lost on average approximately 7% of their body weight by weigh-in and subsequently rehydrated to 3% hypohydration before running to exhaustion. Thus, under typical competitive conditions they would have been competing in a moderately hypohydrated state. VO_2 max was reduced slightly in three of the four wrestlers, but the mean decrement was not significantly different euhydrated vs. hypohydrated. Related observations on these and other wrestlers indicated that aerobic capacity, muscular strength, and isokinetic endurance were little changed over the course of a season probably as a result of the year-round training by the wrestlers. Unfortunately, these measurements were not made when the wrestlers were hypohydrated during the pre-, peak- or postseason testing.

IV. POWER ATHLETES

Caldwell et al.[8] concluded from investigation of power athletes' responses to different dehydration regimens that the ultimate physiological responses to maximal exercise depend not only on the amount of body weight and body fluid loss but also on the way the hypohydration was achieved. For example, among the weightlifters, wrestlers, judokaists, and boxers, maximal oxygen uptake and work load were compromised more when dehydration was achieved by sweating in a sauna or administration of a diuretic (furosemide) than when using submaximal exercise alone. An important variable, however, was the time allowed to achieve the approximately 4% body weight loss. With exercise alone, 48 h was allowed, whereas the sauna and diuretic protocols were for 24 h. Caldwell at al. also concluded that weight loss achieved over a 48-h period was probably less detrimental than that achieved over a 24-h period, but this possible difference was not ascertained using the same procedure for each time period.

In keeping with these results, Torranin et al.[33] have shown diminished endurance of skeletal muscles with acute hypohydration. Although the effects of moderate hypohydration may be perceived at relatively low exercise intensities, perhaps the major impact occurs at or near maximal work intensities that are prolonged, when cardiorespiratory reserves are limited or nonexistent. Thus, performance in competition would be compromised.

V. LIGHTWEIGHT ROWING

Another sport that involves body weight control to meet regulations for competition is lightweight rowing. Lightweight rowers must meet their weight standard at a weigh-in prior to competition but are then allowed to rehydrate if necessary before the actual event. Burge et al.[6] studied eight rowers who had had international competitive experience by dehydrating them through a combination of restricted fluid and food intake plus low-intensity exercise in "sweat gear." With the 24-h dehydration regimen, body weight was decreased about 5% and plasma volume about 12.5% on average. Rehydration with about 1.5 l of water during a 2-h period restored plasma volume about 6%. The rowing test on a rowing ergometer was a maximal one performed up to 4200 revs at 3 kg resistance. The test was designed to simulate the amount of work done during a 2000-m race by a lightweight coxless pair. Performance was assessed as the time to achieve the respective target maximum. The tests were performed in the euhydrated and the partially rehydrated state. Rowing time increased significantly from 7.02 ± 0.17 min with euhydration to 7.38 ± 0.21 min with partial rehydration. Net plasma lactate accumulation was less with partial rehydration than with euhydration, as was glycogen content of the vastus lateralis. The authors concluded that the dehydration/rehydration protocol lessened maximal rowing performance, perhaps due to the compromised plasma volume and the lesser dependence on glycogen utilization. Hypohydration caused a distinct inability to sustain the rowing at a high intensity, which translated into losing a race by about 95 m in a paired-oar event.

There is no doubt that competitive rowing success requires superior strength and muscular endurance as well as aerobic and anaerobic capabilities. That at least some of these attributes can be compromised by rapid weight loss practices and partial rehydration appears probable. It is interesting that in the experiment of Burge et al.,[6] a plot of the increase in rowing time on an interindividual basis was directly related to the decrease in plasma volume from the euhydrated to the partially rehydrated state. The correlation coefficient was r = 0.93 ($p < 0.01$) and the linear regression equation was

$$\text{RT-ET(min)} = 0.094 \cdot \Delta\%PV - 0.243$$

where
RT = partial rehydration trial
ET = euhydration trial
$\Delta\%PV$ = % decrease in plasma volume

In evaluating the PV/hypohydration relationship more closely, Burge et al.[6] concluded that rowing performance was lessened when the plasma volume deficit exceeded 2.6%. Others have suggested that the plasma volume deficit would probably have to exceed 6% before vascular readjustment fails to compensate via peripheral vasoconstriction for the lower blood volume and the reduction in stroke volume and cardiac output.[22]

Another rowing performance time trial was performed with a group of lightweight rowers ($N = 18$), half of whom were requested to lose 3–5% of their pretrial body weight over a 48-h period using water deprivation, exercise-induced sweating, and diet restriction.[23] The average decrease in body weight was 3.6%. Time to complete the 2000-m trial when hypohydrated was 10 s longer. Total power output was also significantly lower (–11.7W ± 8.7) when hypohydrated. The control euhydrated subjects did not experience any reduction in performance when tested before and after the same 48-h period. The investigators pointed out that the respective decrement in performance with hypohydration would constitute the difference between first and last place, or 200 m between boats during an actual 2000-m race.

VI. OTHER RELATED STUDIES

Although concentration in this presentation has been on hypohydration and performance among those engaged in weight-classification sports, it should be pointed out that hypohydration adversely affects runners engaged in endurance events. Armstrong et al.[2] in interpreting their studies concluded that performance in competitive runs of 5000 and 10,000 m is compromised more by hypohydration than shorter runs, including 1500 m. They offered the following explanation for their findings: impaired thermoregulation, increased perception of effort, and compromised anaerobic function — or a combination thereof.

In order to avoid the complications of hypohydration induced before the onset of exercise that decreases plasma volume, stroke volume, and sweat rate during exercise, Walsh et al.[36] induced hypohydration by exercising subjects in the heat and then studying perceived exertion and cycling time to exhaustion. The environmental conditions were 32°C, 60% RH, and windspeed 3km/h. The subjects cycled at 90% of their $\dot{V}O_2$ peak until exhausted. In a control trial, hydration at 10-min intervals with 20 mmol/l NaCl was utilized for the first 50 min of a 70% $\dot{V}O_2$ peak cycling period that lasted 60 min. Thereafter the subjects cycled to exhaustion at a high intensity (> 90% $\dot{V}O_2$ peak). Although hypohydration only averaged 1.8% body weight loss, the decrement in cycling time to exhaustion was significantly decreased and the rating of perceived exertion significantly increased. As with athletes involved with weight classifications, the experiment of Walsh et al. demonstrates the acute effect of even moderate levels of hypohydration on endurance and the perception of exercise intensity.

Hoffman et al.[14] investigated the effects of water restriction on ten basketball players who participated in two-on-two simulated basketball games that lasted 40 min. Thus, the players engaged in what can arbitrarily be termed high-intensity, moderate-duration exercise. Each player participated in two games, one with adequate water and one with restricted water intake. Ambient conditions were 20.8 ± 0.9°C and 0.64 ± 0.05% relative humidity. All players were euhydrated prior to initiation of each simulated game. The players experienced a −1.9 ± 0.4% body weight loss during the game involving water restriction. Testing before and after the games revealed no significant differences associated with water restriction in anaerobic power, squat jump, or countermovement jump overall when comparing pregame, halftime, and postgame results. A 19% lower anaerobic power was observed during the postgame testing with water restriction, which was not quite significant at the 5% level. Similarly an 8.1% decrease in field-goal percentage was seen between the first and second halfs with water restriction. Hoffman et al. concluded that the combination of high-intensity, moderate-duration exercise and water restriction suggested some decrement in skill performance, but the results were not conclusive.

Viitasalo et al.[35] dehydrated men using diuretic administration or 2 h in a sauna and achieved a 3–4% decrease in body weight. They found improved vertical jump performance in the hypohydrated state. They concluded that the reduced body weight was responsible for the improved vertical jump height and that the hypohydration had no discernable physiological effects on the jump performance.

Comparing the vertical jump results obtained by Viitasalo et al.[35] with the squat jump and countermovement jump results of Hoffman et al.,[14] who studied simulated basketball activities, reveals some disparity. The less than 2% weight loss achieved with passive water restriction by Hoffman et al. may not have provided sufficient weight loss to affect vertical jump performance. In addition, partial fatigue following the simulated basketball game may have obscured any potential improvement in jump performance associated with water restriction and weight loss. In any event, results with jumping tests such as the ones employed that involved explosive movement were not adversely affected. The effects on such explosive movement of greater hypohydration remain to be determined.

In an interesting study of the effects of acute hypohydration on some of the variables likely to affect weight-class athletes, Greenleaf et al.[12] depleted nine well-conditioned men up to 6.9% of their body weight and gave them several physical performance tests including: $+G_z-3.0G°/min$ (grayout tolerance) acceleration exposure, reaction time and a modified Harvard step test. In general, performance was normal until hypohydration exceeded 4% body weight loss. In their analysis they point out that the availability of "free circulating water" representing a body reserve may prevent adverse effects until the 4% threshold is reached. They also felt that a key factor between hypohydration and performance is the rate at which body water is lost — that is, the faster the rate the poorer the subsequent performance. Thus, both rate and amount of water loss were cited as being of consequence.

Testing whether the hypohydration might be more acute in young children (ages 10–12) engaged in early exposure to weight-classified sports, Bar-Or et al.[3] concluded that exercising children progressively dehydrate — when not forced to drink — and equal percent body weight loss resulted in a greater rise in core body temperature than in lean adults. Thus, children may have a greater potential for heat injury and possible performance decrement.

On the psychological side, Steen and Brownell[32] concluded that "making weight" was associated with fatigue, anger, and anxiety following their assessment of 63 college wrestlers and 368 high school wrestlers. They also found that 30 to 40% of both groups of wrestlers reported preoccupation with food and out-of-control eating after competition. This emphasized to them the potential incursion of psychopathological effects such as eating disorders. Earlier Morgan[24] had indicated that 4% body weight loss probably had no practical effect on anxiety among collegiate wrestlers, but Ryan et al.[27] pointed out that weight-control methods including acute dehydration have been linked to depression and decreased learning ability, although such findings deserve confirmation. Thus, concern about weight-reduction practices including acute dehydration remains, and such practices in relation to psychological variables deserve further attention and investigation.

VII. INTERPRETATIONS

As noted, a variety of studies have been performed to examine the impact of acute or rapid body weight loss and dehydration on physical performance among athletes competing by weight class. Performance assessments have included strength (isometric, isokinetic, isotonic), muscular endurance, aerobic capacity (maximal or peak oxygen uptake, $\dot{V}O_2$ max), anaerobic capacity, exercise time (endurance), simulated competition, and explosiveness (e.g., vertical jump height). Horswill[15] reviewed the literature and found little or no evidence for reductions in strength, peak oxygen uptake, or anaerobic power following rapid weight loss. He identified possible reasons for the retention of strength and power with hypohydration:

1. muscle energetics are self-contained and not dependent on bloodborne substrates such as glucose, free fatty acids, or oxygen;
2. a decrease in blood flow to the muscle with sustained or brief intense and rapid contractions should not be an impediment;
3. muscle excitability is quite resistant to alterations in electrolyte and water content allowing normal nerve stimulation of muscle for contraction;
4. there is no apparent decrease in muscle energetic essentials such as ATP and creatine phosphate.

Similarly, $\dot{V}O_2$ max appears largely preserved with hypohydration up to a body weight loss of 4 to 5%, or perhaps even more. Reports of a reduction in $\dot{V}O_2$ max with dehydration have been few and have usually involved heat exposure.[7] Examination of the reason for the relative preservation of $\dot{V}O_2$ max is that cardiac output as well as overall cardiopulmonary function is preserved.[29]

In contrast, endurance may well be compromised with hypohydration, i.e., exercise at or near maximal effort for periods exceeding about 30 s. Again Horswill[15] in reviewing the available information cites several reasons for the decrease in endurance:

1. Muscle glycogen may be significantly decreased.
2. Reduced blood flow to muscle may slow substrate exchange, byproduct removal, and heat dissipation, thereby impeding recovery during periods between contractions.
3. Buffering capacity of the muscle may be compromised.

The net effect is that the athlete loses capability as the intense activity continues and inadequate recovery time cumulatively lowers energy reserves.

In a subsequent analysis of the effects of rapid weight loss on performance, Horswill[16] utilized the three primary energy systems as a means of ascertaining effects: (1) the ATP-PC system, which supports maximal strength and anaerobic power; (2) the intermediate energy system (anaerobic glycolysis), which supports maximum muscular contractions for periods of 30 s to 3 min and (3) the oxidative system, which supports sustained exercise whether submaximal or maximal. Based on effects on wrestlers, it was concluded that the ATP-PC system is relatively unaffected by hypohydration. The intermediate energy system may or may not be affected, with most noted effects in anaerobic capacity relegated to periods exceeding 30 s. The oxidative system is regarded as being adversely affected in many studies, particularly endurance time, but $\dot{V}O_2$ max to some extent as well.[7,37] These conclusions are somewhat at variance with Horswill's[15] earlier views but no doubt reflect the paucity of precise mechanistic information. Horswill[16] therefore recommends that in future studies evaluation of the power or maximal workload at peak $\dot{V}O_2$ be encouraged in order to ascertain whether mechanical efficiency is lessened if power is reduced when peak $\dot{V}O_2$ is maintained.

A complication arises regarding interpretation of poorer endurance among those hypohydrated, at least with respect to skeletal muscle. Jensen et al.[20] reviewed the work on prolonged isometric exercise and muscle swelling due to increased water content. These investigators also utilized ultrasound scanning to visualize the accumulation (swelling) of fluid in the supraspinatus muscle with 30° unilateral isometric shoulder abduction to exhaustion. During the test, which averaged 33 min to produce exhaustion in nine healthy women, the thickness of the supraspinatus muscle increased by 14%. Jensen et al. point out that other investigators have noted comparable muscle edema with intense dynamic as well as isometric exercise. What happens with hypohydration and intense prolonged muscular exercise with respect to fluid transfer has not been resolved and probably is not a simple process. One process that may well be operational with sustained isometric contractions is impaired lymph flow or drainage as a result of high intramuscular pressure. With muscle swelling, there would be an increase in intramuscular diffusion distances, which could impair transport of substrates and contribute to fatigue. Again, the partial compromise that might be expected between hypohydration effects on the muscle countered by fluid retention associated with muscular contraction remains to be resolved.

VIII. SUMMARY

After reviewing the various studies on body weight loss and hypohydration and various aspects of physical performance, it is clear that more research is needed. The task of establishing appropriate laboratory simulations to represent actual competition is a daunting one that has only been partially attacked. Judging imposes qualitative analysis of the performance as well as the aesthetics involved. Simulating what the judge perceives poses an additional complication. To a large extent the physiological mechanisms responsible for deterioration in performance, particularly at the cellular level, with hypohydration remain largely unexplored. For example, does hypohydration affect enzyme activity in skeletal muscle? Similarly, what physiological mechanisms are returned toward or to normal that might help explain regained performance following a relatively acute rehydration regimen after hypohydration?

In terms of what is known, muscular strength explosiveness, reaction time, and athletic skills appear to be maintained with hypohydration at least up to 5% body weight loss. Aerobic capabilities may be partially compromised, particularly if heat stress is also involved. Endurance in most instances is negatively affected and anaerobic capabilities may be lessened with repetitive or prolonged anaerobic demands.

REFERENCES

1. Adolph, E. F., *Physiology of Man in the Desert*, Interscience, New York, 1947.
2. Armstrong, L. E., Costill, D. L., and Fink, W. J., Influence of diuretic-induced dehydration on competitive running performance, *Med. Sci. Sports Exer.*, 17, 456–461, 1985.
3. Bar-Or, O., Dotan, R., Inbar, O., Rothstein, A., and Zonder, H., Voluntary hypohydration in 10- to 12-year old boys, *J. Appl. Physiol.*, 48, 104–108, 1980.
4. Bock, W., Fox, E. L., and Bowers, R., The effect of acute dehydration upon cardio-respiratory endurance, *J. Sports Med.*, 7, 67–72, 1967.
5. Bosco, J. S., Greenleaf, J. E., Bernauer, E. M., and Card, D. H., Effects of acute dehydration and starvation on muscular strength and endurance, *Acta Physiol. Pol.*, 25, 411–421, 1974.
6. Burge, C. M., Carey, M. F., and Payne, W. R., Rowing performance, fluid balance and metabolic function following dehydration and rehydration, *Med. Sci. Sports Exer.*, 25, 1358–1364, 1993.
7. Buskirk, E. R., Iampietro, P. F., and Bass, D. E., Work performance after dehydration: Effects of physical condition and heat acclimatization, *J. Appl. Physiol.*, 12, 189–194, 1958.
8. Caldwell, J. E., Ahonen, E., and Nousianinen, U., Differential effects of sauna-, diuretic- and exercise-induced hypohydration, *J. Appl. Physiol.*, 57, 1018–1023, 1984.
9. Craig, F. N. and Cummings, E. G., Dehydration and muscular work, *J. Appl. Physiol.*, 21, 670–674, 1966.
10. Fogelholm, G. M., Koskinen, R., Laakso, J., Rankinen, T., and Ruokonen, I., Gradual and rapid weight loss: Effects on nutrition and performance in male athletes, *Med. Sci. Sports Exer.*, 25, 371–377, 1993.
11. Fogelholm, G. M., Effects of body weight reduction on sports performance, *Sports Med.*, 18, 249–267, 1994.
12. Greenleaf, J, E., Malter, M., Jr., Bosco, J. S., Douglas, L. G., and Averkin, E. G., Effects of hypohydration on work performance and tolerance to +Gz acceleration in man, *Aerosp. Med.*, 37, 34–39, 1966.
13. Herbert, W. G. and Ribisl, P. M., Effects of dehydration upon physical working capacity of wrestlers under competitive conditions, *Res. Q.*, 43, 416–422, 1972.
14. Hoffman, J. R., Stavsky, H., and Falk, B., The effect of water restriction on anaerobic power and vertical jumping height in basketball players, *Int. J. Sports Med.*, 16, 214–218, 1995.
15. Horswill, C. A., Applied physiology of amateur wrestling, *Sports Med.*, 14, 114–143, 1992.
16. Horswill, C. A., Weight loss and weight cycling in amateur wrestlers: Implications for performance and resting metabolic rate, *Int. J. Sports Nutr.*, 3, 245–260, 1993.
17. Horswill, C. A., Scott, J. R., and Dick, R. W., Influence of rapid weight gain after the weigh-in on success in collegiate wrestlers, *Med. Sci. Sports Exer.*, 26, 1290–1294, 1994.
18. Houston, M. E., Marrin, D. A., Green, H. J., and Thomson, J. A., The effect of rapid weight loss on physiological function in wrestlers, *Physician Sports Med.*, 9, 73–78, 1981.
19. Jacobs, I., The effects of thermal dehydration on performance on the Wingate anaerobic test, *Int. J. Sports Med.*, 1, 21–24, 1980.
20. Jensen, B. R., Jorgensen, K., and Sjogaard, G., The effect of prolonged isometric contractions on muscle fluid balance, *Eur. J. Appl. Physiol.*, 69, 439–444, 1994.

21. Kelly, J. M., Gorney, B. A., and Kalm, K. K., The effects of a collegiate wrestling season on body composition, cardiovascular fitness and muscular strength and endurance, *Med. Sci. Sports*, 10, 119–124, 1978.
22. Klinzing, J. E. and Karpowicz, E., The effects of rapid weight loss and rehydration on a wrestling performance test, *J. Sports Med.*, 26, 149–156, 1986.
23. Meiggs, R. A., MacConnie, S. E., and Hyland, P. J., Effects of rapid weight loss on a 2000 meter rowing ergometer performance time trial, American College of Sports Medicine, Southwest Chapter, 13th Annual Meeting Publication November 1993, 313 (Abstract).
24. Morgan, W. P., Psychological effect of weight reduction in the college wrestler, *Med. Sci. Sports*, 2, 24–27, 1970.
25. Palmer, W. K., Selected physiological responses of normal young men following dehydration and rehydration, *Res. Q.*, 39, 1054–1059, 1968.
26. Ribisl, P. M. and Herbert, W. G., Effects of rapid weight reduction and subsequent rehydration upon the physical working capacity of wrestlers, *Res. Q.*, 41, 536–541, 1970.
27. Ryan, A., Gable, D., Tipton, C. M., Morgan, W. P., Lewis, R., and Roy, S., Weight reduction in wrestling: A round table, *Physician Sports Med.*, 9, 79–96, 1981.
28. Saltin, B., Aerobic and anaerobic work capacity after dehydration, *J. Appl. Physiol.*, 19, 1114–1118, 1964.
29. Saltin, B., Circulatory response to submaximal and maximal exercise after thermal dehydration, *J. Appl. Physiol.*, 19, 1125–1132, 1964.
30. Serfass, R. C., Stull, G. A., Alexander, J. F., and Ewing, J. L., The effects of rapid weight loss and attempted rehydration on strength and endurance of the handgripping muscles in college wrestlers, *Res. Q. Exer. Sport*, 55, 46–52, 1984.
31. Singer, R. N. and Weiss, S. A., Effects of weight reduction on several anthropometric, physical, and performance measures of wrestlers, *Res. Q. Exer. Sport*, 39, 361–369, 1968.
32. Steen, S. N. and Brownell, K. D., Patterns of weight loss and regain in wrestlers: Has the tradition changed? *Med. Sci. Sports Exer.*, 22, 762–768, 1990.
33. Torranin, C., Smith, D. P., and Byrd, R. J., The effect of acute thermal dehydration and rapid rehydration on isometric and isotonic endurance, *J. Sports Med. Phys. Fitness*, 19, 1–9, 1979.
34. Tuttle, W. W., The effect of weight loss by dehydration and the withholding of food on the physiological responses of wrestlers, *Res. Q.*, 14, 158–166, 1943.
35. Viitasalo, J. T., Kyrolainen, H., Bosco, C., and Allen, M., Effects of rapid weight reduction on vertical jumping height, *Int. J. Sports Med.*, 8, 281–285, 1987.
36. Walsh, R. M., Noakes, T. O., Hawley, J. A., and Dennis, S. C., Impaired high intensity cycling performance time at low levels of dehydration, *Int. J. Sports Med.*, 15, 392–398, 1994.
37. Webster, S., Rutt, R., and Weltman, A., Physiological effects of a weight loss regimen practiced by college wrestlers, *Med. Sci. Sports Exer.*, 22, 229–234, 1990.
38. Zambraski, E. J., Foster, D. T., Gross, P. M., and Tipton, C. M., Iowa wrestling study: Weight loss and urinary profiles of collegiate wrestlers, *Med. Sci. Sports*, 8, 105–108, 1976.
39. Zambraski, E. J., Tipton, C. M., Jordon, H. R., Palmer, W. K., and Tcheng, T. K., Iowa wrestling study: Urinary profiles of state finalists prior to competition, *Med. Sci. Sports*, 6, 129–132, 1974.
40. Zambraski, E. J., Tipton, C. M., Tcheng, T. K., Jordan, H. R., Vailas, A. C., and Callahan, A. K., Iowa wrestling study: Changes in the urinary profiles of wrestlers prior to and after competition, *Med. Sci. Sports*, 7, 217–220, 1975.

Chapter 15

CLINICAL COMPLICATIONS OF BODY FLUID AND ELECTROLYTE BALANCE

James P. Knochel

CONTENTS

I. Clinical Disorders Related to Heat Stress 297
   A. Heat Cramps 297
   B. Heat Exhaustion 298
      1. Treatment of Heat Exhaustion 299
   C. Heat Stroke 300
      1. Laboratory Findings 301
      2. Pathophysiology 302
      3. Complications of Heat Stroke 307
      4. Treatment of Heat Stroke 310

II. Hyponatremia in Long-Distance Runners 312

III. The Risk of Heat Stroke and Exertional Rhabdomyolysis in Athletes with Sickle Cell Trait 313

IV. The Role of Negligence and Punition in Heat Stroke 314

V. Summary 315

References 315

I. CLINICAL DISORDERS RELATED TO HEAT STRESS

A. HEAT CRAMPS

Sustained work in a hot environment may be complicated by painful, excruciating contractions. They are more apt to occur in muscles used during work. Most commonly, cramps appear at the end of the day when activity has ceased and especially if the muscles are cooled down by taking a shower. Cramps of the rectus abdominus may cause frank abdominal rigidity simulating an intraabdominal catastrophe. Usually, physical examination shows rigid muscles that are not particularly tender.

Heat cramps are most common in heat-acclimatized, well-trained persons who have produced voluminous quantities of sweat in response to working in the heat.[47] Characteristically, these people replace their sweat losses with adequate amounts of water but inadequate quantities of salt, thus explaining the findings of hyponatremia and hypochloremia. Training and acclimatization to heat, by increasing the volume of sweat produced in response to a given exercise load, may in some cases lead to increased rather than decreased losses of sodium chloride in sweat.[25,33] Although sweat concentrations of sodium and chloride become frankly lower after acclimatization, levels of both rise in proportion to sweat rate. Because sweat is an ultrafiltrate of plasma, secretion at high rates allows inadequate time for aldosterone-mediated reabsorption of sodium and apparently passive reabsorption of chloride.[41] Under these conditions, a high volume and a relatively high concentration of salt causes salt depletion and hyponatremia if an adequate volume of water is ingested.

Hypothetically, hyponatremia reduces the chemical gradient driving sodium across the sarcolemma, thus reducing sodium extrusion by the sodium–potassium ATPase pump. Decreased 3 Na^+ pumped out for $2K^+$ pumped in reduces transmembrane electrical potential difference. The reduction of intracellular electronegativity reduces passive entry of sodium ions, and in turn, reduces outward movement of calcium ions.[10] The resulting elevation of myoplasmic calcium concentration triggers release of additional calcium from the sarcoplasmic reticulum. The increased myoplasmic calcium concentration disinhibits tropomycin, thereby facilitating interaction of actin and myosin, and contraction follows. Restoration of the normal sodium gradient across the cell by correction of hyponatremia leads to rapid improvement.

Laboratory findings in patients with heat cramps usually consist of hyponatremia and hypochloremia. Rhabdomyolysis may occur in some patients.

Muscle cramps usually respond to administration of salted solutions by mouth or, if necessary, by intravenous infusion of normal saline in a dose of 10–15 ml/kg body weight. Heat cramps may be prevented in most patients by prophylactic administration of hypotonic salt solutions.

B. HEAT EXHAUSTION

Heat exhaustion is the most common clinical syndrome resulting from heat stress. It occurs in persons who are unacclimatized to work in the heat. It may occur in temperate weather by hard work causing large losses of water and salt by sweating. Heat exhaustion usually develops slowly over the course of several days. Predominant dehydration occurs when salt is consumed without adequate water. Healthy, fit persons almost never voluntarily replace total body water losses induced by thermal stress. This problem is magnified in the elderly athlete, whose thirst response to dehydration may be less than that observed in young persons.[7] In the past, water was deliberately restricted during football drills because of the misconception that replacement retarded training. The symptoms of water-depletion heat exhaustion include intense thirst, fatigue, weakness, discomfort, anxiety, restlessness, confusion, impaired judgment, disorientation, paresthesias, and muscular incoordination. The central nervous system manifestations of dehydration are those of a metabolic encephalopathy. Delirium, tachycardia, hyperventilation, fever up to 102°F, and coma represent advanced stages of this disorder. Sweating is usually detectable. The urine is usually scanty, dark, and concentrated, showing a low concentration of sodium and a high concentration of urea reflecting normal renal conservation of salt and water. Hypernatremia is always present with serum sodium values as high as 170 meq/l. Recognition of water depletion and heat exhaustion is critical because if neglected, frank heat stroke and death may supervene.

Heat exhaustion due to predominant salt depletion presents a remarkably different picture from the hypernatremic form. In these cases, sweat losses have been replaced by adequate water but inadequate quantities of salt. The patients display hyponatremia and hypochloremia. Although muscular cramps may occur, these patients are sick. Symptoms include profound weakness, fatigue, severe headache, myalgias, giddiness, anorexia, nausea, vomiting, and in some cases, diarrhea. The skin is pallid, clammy, and inelastic. Hypotension, orthostasis, tachycardia, and syncope may occur. Body temperature remains normal or subnormal. The occurrence of nausea, vomiting, and diarrhea may erroneously suggest a viral syndrome, especially if the patient complains of myalgias and headache. In contrast to viral syndromes, these symptoms markedly improve after rest and administration of salt and water.

Hypercalcemia is observed in some patients with heat exhaustion who are volume depleted and hemoconcentrated. One of the author's recent patients showed a total serum calcium level of 12.5 mg/dl and a serum albumin concentration of 5.8 g/dl. In this patient, total protein concentration before treatment was 9.7 g/dl. His serum phosphorus was 4.5 mg/dl, magnesium 2.5 meq/dl, and uric acid 11 mg/dl. All of these values are elevated and promptly returned to normal following administration of hypotonic saline. This patient also developed rhabdomyolysis. His creatine kinase level rose to 22,000 IU/l, reflecting damage to skeletal muscle (rhabdomyolysis).

1. Treatment of Heat Exhaustion

Athletes training in the heat should be monitored closely, consume abundant water, and salt their food generously at mealtime. Weighing before and after practice will identify those who fail to consume adequate fluids and also enlighten the athlete as to the quantity of sweat produced (weight loss plus volume of fluid consumed approximates sweat volume). Workouts should be conducted during the cool part of the day, taking precautions to adjust activities with respect to heat and humidity, and if possible, avoiding direct exposure to the sun.

Most athletes with heat exhaustion respond to simple measures. These include cooling by application of moist towels to the body surface, fanning, removal of unessential clothing and football gear, and administration of lightly salted fluids. Fluids should never be given to an obtunded or poorly responsive athlete because of the danger of aspiration. Removal from direct sunlight is essential if possible. Heat exhaustion victims who are vomiting, orthostatic, confused, disoriented, or febrile should probably be taken to an emergency room or hospital. It is extremely difficult for a trainer, a coach, or even an experienced physician to ascertain the potential severity of heat exhaustion by simple observation and examination. Laboratory measurements of serum electrolytes are readily available, are low in cost, and can be performed very quickly. Availability of such information helps immensely to assess severity and the subsequent plan of treatment.

In hypernatremic heat exhaustion, one must avoid reducing serum sodium concentration too rapidly. If a patient with hypernatremia is given large quantities of free water (5% dextrose), cerebral edema may potentially result with the risk of uncal herniation and death. Because of the osmotic effects of hypernatremia, cells in the central nervous system initially respond by losing water and reducing their volume. In response to this, there is a signal to synthesize taurine and other osmotically active substances inside the cells, which over a period of 2–3 d serves to increase osmolality, facilitate water uptake, and return cell size to normal.[22] Because the interior of the cell is equally hypertonic to the extracellular fluid, administration of hypotonic fluid leads to a rapid shift of water into the cell, eventually resulting in cerebral edema. When confronted with a hypernatremic athlete who has probably become ill over the course of several days, the best method of treatment is to administer 1–2 l of normal saline intravenously over a period of 3–6 h. This should be followed by cautious administration of 5% glucose solution at a rate such that serum sodium falls no more rapidly than 2 meq/l/h. This will allow time for taurine and other osmotically active solutes to diffuse from the cells or to be metabolized and thereby prevent major shifts in cell volume. It should be appreciated that severe hypernatremia is potentially very serious and requires management by a person knowledgeable in fluid and electrolyte disorders.

Hyponatremic heat exhaustion due to salt or water depletion is very simply managed by administration of salt and water. These patients generally recover fairly rapidly and are generally able to resume their activities after a period of 24 h.

C. HEAT STROKE

Heat stroke is a dire medical emergency that if untreated will generally be fatal. It is fortunately the rarest disorder caused by heat stress. Prevention of morbidity or death from heat stroke depends directly upon anticipation, prompt recognition, and emergent cooling. Complications depend directly upon the degree and duration of hyperthermia. Thus, trainers, coaches, and participants in competitive events must be informed about hazardous environmental situations and the associated risks. Guidelines for appropriate timing of athletic events to avoid heat stress and provision of ice and facilities to allow immediate cooling are of paramount importance. Trained, experienced personnel who recognize the earliest signs of impending heat stroke and respond instantly save lives and prevent organ damage. Except for an occasional case, heat stroke is almost always preventable if appropriate precautions are taken.

The cardinal symptoms of heat stroke are those of central nervous system (CNS) dysfunction, a rectal or core temperature exceeding 105°F, and hot, flushed dry skin. CNS dysfunction is a prerequisite; without this component, the diagnosis can not be made.[3,8,16,43,44,46] The earliest signs of impending heat stroke may be subtle.[37] There may be complaints of weakness, paresthesias, headache, or dizziness. Not uncommonly, a change in performance or mental status may be a tip-off.[2] The football player may miss a block, forget his assignment, become uncharacteristically belligerent, or, for no reason, take a swing at his best friend. He may develop a vacant stare and appear confused. Another may begin to babble or run aimlessly. A runner may become unstable, wander off the course, and appear confused and disoriented. Most victims will collapse and become unconscious. Although a variety of transient findings have been described such as opisthotonus, or unilateral fixed dilatation of a pupil, most cases show flaccid coma. Bowel and bladder incontinence may occur. Convulsive seizures may be seen at presentation but most often appear during active cooling.

The degree of hyperthermia is variable. A core temperature of at least 105°F is usually required for the diagnosis. However, actual temperatures are generally in the vicinity of 107–108°F, with unusual cases ranging up to 115.7°F.[45] Although anhidrosis with a hot, flushed skin is a criterion of heat stroke, most cases of exertional heat stroke are perspiring at the onset. In fact, in such cases vaporization of sweat may deceptively cool the body surface despite frank hyperthermia, and thus lead to delays in treatment.

Other findings at the onset include tachycardia and hyperventilation in all patients and hypotension in nearly half.

1. **Laboratory Findings**

Approximately 50% of patients with acute exertional heat stroke are hypokalemic during the first few hours after onset.[23,26,37] This could be explained by potassium deficiency (to be discussed below), or a shift of potassium from plasma to the intracellular space either as a result of respiratory alkalosis or catecholamines. As a result of tissue injury or acute renal failure, hypokalemia may be supplanted by hyperkalemia after the first 12–24 h.

Patients with classical heat stroke commonly demonstrate pure respiratory alkalosis,[4,16] whereas those with exertional heat stroke most often demonstrate a mixed acid-base disorder dominated by lactic acidosis and respiratory alkalosis.[30] Lactic acidosis in patients with exertional heat stroke generally clears very rapidly in response to administration of glucose and saline. Persistent lactic acidosis suggests circulatory failure.[16]

Volume depletion, hemoconcentration, and hyperalbuminemia may result in mild hypercalcemia early during the course of heat stroke. Later, calcium salts precipitate in injured muscle, sometimes resulting in profound hypocalcemia.[34]

Serum phosphorous levels may be transiently elevated in some patients with acute heat stroke, but often fall to values below 1.0 mg/dl.[29] Hypophosphatemia usually appears to be the result of respiratory alkalosis, which by elevating intracellular pH, activates phosphofructokinase and causes a net shift of phosphorus from serum to intracellular water during the course of phosphorylation of glucose.[33] Urine samples collected at the same time show extremely low concentration of phosphorus.[29] Although it has been suggested that renal loss of phosphorus is responsible for hypophosphatemia, the precise study to validate this hypothesis has not been published. Hyperphosphatemia often appears later in patients with widespread tissue injury, and renal failure and may be directly responsible for hypocalcemia because of tissue deposition of calcium phosphate.

Although unusual, heat stroke may cause abnormalities of liver function as indicated by elevated levels of alanine amino transferase (ALT), aspartate aminotransferase (AST), and lactic dehydrogenase (LDH). ALT, AST, and LDH can also become substantially elevated as a result of rhabdomyolysis. Although a slight elevation of bilirubin may be derived from metabolism of myoglobin, frank jaundice may appear in a small percentage of patients, reflecting hepatic injury.[17]

Severe work in the heat usually results in a modestly concentrated, acid urine that is clearly appropriate for the level of hydration and renal function. Urinary findings of proteinuria, erythrocytes, red cell, or granular casts may be seen in any normal athlete following brisk activity, especially in hot weather. This finding has been termed "athletic pseudonephritis" because it apparently does not necessarily reflect renal injury.[27]

2. Pathophysiology

Virtually all cases of exertional heat stroke are caused by generation of heat in excess of the body's capacity to dissipate heat to the surrounding air. This concept and physical factors modulating heat production, storage, and dissipation are extensively discussed elsewhere in this text. Discussions in this section are limited to those factors that pertain specifically to heat stroke.

a. *CNS Temperature vs. Core Temperature*

Because frank hyperthermia may occur in competitive athletes who show no apparent ill effects,[36] hyperthermia per se may not necessarily be an ominous finding. This is an important consideration because some athletes who collapse after exertion and who demonstrate CNS dysfunction and cessation of sweating may paradoxically show core temperatures as low as 103°F. This explains why the precise core temperature as a criterion of heat stroke varies among different investigators. Accordingly, interest has been directed toward brain temperature, which could be a much more critical determinant of CNS dysfunction and loss of thermoregulation.[6,34] Anatomically, venous blood returning from the face drains directly into venous plexuses between the nasal cavity and the palate and thence into venous sinuses that pass beneath the basilar surface of the brain enroute to the jugular veins. Air movement over mucous membranes in the nose, mouth, and throat cools blood flowing through the submucosal veins, and this in turn presumably cools adjacent brain tissue. Although cerebral temperature cannot be measured directly, some evidence suggests that tympanic membrane temperature, when properly recorded, possibly reflects that of the adjacent brain. Cooling the face reduces tympanic temperature. Everyone who has experienced the discomfort of heat stress clearly appreciates the immediate relief obtained by splashing the face with cool water or by pouring cool water over the head. Perhaps we should concentrate our efforts upon cooling the head as aggressively as we cool the whole body to treat acute heat stroke.

b. Sweat Gland Failure in Heat Stroke

Production of sweat is regulated by hypothalamic thermoregulatory centers and local factors within the sweat gland itself. The finding of hot dry skin in victims of heat stroke led to the notion that sweat gland failure may partially explain their hyperthermia. Anhidrosis is more common in the classic variety of heat stroke. However, persistent sweating in exertional heat stroke occurs in the majority of cases and accordingly, cessation of sweating cannot be the sole factor responsible for hyperthermia in those instances. Clearly, injury of temperature control centers in the hypothalamus may affect thermoregulation and impair reflexes that initiate sweating. There also exists a major role of the autonomic nervous system in thermoregulation, because patients with congenital or acquired autonomic neuropathy may be unable to sweat normally and are at risk of developing heat stroke.[11] Another theory proposes that sweat gland fatigue explains the appearance of anhidrosis in heat stroke victims. Patients with classic heat stroke may not show a sudorific response to cholinergic drugs. Other studies showed a progressive reduction of cholinergic drug-induced sweat rates over time in normal subjects, thus implying "fatigue" of sweat glands. More recent evidence suggests that sweat gland fatigue may reflect mechanical obstruction of the sweat gland orifice caused by epithelial swelling incident to prolonged soaking of the skin. Thus, the fatigue disappears if sweat is not allowed to accumulate on the skin surface, or if sweat gland stimulation is conducted in very low humidity to facilitate rapid evaporation, or if the superficial hydrophilic corneal layer of skin is stripped away.[42] This process of sweat-induced ductal obstruction has been termed hydromeiosis.

c. Circulatory Failure in Heat Stroke

Circulatory failure is one of the most critical factors underlying the development of heat stroke, especially in otherwise healthy subjects and athletes. Observations by Rowell and his associates[39] on unacclimatized volunteers running at 43.3°C dry bulb, 28.3°C wet bulb closely resemble the sequence of events observed in athletes who have collapsed during competitive running in the heat. Thus, early in the race they perspire heavily, become flushed, then begin to stumble and appear disoriented.[31] A transient period of pallor may occur, suggesting a loss of blood flow to the skin. Afterward, sweating may cease. When they collapse, the skin usually resumes its flushed or red appearance. Similar observations were made on Israeli soldiers exercising in the heat.[13] When their rectal temperatures approached 106°–108°F, they demonstrated a grayish color and confusion before the point of collapse. These findings suggest that circulatory failure, implying a reduced cardiac output secondary to decreased venous return, leading to decreased cerebral and cutaneous perfusion, represents a cardinal event in the pathogenesis of exertional heat stroke. All normal subjects exposed to a high ambient temperature hyperventilate and commonly develop respiratory alkalosis.[4] A reduction of arterial carbon dioxide tension produced by hyperventilation causes cerebral vasoconstriction and a substantial reduction in cerebral blood flow.[15] Such events could be at least partially responsible for certain central nervous system disturbances characteristic of heat stroke.

d. Role of Splanchnic Ischemia and Endotoxins in Heat Stroke

Hard work in the heat leads to a reduction of splanchnic blood flow as a result of translocation of blood from the visceral circulation to working muscle and skin in response to exercise and hyperthermia.[39] When mesenteric blood flow is reduced, endotoxins are absorbed from the gut to the portal circulation.[1] Endotoxin and resulting cytokines adversely affect survival during experimental hyperthermia. Thus, germ-free animals do not demonstrate endotoxinemia during hyperthermia and display a marked reduction in morbidity compared to animals with a normal intestinal flora. Sterilization of the gut with antibiotics, immunization against Gram-negative endotoxins, and infusion of endo-toxin antibodies reduce mortality and morbidity from hyperthermia. Trained, heat-acclimatized athletes show higher levels of antibodies against endotoxins than unacclimatized subjects. Infusion of endotoxin or cytokines that result from endotoxin activation of monocytes, as will be pointed out subsequently, reproduce many of the catabolic and destructive organ complications seen in patients with severe heat stroke. Patients with heat stroke clearly show marked elevations of endotoxin levels in their blood. Mucosal damage to the gut and endotoxinemia after hyperthermia may be the result of enhanced nitric oxide production in the splanchnic circulation causing reperfusion injury.[14]

e. Role of Drugs and Medications in Heat Stroke

A number of medications play important roles in the pathogenesis of heat stroke. These include anticholinergics or anti-Parkinsonian drugs, diuretics, and antipsychotics including haloperidol and phenothiazines. In contrast, some athletes with exertional heat stroke have inappropriately used amphetamines, cocaine, or over-the-counter anorexigenic sympathomimetic drugs (phenylpropanolamine) in an attempt to improve their performance. These drugs may increase heat production or blunt recognition of fatigue. They may also intensify lactic acidosis.[5] Other athletes innocently use nasal decongestants, antihistamines, or anticholinergic drugs that reduce sweat production. A number of cardiovascular medications are commonly used by older athletes that could lower the threshold to develop heat stroke. Thus, diuretics employed for hypertension could affect balance of salt, potassium, and water. Spironolactone and triamterine interfere with the action of aldosterone on sweat glands and allow sweat sodium concentration to approach higher levels. Beta-adrenergic blocking agents, especially propranolol, may not only reduce sweat volume but also reduce heart rate, myocardial contractility, and cardiac output. Calcium channel-blocking drugs used for hypertension may also reduce cardiac output. Angiotensin-converting enzyme inhibitors, although theoretically dangerous because they downregulate the renin–angiotensin–aldosterone axis, surprisingly have not been as hazardous in athletic performance as one would have predicted. Similarly, central adrenergic agonists, such as clonidine and guanfacine, that indirectly reduce norepinephrine release from peripheral sites of storage, do not appear to be a formidable problem. The proper recommendations for selecting and adjusting dosages of these drugs during hot weather and during the immediate period preceding athletic events in athletes with hypertension or other cardiovascular disorders have not been delineated.

f. Aging and Heat Stroke

A variety of factors associated with aging could lower the threshold for developing heat-stress injury in elderly athletes. Cutaneous blood flow during heating is lower in elderly persons.[38] The core temperature at which sweating is initiated (thermoregulatory setpoint) is increased.[40] Sweat production in comparison to core temperature is generally less.[20] Thirst perception is decreased for any given level of plasma hypertonicity or volume depletion. Release of antidiuretic hormone from the posterior pituitary gland is reduced for any given level of water depletion or hypertonicity. With aging, there is a downregulation of the renin–angiotensin system.[49] More specifically, for any degree of extracellular volume depletion, the expected rise of plasma renin levels and, in turn, aldosterone production appears to be less in an older than a younger person. There is also a general downturning of autonomic circulatory control.[18] Finally, cardiovascular function is depressed in the aged because of ventricular stiffness, which could conceivably affect both ventricular filling and ejection velocity.

In view of the foregoing effects of aging, it would appear that heat stroke would be rampant among the elderly performing any form of work in the heat. To the contrary, most of these individuals appear wise enough to avoid threatening situations, and it would appear that heat stroke and related disorders are perhaps even less common among elderly athletes than they are in the young.

g. Potassium (K) Deficiency During Training in Hot Weather

Men who perform hard work in the heat for many hours during the day can lose substantial quantities of K in sweat.[24] Although K concentration in sweat secreted at low rates averages around 5 meq/l, when it is produced in large quantities (i.e., at approximately 10 l per day), sweat K concentrations range up to 10 meq/l.[32] A number of investigators have shown that military trainees, trained troops, and football players often produce 10 l or more of sweat per day. Because the usual dietary K intake averages around 100 meq/d, this quantity could easily be lost in the sweat, and any additional quantity of K lost in the urine could result in a substantial cumulative loss. Because of salt and water losses during such activities, brisk renin secretion, resulting in increased production of aldosterone, could contribute to these losses.

Relevant studies on the above possibilities were conducted on normal, healthy military recruits undergoing basic training in hot weather and again during cool weather.[24] While consuming a constant diet containing 106 meq of K daily, control and weekly studies for 5 consecutive weeks showed an average reduction of total body K averaging 517 meq during the first few weeks of training in the heat. Despite the K deficit, urinary K excretion averaged 67 meq/d when K deficiency was at its peak. Although plasma renin activity, aldosterone secretory rates, and aldosterone excretion into the urine were unequivocally elevated, we were unable to establish whether aldosterone played a role in net K loss.

When total body K was at its lowest value in the hot weather study, there also occurred biochemical changes characteristic of rhabdomyolysis.[27] These include elevated serum creatine kinase activity, a disproportionate elevation of the creatinine:urea nitrogen ratio in serum, a reduction of serum calcium and elevation of serum phosphorus, all appearing simultaneously. Although we did not clearly understand or consider what role rhabdomyolysis played in the reduction of total body K at the time these studies were conducted, in retrospect, rhabdomyolysis was almost certainly a key factor. Our subsequent experimental studies showed clearly that muscle cell injury, regardless of its cause, is always associated with loss of K. All men taking part in these activities showed tender, stiff muscles during the first to third weeks of training, which coincided with biochemical evidence of rhabdomyolysis. It is well recognized that intense, repetitive training exercises in hot weather result in more severe injury to skeletal muscle than comparable training in cool weather.[34]

Biochemical as well as physical signs of muscle injury were virtually nonexistent in our subjects who performed identical training in cool weather.[24]

In the latter group, total body exchangeable K values rose progressively from the start in consonance with the rise of lean body mass.

These data indicate that the reduction of total body K observed in men training in the heat was caused by losses from injured muscle as well as losses in sweat. Because K deficiency itself can cause rhabdomyolysis[25] and impair cardiovascular performance as well, the possibility remains that K deficiency per se may play a role in heat-stress injury that occurs in persons performing sustained, intense, and prolonged work in the heat.

3. Complications of Heat Stroke
a. Shock

Hypotension occurs in about half of all patients with exertional heat stroke. Volume depletion incident to losses of salt and water, fever, vasodilatation secondary to metabolic acidosis, decreased cardiac output, translocation of blood from the central circulation to the skin and muscle, and plasma leakage into injured tissue are adequate explanations. Myocardial depression also results from endotoxin-mediated kinins. Cooling and volume repletion correct this abnormality in most cases.

b. Rhabdomyolysis

Rhabdomyolysis is a term defining injury to the plasma membrane and intracellular structures of skeletal muscle cells such that their contents, including myoglobin, contractile proteins, enzymes, adenine nucleotides, K, and phosphorus leak into the venous circulation.[35] Myoglobin is a heme pigment with a molecular weight of approximately 17,000 D. Because it has no important binding protein in serum, it is readily filtered by the glomerulus and appears in the urine, referred to as myoglobinuria. Urine samples may resemble motor oil or cola. All patients with exertional heat stroke have rhabdomyolysis, which in turn may cause major morbidity and mortality. Laboratory findings that positively identify rhabdomyolysis include an elevation of creatine kinase (CK) of the MM isoform, and a disproportionate elevation of serum creatinine compared to urea, which usually has a ratio of 0.1. Creatine phosphate is released from injured muscle cells. Creatine is spontaneously dehydrated to creatinine, thus accounting for an acute disproportionate elevation of the creatinine:urea ratio. Patients with substantial rhabdomyolysis whose CK levels exceed 100,000 IU/l, may show creatinine levels of 3 with serum urea nitrogen levels below 20 mg/dl.

c. Hyperkalemia

Hyperkalemia is an ominous, common, and potentially fatal complication of exertional heat stroke.[3,34,35] Its cause is widespread tissue injury or destruction, especially of skeletal muscle (rhabdomyolysis), which causes release of K ions into the blood, and impaired renal excretion either as a consequence of diminished renal perfusion or acute renal failure. The major effects of hyperkalemia include muscular weakness, paralysis (including paralysis of the diaphragm with respiratory failure), decreased cardiac contractility, cardiac arrhythmias, and cardiac arrest. Cardiotoxicity from hyperkalemia is best detected by electrocardiographic abnormalities. Even modest hyperkalemia — for example, a plasma level of 6.5 meq/l, which would cause only mild electrocardiographic changes in other situations — may be potentially fatal in patients with exertional heat stroke because of rhabdomyolysis. In this instance, hypocalcemia occurs because of calcium crystal deposition in injured muscle. Reduced concentrations of ionized calcium aggravate the cardiotoxic effects of hyperkalemia. These changes are consistently reflected in the electrocardiogram. The sequence of electrocardiographic abnormalities of hyperkalemia consist of peaked T-waves, followed by disappearance of P-waves, broadening of the QRS complex, and eventually the appearance of a sine wave. Such changes demand immediate recognition and intervention to prevent death due to either ventricular fibrillation or cardiac arrest. Treatment consists of ventilation, oxygen, administration of calcium salts intravenously, and infusion of glucose and insulin. In severe cases, dialysis is necessary.

d. Hypocalcemia and Hyperphosphatemia

Leakage of phosphorus from injured muscle causes hyperphosphatemia. Calcium phosphate crystals deposit in injured tissue and cause potentially severe hypocalcemia. Hypocalcemia may further reduce cardiac output and aggravate hyperkalemic toxicity.[3,35]

e. Acute Renal Failure

Approximately 30% of patients with exertional heat stroke will develop acute oliguric renal failure.[26,48] This, along with hyperkalemia, is an ominous complication of this illness and is often responsible for death. Volume depletion and shock play important roles. However, in most cases, rhabdomyolysis is responsible for acute renal failure as a result of pigment nephropathy.[26,35] Pigment nephropathy is characterized by two distinctive lesions. First, acute tubular injury or necrosis occurs as the result of myoglobin absorption by the proximal tubular cells. Myoglobin absorbed into the proximal tubular cell is taken up by lysosomes. Because of the low lysosomal pH, myoglobin dissociates into ferrihemate and globin. The ferrihemate is actively transported from the proximal tubular cell, which consumes oxygen and ATP. Myoglobin apparently binds nitric oxide and induces vasoconstriction. Reduction of oxygen stores and utilization of ATP in the proximal tubular cell in conjunction with ischemia results in proximal tubular necrosis. The second lesion, also characteristically seen in pigment nephropathy, is distal tubular obstruction caused by myoglobin casts. The myoglobin that escapes absorption in the proximal tubule precipitates in the acid pH of the distal tubular urine, becoming a viscous gel that causes intratubular obstruction. The importance of myoglobin in the pathogenesis of acute renal failure in exertional heat stroke is underscored by the relative rarity of acute renal failure in the classic form of heat stroke, in which rhabdomyolysis is seldom of importance.

f. Adult Respiratory Distress Syndrome (ARDS)

ARDS, or pulmonary capillary leak syndrome, in patients with exertional heat stroke is a serious complication that generally does not occur until the second or third day of the illness. The cause of this complication is poorly understood but is likely the result of kinin-induced hyperpermeability of pulmonary capillaries. The cardinal features are hypoxia, accumulation of proteinaceous fluid in pulmonary alveoli, and radiographic changes resembling pulmonary edema. Capillary wedge pressures are normal, which excludes cardiogenic pulmonary edema. It is more apt to occur in severe cases, especially when shock and the multiple organ failure syndrome have been prominent parts of the illness. Although this complication is usually fatal, some patients have recovered.

g. Myocardial Necrosis

Apparently normal young men with exertional heat stroke have developed acute, transmural myocardial infarction as a complication of this illness. In Malamud's classic pathological description of young soldiers dying with heat stroke, patchy myocardial necrosis and hemorrhage were commonly found in the interventricular septum.[26] One of this author's patients with exertional heat stroke showed transmural myocardial infarction. At autopsy, this patient's coronary arteries were perfectly normal.[23] Apparently, myocardial necrosis can result from extreme metabolic demands on the heart produced by hyperthermia, poisonous levels of catecholamines, excessive calcium entry into the cytoplasm of myocardial cells, and ischemia. Many patients with heat stroke show transient electrocardiographic changes suggesting ischemia, myocardial injury, or conduction defects. It is often difficult to differentiate these changes from those caused by abnormalities of serum electrolyte concentrations. Further confusion may occur due to elevation of CK–MB, which ordinarily indicates myocardial infarction. However, in highly trained athletes, CK-MB may derive from skeletal muscle as well as the heart.[30] In these instances, other tools to identify myocardial infarction, such as nuclear scans and echocardiography, may be helpful.

h. Liver Injury

Mild levels of hepatic damage in acute exertional heat stroke are common. When significant hepatocellular injury occurs, most patients have been severely ill with multiple organ injury. In those who have survived, recovery from hepatic damage is the rule. Hypoglycemia may reflect impaired glucose production by an injured liver[8] or the result of insulin administration for hyperkalemia.

i. CNS and Peripheral Nervous System Damage

CNS damage is common in patients with severe, prolonged, or improperly treated hyperthermia. It seems clear that immediate recognition of heat stroke and aggressive rapid cooling sharply reduce this complication. The characteristic

CNS damage most often occurs in the cerebellum, producing clinical manifestations of dysmetria, incoordination, and gait disturbances. However, almost any part of the brain may be damaged, including thermoregulatory centers in the hypothalamus. Residual injury may range from isolated cognitive or functional disorders without motor dysfunction, to a persistent vegetative comatose state. Isolated episodes of spinal cord infarction or peripheral nerve damage have also been described.

j. Hemorrhagic Disorders

Virtually all patients with exertional heat stroke are susceptible to major bleeding. This is characterized by endothelial injury,[34] and intravascular coagulation, which by consumption of platelets and clotting factors leads to hemorrhage. Direct thermal activation of platelets may also contribute to thrombocytopenia.[12] Generally, thrombocytopenia is most severe after the first 24 h and is responsible for petechial hemorrhage or gross bleeding. Hepatic injury may impair synthesis of coagulant proteins. Fibrinolysis has also been described.[44]

k. Intestinal Infarction

Necrosis of the small intestine has been a rare but serious complication in patients with severe illness complicated by multi-organ damage. To my knowledge, it has been universally fatal. Patients with intestinal infarction appear critically ill and demonstrate generalized, vague abdominal tenderness, distension, rebound tenderness, a loss of bowel sounds, lactic acidosis and disproportionate hyperphosphatemia, shock, and eventually death. Abdominal X-ray findings are characteristic, showing dilated and edematous loops of small bowel.

l. Pancreatic Injury

Elevation of pancreatic amylase and lipase occur rather commonly in patients with severe heat stroke. This is probably just another manifestation of severe multi-organ damage as a result of decreased perfusion and hyperthermia. Generally, this is not a severe complication of this illness.

4. Treatment of Heat Stroke

All victims of frank heat stroke require evaluation by a physician and generally require hospitalization.

The most critical factors determining survival in a patient with acute heat stroke, whether of the classical or exertional variety, is anticipation, prompt recognition, and immediate reduction of body temperature. Rapid cooling is critical if one is to reduce morbidity and mortality in patients with this disorder. If possible, heat stroke patients should be placed in the shade. Clothing should be removed and the body surface, including the face and head, should be wet down. Air movement, to facilitate cooling of the skin by vaporization, should be promoted by fanning or treatment in a well-ventilated, air-conditioned room. Conventional treatment consists of immersion in ice water and brisk rubbing of the body surface with ice. Because icing causes cutaneous vasoconstriction, and shivering, some authorities believe that this technique may actually impair heat loss. Accordingly, some believe that application of cool or tepid aerosolized water to the body surface may satisfactorily reduce body temperature.[21] However, applications of ice, massage, and fanning remain the gold standard.[9] An initial core temperature of 108°F may be reduced to 102°F within a period of about 45 min by these measures. Cooling should be stopped when rectal temperature reaches 102°F because invariably body temperature will continue to fall after that point. Although convulsive seizures may occur before treatment, most commonly muscle tremors, chills, and seizures appear during the cooling process. Diazepem, 5 mg intravenously, may prevent tremors or seizures. Because of the threat of vomiting during convulsive seizures, it is wise to intubate the trachea in comatose patients and place a nasogastric tube into the stomach, aspirate the contents, and instill sodium bicarbonate to neutralize gastric acid as early as possible during the treatment process. This will help avoid aspiration pneumonia and lung injury, which can be a very serious complication. Although severe hypotension is present in about half of these patients, it very often responds to simple cooling that results in translocation of blood from the skin surface back to the central circulation, improving venous return to the heart and thereby improving cardiac output and blood pressure. In patients whose blood pressure does not respond to cooling within 10–15 min, 500 ml of normal saline should be administered over a period of 15 min. If this does not result in elevation of blood pressure, one should suspect myocardial damage as a cause of hypotension. The dangers of administering large volumes of saline or other intravenous fluids before initiation of cooling is pulmonary edema. Thus, while there is a volume deficit in the central circulation in these patients before body temperature falls, if a large volume of saline is administered and then the patient is cooled, blood in the skin is shifted to the central circulation, and pulmonary edema can occur as a result of volume overload. Management of such cases can be greatly improved by employing right-heart catheterization to monitor cardiac filling pressures, left ventricular end-diastolic pressure (wedge pressure), and cardiac output as a means to optimize fluid replacement. The hypokalemia that is present in about half of these patients at the onset of heat stroke usually does not require treatment. Similarly, lactic acidosis, which exists in virtually all patients with exertional heat stroke at the time of onset, clears rapidly upon administration of sufficient fluids to restore circulatory volume. Apparently, restoration of hepatic perfusion results in rapid conversion of lactate to glucose. In some patients with severe shock, lactic acidosis initially disappears during infusion of saline, and then, apparently as fluids are more completely replaced, there follows muscle reperfusion, leading to a second-wave of lactic acidosis. Apparently, this is the result of muscle washout of lactic acid. Usually, the second wave type of lactic acidosis also resolves promptly as lactate is metabolized by the liver. Hypoglycemia may occur and should receive prompt treatment with dextrose.

In an attempt to prevent acute renal failure, intravenous fluids, either normal or hypotonic saline, should be infused to maintain renal perfusion. Mannitol, 12.5–25 g, should be administered as a 50 or 20% solution, over a period of 15–30 min. A single dose of furosemide, 200 mg intravenously, is also recommended. Mannitol, by accelerating urine output, serves to accelerate removal of myoglobin from kidney. Furosemide, by interfering with sodium reabsorption, reduces urine concentration and thereby reduces the concentration of myoglobin in the renal tubular lumen in the hope of preventing precipitation. Furosemide also acts on the proximal nephron and hopefully, by blocking sodium reabsorption, decreases oxygen consumption by the proximal tubular cells, which should help maintain vital supplies of ATP. Finally, because precipitation of myoglobin in distal nephrons is accentuated by an acid urine pH, sodium bicarbonate in doses of 90–140 meq should be administered cautiously over the course of an hour or two with the intent of alkalinizing the urine. Unfortunately, the severity of metabolic acidosis and capillary injury in many of these patients increases bicarbonate space sufficiently such that alkalinization of the urine may be difficult to achieve. Some evidence suggests that administration of bicarbonate may actually accentuate intracellular acidosis.

DIC, fibrinolysis, and consumption of coagulant proteins may result in major, life-threatening hemorrhage in these patients. Frank purpura and gastrointestinal hemorrhage are common. In most instances, DIC clears spontaneously without specific treatment. However, if this is severe and significant hemorrhage appears, administration of fresh frozen plasma, platelets, or specific coagulant proteins may be necessary.

Patients with acute heat stroke are critically ill and liable to develop major complications of all organ systems. The most important and preventable causes of death in these patients are hyperkalemia, volume overload in patients with sepsis, major hemorrhage, acute renal failure, and ARDS. Patients with acute exertional heat stroke who do not recover immediately upon cooling should be hospitalized and managed by a physician who is knowledgeable in management of these disorders. Early and intense hemodialysis is often necessary for treatment of hyperkalemia or volume overload.

II. HYPONATREMIA IN LONG-DISTANCE RUNNERS

Whenever severe hyponatremia occurs rapidly, symptoms and complications are usually much more severe and potentially life-threatening. Hyponatremia that develops more slowly allows time for adaptation by brain cells and is less dangerous.

A number of case reports describe acute, severe hyponatremia early, toward the end, or shortly after completion of long-distance running events. The symptoms demonstrated by these athletes include mental confusion, disorientation, transient neurological deficits, seizures, and coma. The absence of hyperthermia serves to exclude the diagnosis of heat stroke. Serum sodium concentration is usually below 125 meq/l. This illness is not a variant of heat exhaustion, but rather water intoxication. Generally, these runners have consumed unusually large quantities of water or hypotonic fluids before and during their races. In some, the sudden appearance of symptomatic hyponatremia after completion of the event is difficult to explain but suggests that fluid had pooled within the gut and was suddenly absorbed when running ceased. During intense physical activity, blood is translocated to muscle and skin and there may be a major reduction in visceral and intestinal blood flow.[31] In the presence of reduced intestinal blood flow, it would seem possible that intestinal absorption would become extremely limited. Reestablishment of intestinal blood flow upon completing a race could explain rapid absorption of the ingested water from the intestine and the development of acute hyponatremia. All of the symptoms demonstrated by these individuals are those seen in nonathletes with acute hyponatremia or acute water intoxication. In runners, this would be aggravated by release of antidiuretic hormone from the posterior pituitary gland, which would impair the ability to excrete free water. Most of these individuals have responded quickly following administration of saline intravenously.

III. THE RISK OF HEAT STROKE AND EXERTIONAL RHABDOMYOLYSIS IN ATHLETES WITH SICKLE CELL TRAIT

Studies by Kark et al.[19] have shown that the risk of sudden death during physical training of military recruits with sickle cell trait is approximately 30 times greater than that of the unaffected population. There have been a number of instances of exertional rhabdomyolysis with or without hyperthermia in young men with sickle cell trait. The severity of exertional heat stroke is unquestionably greater than in unaffected individuals. Thus, the extent of tissue destruction, multiple organ failure, and mortality appears to be more severe. Certain complications, such as lactic acidosis, rhabdomyolysis, intestinal necrosis, and infarction of the spinal cord appear to be much more common in these persons. Presumably, volume depletion, dehydration, metabolic acidosis, and sludging of circulatory flow promote endogenous sickling, which is likely the fundamental defect in this illness. The risk is increased if activities are conducted in high altitude, because sickling is aggravated by hypoxia.

Eight percent of the African-American population in the United States has sickle cell trait. There is no need to deny these persons the opportunity to participate in any form of athletics. If athletes with sickle cell trait take due precautions to protect themselves against volume depletion and overheating, the risk of injury should become essentially equal to that of athletes without sickle cell trait. However, for any given degree of salt and water depletion, injury is much more likely to occur. Accordingly, black athletes with sickle cell trait should learn how to assess in quantitative terms their anticipated salt and water losses and take every precaution to avoid volume loss and excessive heating.

IV. THE ROLE OF NEGLIGENCE AND PUNITION IN HEAT STROKE

Until the late 1950s, there was a misconception among many athletic trainers and coaches that an athlete could not become physically trained or fit if allowed to consume water during training exercises.[28] Another view, possibly dating from times of Napoleon I, asserted that the development of toughness and self-discipline would be compromised if trainees were allowed to consume water. Obviously, these misconceptions had no basis in fact and indeed, compelling evidence shows that avoidance of salt and water depletion during training not only reduces the incidence of heat-stress catastrophes but also results in a healthier and more successful athlete.

The American College of Sports Medicine has established a number of guidelines that are very practical and effective if followed. These guidelines have been disseminated to administrators in high schools and colleges, where they have become quasi-regulations to protect athletes from harm. Clearly, there remain pockets of resistance to these guidelines where they are ignored or bypassed. Both death and permanent disabling injury continue to occur from exertional heat stroke and its complications. As a result, there have been some formidable rewards stemming from lawsuits filed against school districts, school administrators, and other officials consequent to violation of these recommendations. Failure to provide water on the practice field, scheduling practice or events during the hottest part of the day, failure to record temperature and humidity or to observe guidelines for restriction of activity, failure to heed guidelines concerning clothing, failure to acquire adequate skills to recognize and treat athletes with heat injury, and imposition of punitive drills that have even included deliberate water deprivation continue to occur. Until the past few years, most of these catastrophes were written off as unfortunate, unavoidable events. However, because of the monumental increase in the cost of medical care and steadily increasing litigiousness of our society, such negligence and irresponsibility are becoming very costly. In certain areas of the country, insurance carriers have opted to exclude liability for medical costs related to heat stroke if they have identified failure to heed appropriate guidelines. In others, increasing cost of insurance has led to elimination of insurance coverage altogether in some high school districts because of events like heat stroke or other injuries. Physicians, trainers, and other officials should do their utmost to assure that coaches and their assistants are properly instructed to prevent, recognize, and avoid such catastrophes because at the present time they can be held personally liable for such tragedies. In this author's experience, the most effective means to assure compliance with the foregoing guidelines has been to solicit help from Parent-Teacher Associations because for some peculiar reason, coaches often listen to concerned mothers more seriously than other individuals. In the workplace, heat stroke and its complications have been markedly reduced following intervention by the Occupational Safety and Health Administration with a backbone of penalties for infringements. Hopefully, it will never become necessary to have OSHA become involved in organized athletics, although such an action could be conceivable.

V. SUMMARY

Fluid and electrolyte derangements are among the most common medical disturbances of the athlete. This chapter emphasizes those disorders related to physical work in the heat, especially heat cramps, heat exhaustion, and heat stroke, and their complications. The author hopes that this chapter will help trainers, team physicians, and participating athletes to become lucidly aware of precautions to prevent heat-related injuries and how to recognize their earliest signs. Detection of a heat-stress-related disorder can prevent transition from easily managed heat exhaustion to potentially fatal heat stroke. Advice is presented concerning management of these problems. Current information is also presented on rhabdomyolysis or skeletal muscle injury, a common and potentially important complication of heat-stress injury.

Finally, and of practical importance, the climate of litigiousness in the United States is imposing an ever-increasing cost for negligence in the conduct of practice and competitive events when athletes fall victim to the derangements discussed in this chapter. This can only be controlled by understanding the pathophysiology of these disorders and following well-established precautions for their prevention.

REFERENCES

1. Anon., Endotoxins in heatstroke, *Lancet*, 2:1137–1138, 1989.
2. Baxter, C. R. and Teschan, P. E., Atypical heatstroke, with hypernatremia, acute renal failure, and fulminating potassium intoxication, *Arch. Intern. Med.*, 101:1040, 1958.
3. Beller, G. A. and Boyd, A. E., Heatstroke: A report of 13 consecutive cases without mortality despite severe hyperpyrexia and neurologic dysfunction, *Mil. Med.*, 140:464, 1975.
4. Boyd, A. E. and Beller, G. A., Heat exhaustion and respiratory alkalosis, *Ann. Intern. Med.*, 83:835, 1975.
5. Braiden, R. W., Fellingham, G. W., and Conlee, R. K., Effects of cocaine on glycogen metabolism and endurance during high intensity exercise, *Med. Sci. Sports Exer.*, 26:695–700, 1994.

6. Cabanac, M., Keeping a cool head, *News Physiol. Sci.,* 1:41–44, 1986.
7. Collins, K. J., The autonomic nervous system and the regulation of body temperature, in *Autonomic Failure,* 3rd ed., Bannister, R. and Mathias, C. J., Eds., Oxford Press, Oxford, England, 1992, chap. 12.
8. Costrini, A., et al., Cardiovascular and metabolic manifestations of heatstroke and severe heat exhaustion, *Am. J. Med.,* 66:296, 1979.
9. Costrini, A., Emergency treatment of exertional heatstroke and comparison of whole body cooling techniques, *Med. Sci. Sports Exer.,* 22:15–18, 1990.
10. Curtis, B. A., Na/Ca exchange and first messenger Ca in skeletal muscle excitation-contraction coupling, *Adv. Exp. Med. Biol.,* 311:1–17, 1992.
11. Freeman, R., Case record no. 29-1994, Case records of the Massachussetts General Hospital, *New Engl. J. Med.,* 331:259–265, 1994.
12. Gader, A. M. A., Al-Mashhadani, S. A., and Al-Harthy, S. S., Direct activation of platelets by heat is the possible trigger of the coagulopathy of heat stroke, *Br. J. Haematol.,* 74:86–92, 1990.
13. Gilat, T. S., et al., Mechanisms of heat stroke, *J. Trop. Med. Hyg.,* 66:204, 1963.
14. Hall, D. M., Buettner, G. R., Matthes, R. D., and Gisolfi, C. V., Hyperthermia stimulates nitric oxide formation: Electron paramagnetic resonance detection of NO-heme in blood, *J. Appl. Physiol.,* 77:548–553, 1994.
15. Harper, A. M., The inter-relationship between pCO^2 and blood pressure in the regulation of blood flow through the cerebral cortex, *Acta. Neurol. Scand.,* Suppl. 14:94–103, 1965.
16. Hart, G. R., et al., Epidemic classical heatstroke: Clinical characteristics and course of 28 patients, *Medicine,* 61:189, 1982.
17. Herman, R. H. and Sullivan, B. H., Jr., Heatstroke and jaundice, *Am. J. Med.,* 27:154, 1959.
18. Johnson, R. H., Aging and the autonomic nervous system, in *Autonomic Failure,* 3rd ed., Bannister, R. and Mathias, C. J. (Eds.), Oxford Press, Oxford, England, 1992, 882–903.
19. Kark, J. A., Posey, D. M., Schumacher, H. R., and Ruehle, C. J., Sickle-cell trait as a risk factor for sudden death in physical training, *N. Engl. J. Med.,* 317:781–787, 1987.
20. Kenney, W. L. and Fowler, S. R., Methacholine-activated eccrine sweat gland density and output as a function of age, *J. Appl. Physiol.,* 65:1082–1086, 1988.
21. Khogali, M. and Weiner, J. S., Heat stroke report on 18 cases, *Lancet,* 2:276–278, 1980.
22. Kleeman, C. R., Metabolic coma, *Kidney Int.,* 36:1142–1158, 1989.
23. Knochel, J. P., et al., The renal cardiovascular, hematologic and serum electrolyte abnormalities of heatstroke, *Am. J. Med.,* 30:299, 1961.
24. Knochel, J. P., et al., Pathophysiology of intense physical conditioning in a hot climate: I. Mechanisms of potassium depletion, *J. Clin. Invest.,* 51:242, 1972.
25. Knochel, J. P. and Schlein, E. M., On the mechanism of rhabdomyolysis in potassium depletion, *J. Clin. Invest.,* 51:1750, 1972.
26. Knochel, J. P., Environmental heat illness, *Arch. Intern. Med.,* 133:841, 1974.
27. Knochel, J. P., et al., Heat stress, exercise and muscle injury: Effects of urate metabolism and renal function, *Ann. Intern. Med.,* 81:321, 1974.
28. Knochel, J. P., Dog days and siriasis. How to kill a football player, editorial, *J. Am. Med. Assoc.,* 233:513, 1975.
29. Knochel, J. P. and Caskey, J., The mechanism of hypophosphatemia in acute heatstroke, *J. Am. Med. Assoc.,* 238:425, 1977.
30. Knochel, J. P., Heat stroke and related heat stress disorders, *Disease of the Month, Year Book Medical Publishers,* 35:303–377, 1989.
31. Knochel, J. P., Catastrophic medical events with exhaustion exercise: White collar rhabdomyolysis, *Kidney Int.,* 38:709, 1990.
32. Knochel, J. P., Potassium deficiency as a result of training in hot weather, in *Fluid Replacement and Heat Stress,* Proc. Workshop, Institute of Medicine, National Academy of Sciences, Marriott, B. M. and Rosemont, C., Eds., National Academy Press, Washington, DC, 1991, chap. 10.

33. Knochel, J. P., The clinical and physiological implications of phosphorus deficiency, in *The Kidney. Physiology and Pathophysiology,* 2nd ed., Seldin, D. W. and Giebisch, G., Eds., Raven Press, New York, 1992, 2533-2562.
34. Knochel, J. P. and Reed, G., Disorders of heat regulation, in *Clinical Disorders of Fluid and Electrolyte Metabolism,* Narins, R., Ed., McGraw-Hill, New York, 1994, chap. 47.
35. Knochel, J. P., Pigment nephropathy, in *Primer on Kidney Diseases,* Greenberg, A., Ed., Academic Press, San Diego, 1994, chap. 26.
36. Maron, M. B., Wagner, J. A., and Horvath, S. M., Thermoregulatory responses during competitive marathon running, *J. Appl. Physiol.,* 42:909–914, 1977.
37. O'Donnell, T. F., Jr., Acute heatstroke: Epidemiologic, biochemical, renal and coagulation studies, *J. Am. Med. Assoc.,* 234:824, 1975.
38. Rooke, G. A., Savage, M. V., and Brengelmann, G. L., Maximal skin blood flow is decreased in elderly men, *J. Appl. Physiol.,* 77:11–14, 1994.
39. Rowell, L. B., Human circulation during physical stress, in *Thermal Stress,* Oxford Press, New York, 1986, chap. 8.
40. Sagawa, S. K., Shiraki, M. K., Yousef, J. K., and Miki, K., Sweating and cardiovascular responses of aged men to heat exposure, *J. Gerontol.,* 43:M1–M8, 1988.
41. Sato, K., The physiology, pharmacology, and biochemisty of the eccrine sweat gland, *Rev. Physiol. Biochem. Pharmacol.,* 79:52–123, 1977.
42. Sawka, M. N. and Wenger, C. B., Physiological responses to acute exercise-heat stress, in *Human Performance Physiology and Environmental Medicine at Terrestrial Extremes,* Pandolf, K. B., Sawka, M. N.,and Gonzalez, R. R., Eds., Benchmark Press, Indianapolis, 1988, chap. 3.
43. Shapiro, Y. and Seidman, D. S., Field and clinical observations of exertional heat stroke patients, *Med. Sci. Sports Exer.,* 22:6–14, 1990.
44. Shibolet, S., et al., Heatstroke: Its clinical picture and mechanism in 36 cases, *Q. J. Med.,* 36:525, 1967.
45. Slovis, C. M., et al., Survival in a heatstroke victim with a core temperature in excess of 46.5°C, *Ann. Emerg. Med.,* 11:269, 1982.
46. Sutton, J. R., Heat Illness, in *Sports Medicine,* Strauss, R. H., Ed., W. B. Saunders Co., Philadelphia, 1991, chap. 20.
47. Talbott, J. H., Heat cramps, *Medicine,* 14:232–252, 1935.
48. Vertel, R. M. and Knochel, J. P., Acute renal failure due to heat injury: An analysis of ten cases associated with a high incidence of myoglobinuria, *Am. J. Med.,* 43:435, 1967.
49. Weidmann, P., De Myttenaere-Bursztein, S., Maxwell, M. H., and De Lima J., Effect of aging on plasma renin and aldosterone in normal man, *Kidney Int.,* 8:325–333, 1975.

INDEX

A

Absorption. *See* Intestinal absorption
Acceleration exposure, 291
Acclimation. *See* Cold acclimation; Heat acclimation
Acetylene rebreathing method, 199
Acid-base disturbances. *See* Acidosis; Alkalosis
Acidosis, 302, 305, 310, 311
Actin, 298
Actomyosin, 31
Acute mountain sickness (AMS), 126, 190, 192
Adaptation, gastrointestinal, 42–43
ADH. *See* Antidiuretic hormone
Adolescents, fluid volume in, 218–222
Adrenaline, and gastrin, 40
Adrenergic agonists, 305
α-Adrenergic receptors, 77, 240
Adrenocorticotropic hormone (ACTH), 234
Adult respiratory distress syndrome (ARDS), 309, 312
Adults, fluid volume in, 223–228
Aerobic capacity. *See* Exercise capacity
Aerobic exercise, 145–147, 232
Aerobic power, 145, 146
Afferent nerves, 26
Afferent stimuli, 9
Age, 66, 122
    body fluid volume
        infancy, childhood, and adolescence, 216–223
        young, middle-aged, and older adults, 223–228
    and cold-induced diuresis, 168
    and heat stroke, 305–306
    and response to hypoxia, 191
    and thermoregulation, 165
    thirst response in the elderly athlete, 299
Alanine amino transferase, 302
Albumin, 208, 299
Aldosterone, 8
    changes during menstrual cycle, 233–234, 235, 244, 246, 250
    during dehydration, 264
    effect of ANP on, 123

    effect of AVP on, 63
    effect of estrogen on, 238
    effect of renin on, 57
    hormonal integration of, 124–127
    levels after drinking, 68–69
    levels during exercise, 58, 67
    and natruiresis, 200
    production, and age, 305
    regulation of sodium by, 64, 65, 84
    and sodium reabsorption, 202, 298
    during water immersion, 203
Alkalosis, 191, 301–302, 304
Alliesthesia, 260, 264, 273
Altitude, 66, 100, 183–192
    hypohydration at, 184–185
    mountain sickness, 126, 190, 192
    speed of ascent, 192
Altitude sickness, 126, 190, 192
Alveolar epithelium, 100, 109
Amenorrhea, 232, 249, 250
American College of Sports Medicine, fluid replacement guidelines, 263, 314
Amino acids, in water transport, 31
4-Aminoantipyrine, 185
p-Aminohippuric acid, 5
Amphetamines, 305
Anaerobic exercise, 145–147
    and hypohydration, 286, 287, 290, 291
    and muscle endurance, 144
Anemia, 191
Angiotensin-converting enzyme inhibitors, 305
Angiotensin I, 64
Angiotensin II, 7, 39. *See also* Renin-angiotensin-aldosterone axis; Renin-angiotensin system
    blood volume and, 120
    as dipsinogen, 240
    effect of estrogen on, 238, 240
    and glomerular membrane permeability, 77
    regulation by renin, 57, 64–65
Angiotensinogen, 64
Anhidrosis, 303
Anions, and body fluid homeostasis, 4
Anorexia, 42, 189–190, 299
ANP. *See* Atrial natriuretic peptide
ANS. *See* Sympathetic nerves

Anterior hypothalamic area, 5
Anteroventral third ventricle (AV3V) neurons, 7
Anticholinergics, 305
Antidiuretic hormone (ADH), 199, 209. *See also* Arginine vasopressin
   and age, 305
   in endocrine control, 83–85
   secretion, 9
   and urine osmolality, 79
   during water immersion, 204
Antihistamines, 305
Anti-Parkinsonian drugs, 305
Antiport (exchange), 33
Antipsychotics, 305
Appetite. *See* Food intake; Salt appetite; Sodium appetite
Aquaporins, 108
ARDS (adult respiratory distress syndrome), 309, 312
10-Arginine methyl ester (1-NAME), 92
Arginine vasopressin (AVP), 7, 54
   changes during menstrual cycle, 233–234, 244, 246
   effect of estrogen on secretion of, 237, 238–239, 240
   and glomerular membrane permeability, 77
   hormonal integration of, 124–127
   levels after drinking, 68–69
   list of effects, 124
   plasma concentration, 8
   release of, 119–120
   response to exercise, 57–59, 61–62
   suppression, 8, 204
Arterial baroreflex, 62
Arterial pressure, and exercise, 34
Ascent to altitude, 192
Aspartate aminotransferase, 302
Aspirin, 85
"Athlete's amenorrhea," 232, 249, 250
Athletic pseudonephritis, 302
Atmospheric air, water content, 161
ATP, 144, 292, 308, 312
ATPase, 106
Atrial natriuretic factors (ANF)
   changes during menstrual cycle, 233–234
   in diuresis, 199–200
   in natriuresis, 202
Atrial natriuretic peptide (ANP), 7, 54, 123–124, 129
   effect on AVP release, 63
   levels during exercise, 58–59, 63, 69, 85–86
   and renal failure, 92
   and tubular reabsorption, 78
Atrial natriuretic peptide receptor antagonist, 86
Atrial natriuretic peptides (ANF), during water immersion, 205, 206, 209
Atrial pressure, 63, 98, 99, 104, 199
Atrium, 9, 63, 104, 207
Atropine, 128
AVP. *See* Arginine vasopressin
AV3V, 7

B

Balloon, intragastric, 27, 28, 29
Baroreceptors, 9
   and core temperature, 150
   in the elderly, 122
   relationship with chemoreceptors, 191
   sensitivity to blood volume, 57, 61–62, 120
Barrier function of gastrointestinal tract, 44–46
Basal (resting) metabolic rate, 241, 243
Basketball, 290
Beta adrenergic agents, 107, 305
Beta receptors, 56
Bicarbonate, 40, 119, 312
Bile
   acids, 44
   salts, 40
   volume per day, 28
Bleeding of gastrointestinal tract, 44–46
Blood-brain barrier, 5
Blood flow
   cerebral, 304
   cutaneous, 305, 310
   femoral, 239
   gastric mucosal, 41
   heart, 55
   intestinal, 313
   to muscles, 55
   reduction of. *See* Vasoconstriction
   renal. *See* Renal blood flow; Renal venous blood flow
   skin. *See* Skin blood flow
   splanchnic. *See* Splanchnic blood flow
Blood-gas barrier, 98, 109
Blood homeostasis. *See* Serum osmolality
Bloodletting, 284
Blood pressure
   changes during menstrual cycle, 239
   decrease with kaliuretic peptide, 206
   and heat stroke, 311
   and oral contraceptives, 241

Blood viscosity, 146, 244, 246, 310
Blood volume, 11, 120, 232
    acute isoosmotic central, 204
    and ANP levels, 123
    changes during menstrual cycle, 235, 250, 251
    effect of AVP on, 57
    effect of estrogen on, 237
    effect of sweating on, 54
    effect of training on, 66
    and natriuretic effects of hypoxia, 191
    during pregnancy, 241–242
    redistribution, 55, 198
    regulation of, in women, 244–245
BNP (brain natriuretic peptide), 7
Body building, 284
Body fat, 164–165, 249
Body fluid. *See* Fluid
Body fluid compartments, 6–7, 119, 216
Body heat, 54, 175
Body morphology, 164–165
Body position, 66
    and cold-induced diuresis, 168
    seated, during water immersion, 209
Body temperature, 146, 174, 242
Body weight. *See also* Total body water, to body weight ratio; Water, percent of body weight
    changes during menstrual cycle, 233
    loss of, in weight-controlling athletes, 283–294
Boxing, 284, 288
Brain
    damage during heat stroke, 309–310
    peptide release from the, 39, 41
Brain natriuretic peptide (BNP), 7
Bronchi, 104
Brush border, 43

C

Calcium antagonists, 208
Calcium channel blocker, 128, 305
Calcium ions, 298, 302
Caloric density, 23
cAMP, 107
Capillary endothelium, 6, 108–109
Capillary filtration coefficient, 236–237
Capillary permeability. *See* Permeability, capillary
Capillary transmural pressure, 109
Captopril, 85
Carbohydrate (CHO), 20. *See also* Glucose absorption. *See* Intestinal absorption

effect on gastric emptying, 21, 22, 23–24, 26
in fluid replacement during exercise, 262–263, 267–270
gender differences in utilization, 248
intake, 241
rate of consumption, 268
and recovery during exercise, 270–272
and water absorption, 29–30
Carbohydrate-electrolyte solution (CHO-E), 10, 29
    absorption, 32–34
    carbohydrate concentration, 271
    gender differences in glucose content of, 248
    glucose-electrolyte absorption, 32–34, 267, 270–271
    during heat acclimation, 125
    Na^+-glucose ratio, 33
    and plasma volume, 271
    salt concentration, 271
Carbon dioxide, 186, 304
Carbonic anhydrase inhibitors, 141
Cardiac arrhythmia, 308
Cardiac asthma, 104
Cardiac contractility, 308
Cardiac index, 199
Cardiac output, 99, 146
    effect of hypohydration on, 146
    effect of water immersion on, 199, 209
    and heat stroke, 304, 311
    increase with exercise, 99
    and oral contraceptives, 241
    RBF percent of, 87–88
Cardiac transplant, 57, 63
Cardiac volume receptors, 11, 13
Cardiopulmonary adjustments during exercise, 98
Cardiopulmonary receptors, 203
Cardiotoxicity, 308
Cardiovascular drift, 63
Cardiovascular system, 40, 305
Carotid body deactivation, 190
Catecholamines, 39, 54, 56–57
    and active transport of fluid, 107
    effect of cold exposure on, 166
    effect of water immersion on, 207
    and glomerular membrane permeability, 77
    and myocardial necrosis, 309
    and renal nerves, 86
CCK (cholecystokinin), 39, 41
Cell mass, 216
Cell membranes, 5

Cellular dehydration. *See* Dehydration, cellular
Cellular water, 5, 300
Central acute isoosmotic blood volume, 204
Central nervous system (CNS)
    damage during heat stroke, 309–310
    effect of estrogens on, 237
    effect of heat stroke on, 301
    osmoreceptors, 38, 127–129
    regulation of gastrointestinal function, 38
    release of peptides from, 41
    temperature of, *vs.* core temperature, 302–303
Central venous pressure (CVP), 9, 13, 199
Cerebellum, 310
Cerebral blood flow, during heat stroke, 304
Cerebral edema, 190, 300
Cerebral osmoreceptors, 5, 120, 122
Cerebral temperature, 303
cGMP excretion, 205
Channel-forming integral membrane protein, 108
Chemical maturity in humans, 223
Chemoreceptors
    and gastric emptying control, 26
    relationship with baroreceptors, 191
    and renal excretory function, 190–191
Children
    fluid volume, 217–218, 220, 221–222
    hypohydration and, 291
CHIP28, 108
Chloride, 35, 119, 298
CHO. *See* Carbohydrate
Cholecystokinin (CCK), 39, 41
Cholinergic neurotransmission, 9
Chyme
    monitoring, 38
    motility of, 36
    osmolality of, 29
Circulatory failure during heat stroke, 304
Circumventricular organ, 5
Cirrhosis, 208, 209
Clearance, 79
    free water. *See* Free water clearance
    lithium, 202
    lymphatic, 103–104
    osmotic, 61, 199
    renal, 5
    uric acid, 202
Clinical complications, of body fluid and electrolyte balance, 297–315
Clonidine, 305
Clothing, 160
    effect on sweat loss, 172

insulating effect, 161, 170–171, 189
removal during treatment of heat stroke, 310
vapor-impermeable, 284, 286
CNS. *See* Central nervous system
Cocaine, 305
Cognitive performance, 174–175
Cold acclimation, 166–167
Cold exposure, 159–177
    fluid balance during, 167–173
    thermoregulation during, 160–167
Cold-induced diuresis (CID), 167–169, 174, 177
Cold injuries, 175–176
Cold-sensitivity, 8
Colitis, 44
Colloid injection, 9
Colon, 20, 28, 29
Coma, 299, 310, 311, 313
Compartments
    body fluid, 6, 216
    extracellular, 119
    volume of, change during exercise and heat stress, 6–7
Conduction, 161
Congestive heart failure, 102
Contraception. *See* Oral contraceptives
Contractions
    gallbladder, 39
    intestinal, 36
    muscle, 62, 162, 267
Convection, 161
Cooling, in treatment for heat stroke, 311
Coordination, 174, 272
Core temperature, 24, 249
    and age, 305
    and AVP concentration, 124
    and body water loss, 147–148
    effect of heat stroke on, 301
    during hyperhydration, 150, 151
    during luteal phase, 243
    vs. CNS temperature, 302–303
Corn syrup solids, 34
Cortisol, 233–234, 264
Cotransport, 31, 32, 33
Cramps, abdominal, 44, 45
Creatine kinase, 299, 306, 307
Creatine phosphate, 144, 307
Cuffs, 104
Cutaneous blood flow, 305, 310
Cutaneous evaporative water loss, 187, 189
CVP (central venous pressure), 9, 13, 199
Cycle ergometry, 123, 125

Index

Cycling, 146–147, 152, 268, 273, 290
Cystic fibrosis, 10
Cytokines, 304

D

Dancing, 284
Dehydration. *See also* Heat exposure; Heat stroke
   cellular, 4, 5, 6–9, 10, 12, 273. *See also* Osmoreceptors
   during cold exposure
      countermeasures, 176–177
      effect on exercise, 160
      minimization of, 160
      physical and cognitive performance, 174–175
   endocrine control during, 83
   extracellular, 6, 9, 12
   gender differences in, 247–248
   involuntary, mechanism of, 10–12
   renal function during, 81–83
   and response to hypoxia, 191
   thermal, 10, 11, 12
   and thirst response, 261–262
   and vasopressin-osmoregulatory system, 4
   voluntary, 9, 118
      causes of, 121
      during cold exposure, 172
      percent of total fluid loss, 54
      weight loss procedures, 284
   water *vs.* no fluid replacement, 263–264
Delirium, 299
Depression, 291
Deuterium oxide, 35
Dextrose, 312
DHPG (dihydroxyphenylglycol), 207
Diamox, 141
Diarrhea, 20, 33, 44, 299
Diazepam, 311
DIC, 312
Dietary factors, 66. *See also* Food intake
   and cold-induced diuresis, 168
   sodium-restricted, 125
Diffusion, 32, 33, 103
Digitalis receptor, 206
Dihydroxyphenylglycol (DHPG), 207
Dipsogenic agents, 5, 9, 65
Disaccharides, 23, 34
Disease, presence of, 66
Disseminated intravascular coagulation, 312
Distal intestine, percent fluid absorbed by, 28
Distention, gastric, 26–27, 262, 273, 310
Diuresis, 123
   as adaptation to altitude, 184, 190
   cold-induced, 167–169
   effect of AVP on, 204
   in gravity-free environment, 198
   and kaliuretic peptide, 206
   mechanisms of, 199–200
   pressure, 167, 169, 190
   in water immersion, 198
Diuretics, 141, 284, 288, 290, 305
Diuril, 141
Diving, 284
Dizziness, 301
DLW (doubly labeled water), 186
D_2O, 185
Dopa, 207
Dopamine, 78, 207
Doubly labeled water (DLW), 186
Drinking. *See also* Fluid, intake; Fluid, replacement
   angiotentin II-induced, 7
   and gastric emptying, 21–22
   reduced, in the elderly, 122
Drinking behavior, 6, 10, 55, 120–121. *See also* Dehydration, voluntary
   during cold exposure, 173
   definition, 260
   effect of exercise on, 272–273
   learned, 260
Drink taste, 8, 10, 12, 121
Drugs and medications, role in heat stroke, 305
Dry mouth, 4, 8, 262, 272
Duodenal brake, 25
Duodenal osmoreceptors, 9
Duodenojejunum, 28, 34
Duodenum, 23
   release of peptides, 39, 40
   signal transducer in the, 25
Dysmetria, 310

E

Eating. *See* Dietary factors; Food intake
Eating disorders, 42, 189–190, 291
ECF. *See* Extracellular fluid
Edema, cerebral, 190, 300. *See also* Pulmonary edema
EDRF (endothelial-derived relaxing factor), 92
Effort, perception of, 175, 289
Electrocardiograph, 308, 309
Electrochemical diffusion. *See* Diffusion
Electrolytes, 6–7
   absorption. *See* Intestinal absorption
   balance during exercise, 54–55

clinical complications of body fluid and, 297–315
in the kidney, 75–93
in the lung, 97–110
hormonal control of homeostasis, 53–54
loss in weight-controlling athletes, 287
in sport drinks. *See also* Carbohydrate-electrolyte solution
and gastric emptying, 21, 22
and salt, 265
Endocrine cells, release of peptides from, 39, 40, 41
Endocrine function
and athlete's amenorrhea, 250
control of renal function during exercise, 83–86
Endocrine secretion, 26
Endorphins, 41
Endothelial cells, 6, 108–109
Endothelial-derived relaxing factor (EDRF), 92
Endotoxemia, 45, 304
Endotoxins, 304
Endurance. *See* Exercise endurance; Muscular endurance
Energy content, 23
Energy expenditure
effect of altitude on, 185–186, 187, 188, 189
by terrain type, 173
vs. metabolic water production, 188
vs. respiratory evaporative loss, 188
Enkephalins, 41
Enteric nervous system (ENS), 38
fine-tuning of ionic transport, 38
release of peptides from, 41
Enterocytes, glycolytic enzyme activity, 43
Enterogastric inhibitory reflex, 26
Enteroglucagon, 25
Environmental factors, 66
altitude, 66, 100, 183–192
atmospheric air, water content, 161
cold exposure during exercise, 10, 21, 159–177
effect on gastric emptying, 24–25
and fluid replacement, 260–262
heat exposure during exercise, 5, 10, 12, 13, 121, 124–125
Epinephrine
effect of estrogen on, 240
in fetus, reversal of fluid flow near birth, 106
levels during exercise, 56, 58–59
during water immersion, 207

Epithelial lining fluid, 101
Erythrocytes. *See* Red blood cells
Erythrocythemia, 26
Erythropoietin, during pregnancy, 242
17-β Estradiol, 233, 237
Estradiol monobenzoate, 238
Estriol, 233
Estrogen receptors, 240
Estrogens
changes during menstrual cycle, 233–234, 237, 250
effect on fluid intake, 240
effect on temperature regulation, 242–243
and fluid retention, 237–238
and the kidney, 238–239
and peripheral vasculature, 239–240
during pregnancy, 242
Estrone, 233
Ethylenediaminetetracetic acid, 44
Euhydration, 118, 123
definition, 140
maintaining, in the cold, 176–177
Evaporation, heat loss during, 140. *See also* Respiratory evaporative water loss
Exchange, 33
Exercise
acute, 246–248
aerobic, 145–147, 232
anaerobic, 144, 286, 287, 290, 291
change in compartment volumes during, 6–7
changes in renal function, 79–83
chronic, 248–250
effect on intestinal absorption, 34–36
effect on sympathetic tone, 38
to exhaustion, 126, 147, 290
fluid balance during, 54–55
integrated control of, 117–130
in women, 246–250
and gastric emptying, 21, 24
gastrointestinal adaptation to, 42–43
gastrointestinal physiology during, 19–46
under heat stress. *See* Dehydration; Exercise-heat performance; Heat stroke
hormonal responses to, 55–69
control of fluid balance, 231–251
integration of body fluid balance, 123–127
isometric, 293
metabolic heat production of, 162, 164
mode of, 66
performance and tolerance, 142–147
during cold exposure, 174

Index

with hypohydration, 283–294
during pregnancy, 242
recovery from, 270–272, 275
weight-bearing, 249
Exercise capacity
in amenorrheic athletes, 250
and hypohydration, 283–292
and VO_2, 34–36, 123, 174
effect of menstrual cycle on, 247
gender differences, 249
during hypohydration, 285, 292
and oral contraceptives, 241
Exercise duration, 66, 123
Exercise endurance, 248, 251–252, 263
questionable role of carbohydrates in, 267–270
in weight-controlling athletes, 286, 288, 293–294
Exercise-heat performance, 5, 10, 12, 13, 121, 124–125. *See also* Dehydration; Heat stroke
Exercise intensity, 123
Exhaustion, 126, 147, 290
Explosiveness, 291, 293
Extracellular fluid (ECF), 6, 141, 218
osmotic stimuli, 7
percent of body weight, 216–217, 226–227, 228–229
volume, 5
and acute saline administration, 199
effect of hypoxia on, 184, 185
Extracerebral osmoreceptors, 5, 8–9

F

Fat
effect on gastric emptying, 21, 26
stimulation of peptide release, 40
and thermoregulation, 164–165, 166
water from oxidation of, 187
Fat-free mass (FFM), 215, 217, 220, 224–225, 228
Fatigue, 143, 144. *See also* Muscular endurance
perception of, 305
Fat mass (FM), 222
Femoral blood flow, effect of estrogen on, 239
Femoral vein, 127
Fertility, 250
Fever, 299
FFM. *See* Fat-free mass
Fibrinolysis, 310, 312
Figure skating, 284
Fitness, 8, 165, 207

Fluid
availability, 172–173
distribution during menstrual cycle, 237
excretion, hormonal control of, 232
intake, 3–13, 67, 260. *See also* Fluid, replacement
definition, 260
environmental factors, 260–262
equation for, 5
factors limiting, 171–173
and food intake, 121, 172–173, 261
hormonal control of, 232
and rehydration, 272
voluntary, 10
loss of, 54. *See also* Water, loss of
overload, 152. *See also* Hyperhydration
replacement. *See also* Fluid, intake
definition, 260
environmental factors, 260–262
during exercise, 262–270, 272–275
guidelines for, 263
retention, 176, 236, 237
mechanisms for, 237–241
during menstrual cycle, 250
and oral contraceptives, 241
transport of
across the endothelium, 101–102
active, 106–107
passive, 104–106
Fluid balance
during cold exposure, 167–173
during exercise, 54–55
clinical complications of, 297–315
integrated control of, 117–130
women, 231–251, 246–250
in gastrointestinal tract, 38–42
role of kidneys in, 75–93
role of lungs in, 97–110
Follicular phase, 234, 236
body temperature during, 242
plasma volume during, 248
Follicular stimulating hormone, 233
Food antigens, 44
Food intake. *See also* Anorexia; Dietary factors
caloric deprivation, 66
changes during menstrual cycle, 240–241
with exposure to hypoxia, 189–190
flow and delivery of nutrients, 25
and fluid intake, 121, 172–173, 261
and gastric distention, 27
and gastrointestinal peptides, 39, 40
GI adaptation to changes in, 42–43

Fraction of water in fat-free mass (FWFFM), 221, 222, 223, 224–225
Free water clearance, 81, 85
  rate during exercise, 61, 62
  during water immersion, 199
Fructose, 270
  effect on gastric emptying, 23
  transport of, 30
Fullness, feeling of. See Gastric distention
Furosemide, 141, 288, 312
FWFFM. See Fraction of water in fat-free mass

G

Gait disturbances, 310
Gallbladder contractions, 39
Gastric distention, 26–27, 262, 273, 310
Gastric emptying (GE), 20–22
  acute and chronic exercise, 24
  control of, 25–26
  dietary history, 42–43
  environment and hydration state, 24–25
  exercise, 35, 46
  maximum rate, 32, 118–119
  methodologies, 20–21
  osmolality and carbohydrates, 23–24
  peptides, 41
  rate, at rest, 22
  volume, 21–22
Gastric mucosal blood flow, effect of peptides on, 41
Gastric reflux, 20
Gastric secretions, volume per day, 28
Gastric sensations, 26–27
Gastrin, 39–40
Gastritis, 44
Gastrointestinal adaptation, 42–43
Gastrointestinal (GI) tract, 8. See also Intestinal absorption
  feedback inhibition in the, 25
  function of
    bleeding and barrier function, 44–46
    neural and hormonal control, 38–42
  gut motility, 36–38, 40, 41
  pain in the, 26
  release of NO from, 41
  VIP in, 40
Gastrointestinal osmoreceptors, 9, 129
Gastrointestinal physiology, during exercise, 19–46
GE. See Gastric emptying
Gender differences, 66
  and cold-induced diuresis, 168
  in fluid requirements, 247
  in plasma volume, 247
  in sweating, 243–244
  VO_2, 249
G forces, 123
GFR. See Glomerular filtration rate
Glomerular filtration, 76, 77
Glomerular filtration rate (GFR), 57, 61, 65, 67
  during acute exercise, 80
  and renal excretion, 191
  and renal water loss, 118
Glucose, 122. See also Carbohydrate-electrolyte solution (CHO-E)
  blood, 269, 270
  effect on gastric emptying, 23, 25
  in fluid replacement drinks
    gender differences, 248
    role of, 33, 268, 269, 270
  in plasma, 267
  supplementation, for glycogen restoration, 270
  in water transport, 31, 32
D-Glucose, 31
Glucose receptor, 23, 26
GLUT2 exit mechanism, 30
GLUT5 transport, 30
Glycerol, 120, 152, 176
Glycogen, 141
  depletion, 26, 292
  formation, gender differences in, 248
  repletion, 270–271
  storage, 20, 166, 270
Glycolysis, 144, 292
Gravity-free environment, 198
Greyhounds, 109
Greyout tolerance, 291
Growth hormone, 242, 248
Guanfacine, 305
Guanosine 3',5'-cyclic monophosphate (cGMP), 205
Gut barrier function, 44–46
Gut motility, 36–38, 40, 41
Gymnastics, 284

H

Habituation. See Cold acclimation; Heat acclimation
Haloperidol, 305
Harvard step test, 291
Heart, blood flow to the, 55
Heart rate, and rehydration, 266
Heat acclimation, 35, 124–126

and ANP, 123
and drinking behavior, 273–274
and heat cramps, 298
and hyperhydration, 151
and lack of effect on GI function, 10
and sodium content of sweat, 10
in women, 245–246, 251
Heat balance, 140, 161. *See also*
  Thermoregulation
Heat cramps, 267, 297–298
Heat exhaustion, 263, 264, 267. *See also* Heat
  stress; Heat stroke
  pathophysiology, 298–299
  symptoms, 299
  treatment, 299–300
Heat exposure, 5, 121, 139–152. *See also*
  Dehydration
  and heat acclimation, 124–125
  involuntary dehydration during, 10, 12, 13
  in women, 242–246
Heat illness, 263
Heat production, 162, 164, 243
Heat storage, 54, 175
Heat stress, 83. *See also* Heat exposure; Heat
  stroke
  change in compartment volumes during,
    6–7
  and gastric emptying, 21, 24–25
  gender similarities under, 244
Heat stroke, 140, 299, 300–312
  in athletes with sickle cell trait, 313–314
  laboratory findings, 301–302
  pathophysiology, 302–307
  role of negligence and punition in,
    314–315
  symptoms, 301
  treatment of, 310–312
Heat tolerance, 147, 152
Height, and total body water, 222
Hematocrit
  in amenorrheic athletes, 250
  changes during menstrual cycle, 235, 236
  effect of estradiol on, 238
  levels after drinking, 68–69
Hemoconcentration, 302
Hemodilution, 12, 244, 246
Hemoglobin, 98, 250
Hemorrhage, 7
  capillary, 109–110
  and heat stroke, 312
  pulmonary, 109
  reduction in plasma volume, 9
Hemorrhagic disorders, 310
Hepatic damage during heat stroke, 309

Hepatic portal vein, 127
Hepatoportal osmoreceptors, 8, 12, 127,
  128
Hexose, 34
Hikers, 184
Historical background, 4–5
  dehydration and performance research,
    284–285
  of fluid balance during exercise, 118–120
Hobbling effect, 171, 173
Homeostatic drinking, 10
Hormonal control
  of electrolyte homeostasis, 53–54
  feedback, and athlete's amenorrhea, 250
  of fluid balance in women during exercise,
    231–251
  of fluid intake/excretion, 232
  in gastrointestinal tract, 38–42
  of kidneys, 54, 55
Hormones, 7. *See also* Individual hormones
  response to exercise, 55–69
  role in thirst, 55
Horseradish peroxidase, 101
Humidity, 187, 260
Humoral natriuretic factor (OLF), 202,
  206–207
Hydration status, 24–25, 66
Hydrochloric acid, 40
Hydromeiosis, 243, 303
Hydrostatic pressure, 6, 208
  in the lungs, 101, 102
Hydrotherapy, 198
Hyperaldosteronism, 210
Hypercalcemia, 299
Hyperhydration, 118, 150–152
Hyperkalemia, 307–308
Hypernatremia, 126, 299, 300
Hyperosmolality, 6, 11, 122, 128
  from environmental factors, 260
  extracellular fluid, 11, 119, 273
Hyperphagia, 43
Hyperphosphatemia, 302, 308, 310
Hyperpnea, 104
Hypertension, 208
Hyperthermia, 24, 26, 41, 273
  during heat stroke, 301, 302, 303
Hypertonicity, 119
Hyperventilation, 299, 304
Hypervolemia, 11, 208, 209
Hypobaric hypoxia, 184
Hypocalcemia, 302, 308
Hypochloremia, 298, 299
Hypodipsia, 122, 189–190
Hypoglycemia, 166, 268, 309, 312

Hypohydration, 121, 263
  and aerobic power, 145, 146, 152
  at altitude, 184–185
  by athletes, 81, 82, 140, 284–285
  and cognitive performance, 174–175
  effect on aerobic capacity, 145
  and gastric emptying, 24
  isotonic, 150
  and muscle strength, 143–144, 152, 286
  reasons for retention of strength and power during, 292
  as stimulus for thirst, 119
  and thermoregulation, 148–150
  and work capacity, 145, 284–285
Hypokalemia, during heat stroke, 301, 311
Hyponatremia, 270
  and ANP, 124
  due to sweating, 20, 91
  in heat cramps, 298
  in heat exhaustion, 299
  in long-distance runners, 312–313
  symptoms of, 265
Hypotension, 299, 311
Hypothalamus, 7, 127
  and athlete's amenorrhea, 250
  AVP production, 57
  estrogen receptors in the, 240
Hypothermia, in the eldery, 165
Hypovolemia, 126. *See also* Plasma volume
  and cardiac volume receptors, 11, 13
  in the elderly, 122
  from environmental factors, 260
  and exercise performance, 152
  mediation of sweating response, 149
  response to hypoxia, 191
  and stretch receptor stimulation, 9
Hypoxemia, 109, 184
Hypoxia, 98, 99
  effect of, 184–192
  hypobaric, 184, 191
  hypoxic, 184
  and sickle cell trait, 313

I

ICF. *See* Intracellular fluid
Ileal brake, 25
Ileum, release of peptides from, 40, 41
Immersion model
  "afferent limb of the," 198–199
  "efferent limb of the," 199–207
  salient features of the, 208, 209
Indomethacin, 85, 204
Infants, fluid volume in, 216–217, 218, 220

Inflammatory response, 44–45
Ingestion of fluid. *See* Drinking; Fluid, intake; Fluid, replacement
Injury, susceptibility during cold exposure, 175–176
Insensible water loss, 118
Insulation, 162, 164, 166, 170–171, 189
Insulin, 270, 309
Interstitial fluid (ISF), 6, 13, 216
Interstitium, 98, 101
  edema formation, 99, 100
  protein concentration in, 102, 103
  storage of fluid, 106
Intestinal absorption, 20, 27–38
  effect of exercise on, 34–36
  maximal capacity for water transport, 21
  role of gut motility, 36–38
  role of osmolality and solute transport, 29–30
  volume per day, 28
  water, 28–32, 35
Intestinal blood flow, 313
Intestinal infarction, 310
Intestinal sensory receptors, 25–26
Intoxication, water, 90–91, 124, 313
Intracarotid infusion, 5
Intracellular fluid (ICF), 6, 141, 218
  percent of body weight, 216, 217, 226–227, 228–229
  water transport of, 31–32
Intracellular volume, effect of hypoxia on, 184, 185
Intravascular coagulation, 310
Intravascular fluid, percent of body weight, 216
Intrinsic factor, 40
Inulin, 5
Involuntary dehydration, 10–12
Ischemia, 44
ISF (interstitial fluid), 6, 13, 216
Isometric exercise, 293
Isoosmotic central volume expansion, 204
Isotonic solutions, 11, 34
I.V. infusion, 5

J

Jaundice, 302
Jejunum, 25, 35, 36
  glycolytic enzyme activity in the, 43
  release of peptides, 40
Jockeys, 284

Index

J-receptors, 99
Judo, 284, 286–287, 288
Jugular vein, 128
Jumping, 174, 290–291

K

Kaliuresis, 200
Kaliuretic peptide, 205–206
Karate, 284
Kidneys
  and body fluid balance during exercise, 75–93
  estrogen-progesterone and the, 238–239
  hormonal regulation of, 54, 55

L

Lactate, 247, 248, 249, 288
Lactation, 43
Lactic dehydrogenase, 302
Large intestine, 39
Lasix, 141
Laxatives, 284
Lean body mass (LBM), 215
Learned behaviors, 260
Learning ability, 291
Leg volume and distensibility, 235
Lightweight rowing, 146, 284, 288–289
Lipids, effect on gastric emptying, 25
Lithium clearance, 202
Liver
  glycogen stores in, 270
  hepatoportal receptors, 8, 12, 127, 128
  injury during heat stroke, 302, 309
Lower body negative pressure, 123
Lungs
  angiotensin in the, 64
  fluid and electrolyte balance during exercise, 97–110
  structure, 100–101
  VIP in, 40
  water transport in the, 107–108
Luteal phase, 233, 234, 236, 238
  and blood-lactate levels, 248
  body temperature, 242–243
  delay of sweating response during, 244
  metabolic rate during, 241, 243
  and resting muscle glycogen, 248
  urine flow during, 246
Luteinizing hormone, 233
Lymphatic clearance, 103–104
Lymph flow, 103–104

M

Magnesium, 119
Malaise, 26
Maltodextrins, 23, 24, 34, 270
Maltrin, 270
Manned space flights, 198, 210
Mannitol, 8, 128, 208, 312
Manual dexterity, 162, 175
Marathoners, 44, 45, 249, 267. *See also* Running
Markers, for intestinal absorption, 28
Maximal capacity for water absorption, 32
Maximal exercise capacity. *See* Exercise capacity, and VO_2
Mechanical trauma, 44
Mechanoreceptors, 9
Menstrual cycle, 192, 232–250
Mercury bag, 28, 29
Metabolic heat production, 162, 164, 243
Metabolic rate, 148, 241
  and respiratory water loss, 169, 170
Metabolic water production, 186, 187, 188
3-O-Methyl-D-glucose (3MG), 35
3MG, 35
Mineralocorticoids, 78, 238. *See also* Aldosterone
Missing osmols, 121
Mitral stenosis, 102
Mode of exercise, 66
Motilin, 40
Motility, gut, 36–38, 40, 41
Mountaineers, 184. *See also* Altitude
Mountain sickness, 126, 190, 192
Mouth dryness, 4, 8, 262, 272
mRNA of CHIP28, 108
Multiple-factor theory of thirst, 5
Muscle contractions
  and AVP, 62
  during heat cramps, 267
  and metabolic heat production, 162
Muscle glycogen. *See* Glycogen
Muscles
  blood flow to, 55
  handgripping, 286
  and potassium deficiency, 306–307
  skeletal, 293. *See also* Rhabdomyolysis
  temperature of, 174
Muscular endurance, 143–144, 288, 291
Muscular strength, 142–143, 152, 174, 286
Myalgia, 299
Myocardial infarction, 309
Myocardial necrosis, 309

Myoglobin, 307, 308, 312
Myoglobinuria, 307
Myosin, 298

N

Nasal decongestants, 305
Natriuresis, 81, 123
  as adaptation to altitude, 184, 190
  ANF as effector of, 205
  changes during menstrual cycle, 235
  dissociation of, from diuresis, 200
  effect of immersion on, 201
  effect of indomethacin on, 204
  effect of kaliuretic peptide on, 206
  in gravity-free environment, 198
  mechanisms of, 200
Nausea, 26, 44, 299
NCAA, 285, 286
Nephron sites, 200, 202
Nephrotic syndrome, 208, 209
Neural control, of gastrointestinal tract, 38–42
Neuromodulators, 38
Neuronal factors, 7
Neuropeptides, 38–42
Neurotensin, 25, 41
Neurotransmitters, 38
NI. See Water immersion
Nitric oxide (NO), 41–42, 78
  during acute renal failure, 308
  effect of estrogen on, 239
  during hyperthermia, 304
  and renal failure, 92
Nonhomeostatic drinking, 10
Nonregulatory drinking, 10
Nonsteroidal antiinflammatory drugs (NSAIDS), 44, 45, 92
Norepinephrine, 38–39, 65, 305
  effect of estrogen on, 240
  levels during exercise, 56, 57, 58–60
  organ responsible for, 89–90
  during water immersion, 207
NSAIDS, 44, 45, 92
Nutrient intake. See Dietary factors; Food intake
Nutrition status, 166

O

Occupational Safety and Health Administration, 315
OLF (humoral natriuretic factor), 202, 206–207

Oncotic pressure, 4
Opiate peptides, 41
Oral contraceptives, 240, 241, 246, 248, 251
Oral pharyngeal reflex, 20, 67, 262
Oral rehydration solution, 29. See also Carbohydrate-electrolyte solution; Sport drinks
Organic phosphates, 119
Organum vasculosum laminae terminalis, 5
Orocecal transit time, 46
Oropharyngeal receptors, 8, 12
Oropharyngeal reflex, 20, 67, 262
Oropharyngeal tract, 8
ORS (oral rehydration solution), 29
Orthostasis, 299
Osmolality, 6, 8. See also Hyperosmolality
  body water loss effects on, 141, 142
  during dehydrated state, 82
  effect of sweating on, 10, 149
  effect on gastric emptying, 23–24
  during pregnancy, 242
  range of, 119
  in water absorption, 29–30
  in water transport, 31–32
Osmoreceptor dehydration. See Dehydration, cellular
Osmoreceptors, 5, 7–9
  cerebral, 5, 120, 122
  CNS and peripheral, 127–129
  extracerebral, 5, 8–9
  hepatoportal, 8, 12, 127, 128
  intestinal, 9, 129
  portal-bed, 9, 127–128
  renal, 12
  stimulation of, 9, 119
Osmoregulation, 11, 119–120
Osmotic clearance, 61, 199
Osmotic factors, 5
Osmotic fluctuations, 5
Osmotic pressure, 6, 101, 237
Osteoporosis, 250
Ouabain, 120, 206
Ouabain-like factor, 202, 206
Ovulation, 232–233, 239, 241
Oxidative system, 292
Oxygen availability, 184. See also Altitude
  hypobaric hypoxia, 184, 191
Oxygen consumption, rate during exercise, 98
Oxygen production (VO_2)
  effect of cold exposure on, 164
  and exercise capacity. See Exercise capacity, and VO_2

Index

gender differences, 249
maximum, 34–36, 38
at rest and during exercise, 99

P

Palatability of fluid, 8, 10, 12, 120–121, 261, 273
Pancreas, 39, 40, 310
Pancreatic and intestinal secretions, volume per day, 28
Paracrine activity, 41
Paralysis, 307–308
Parent-Teacher Associations, 315
Passive fluid transport, 104–106
Pepsin, 40
Peptides, 39–42
Peptide YY, 25
Perception of effort, 175, 289
Perception of fatigue, 305
Performance
  and carbohydrates in fluid replacement, 269
  cognitive, 174–175
  during cold exposure, 174–175
  during exercise, 142–147
  under heat stress. *See* Exercise-heat performance
  during hypohydration, 283–294
  with hypovolemia, 152
  during pregnancy, 242
Peripheral cold injury, 175–176
Peripheral osmoreceptors, 5, 8–9
Peripheral vasculature
  arterial chemoreceptors and renal excretory function, 190–191
  and estrogen-progesterone, 239–240
Permeability
  capillary, 101–102, 103, 309
    changes during menstrual cycle, 235, 240, 244
  glomerular membrane, 77
  pulmonary epithelium, 106
  red cells, 107
Perspiration. *See* Sweating
PGE_2, 77
PGE (renal prostaglandins), 199, 202, 204–205, 209
PGI_2, 77
pH, arterial, 99
Pharyngeal receptors, 8, 12
Phenothiazines, 305
Phenylpropanolamine, 305
Phosphate
  absolute and fractional excretion, 202
  during heat stroke, 302
  organic, 119
  renal, 202
Phosphofructokinase, 302
Phosphorous, serum, 299
Physical activity. *See* Exercise
Physical fitness, 8, 165, 207
Physical work capacity, 13, 145, 174, 285
Physiology
  gastrointestinal, 19–46
  renal, 75–79
Pigment nephropathy, 308
Pilocarpine, 4
Plasma osmolality, 232
  and AVP, 57, 62, 120
  effect of sweating on, 20, 54
  as stimulus for thirst, 240
Plasma proteins, 4, 102
Plasma renin activity (PRA), 8, 58–59, 64–65, 120, 264
  hormonal integration of, 124–127
  during water immersion, 203, 209
  in women, 246
Plasma volume (PV), 6, 12, 13. *See also* Hypovolemia
  and ANP, 124
  changes during exercise, 249, 273
  changes during menstrual cycle, 235, 236, 247–248, 250
  effect of body water loss on, 141, 142, 247
  effect of sweating on, 20
  and hemorrhage, 9
  and hypohydration in weight-controlling athletes, 288, 289
  with hypoxia-induced loss in TBW, 184
  and oral contraceptives, 241
  during pregnancy, 241–242
  and rehydration, 265, 266, 267, 271, 272
  and thirst stimulation, 121
  in women, 244–245, 247
Pleura, 104
PMS, 233, 236–237
Polyethylene glycol, 28
"Pores," in red cell membranes, 107
Portal-bed osmoreceptors, 9, 127–128
Portal vein, 9, 127–128
Position. *See* Body position
Potassium, 119
  absorption, 35
  deficiency, and heat stroke, 306–307
  during dehydrated state, 81, 82
  excretion
    kaliuresis, 200

kaliuretic peptide, 205–206
plasma concentration, 8, 124
urine concentration of, 5, 77
Potassium chloride, 4
Potassium deficiency, and rhabdomyolysis, 306
Power athletes, 287–288
Pregnancy, 43, 232, 241–242
Premenstrual syndrome (PMS), 233, 236–237
Preoptic-anterior hypothalamic neurons, 8, 149
Preoptic area, 5
Pressure baroreceptors. See Baroreceptors
Progesterones
  changes during menstrual cycle, 233–234, 237, 246, 247, 250
  effect on food intake, 241
  effect on temperature regulation, 242–243
  and the kidney, 238–239
  and peripheral vasculature, 239–240
  during pregnancy, 242
Prolactin, 233–234, 242
Propranolol, 305
Prostaglandins, 77, 78
  inhibition of ADH, 81
  renal, 199, 202, 204–205, 209
  and renal failure, 92
  and renal function, 85
Protein
  and athlete's amenorrhea, 249
  effect on gastric emptying, 21, 119
  in interstitium, 102, 103
  plasma, 102
  serum, 238
Proteinuria, 90, 302
Pseudonephritis, 302
Psychological factors
  of athlete's amenorrhea, 249, 250
  calm vs. excited, 262
  to heat stress, 245
  personal opinions, 261
  social customs, 260–261
  symptoms of heat stroke, 301
  in weight-controlling athletes, 291
Pulmonary arterial pressure, 99, 199
Pulmonary capillaries
  filtration across, 101–103
  stress failure in, 108–110
Pulmonary capillary leak syndrome, 309
Pulmonary edema, 98–100, 106, 190
  factors that contribute to, 102
  during heat stroke treatment, 311

Pulmonary epithelium
  active transport across, 106–107
  aveolar, 100, 108
  fetal, 106
  passive transport of fluid across, 104–106
  permeability, 106
Pulmonary hemorrhage, exercise-induced, 109
PV. See Plasma volume

R

Racehorses, 109
Radioimmunoassay, 204
RBF. See Renal blood flow
Reaction time, 291, 293
Recovery, from exercise, 270–272, 275
Rectal temperature, 8, 266, 304
Red blood cells, 107–108, 126
  mass, during menstrual cycle, 235
  permeability, 107
  volume, 249. See also Blood volume
Regulatory drinking, 10
Rehydration, 6, 11, 121. See also Hypohydration
  effect on plasma volume, 265, 266, 267, 271, 272
  gender differences in, 247–248
  oral solutions, 29. See also Carbohydrate-electrolyte solution; Sport drinks
  and sweating, 22
  in weight-controlling athletes, 287, 288
Renal artery, 8
Renal blood flow (RBF), 77, 79–80
  redistribution of, 87–88
  stimulation of renin release by, 120
Renal clearance, 5
Renal failure, acute, 91–92, 307, 308, 312
Renal function
  changes with acute exercise, 79–83
  in dehydrated state, 81–83
  factors controlling, 83–87
  problems during exercise, 90–92
Renal natriuretic peptide (urodilatin), 199, 205, 209
Renal nerves, 9, 86–87
Renal osmoreceptors, 12
Renal physiology, 75–79
Renal plasma flow (RPF), 79
Renal prostaglandins (PGE), 199, 202
  and water immersion, 204–205, 209
Renal sodium handling, in the immersion model, 200–202, 209
Renal tubules, 31, 76, 77, 78, 90, 238

Renal venous blood flow (RVBF), 56, 57, 60
Renal water handling, in the immersion model, 199–200
Renal water loss, 118–119
Renin, 57, 129. *See also* Plasma renin activity
 effect of ANP on, 123
 effect of estrogen on, 240
 effect of oral contraceptives on, 241
 levels during exercise, 60, 89
 renal blood flow and, 120
Renin-angiotensin-aldosterone axis, 38, 54
 during exercise, 64–65, 84–85
 and heat stroke, 305
 during water immersion, 202–203, 209
Renin-angiotensin system, 9, 120, 242
Reperfusion injury, 304
Resistive exercise, 232
Resorption, 78–79
Respiratory evaporative water loss, 118, 169–170
 calculation of, 186
 effect of altitude on, 186–187, 192
 vs. energy expenditure, 188
Rest, and fluid intake, 262
Resting metabolic rate, 241, 243. *See also* Metabolic rate
Rhabdomyolysis
 in athletes with sickle cell trait, 313–314
 with heat cramps, 298
 with heat exhaustion, 299
 with heat stroke, 307, 308
 induction of renal failure, 91
 LDH levels and, 301
 and potassium deficiency, 306
Rowing, lightweight, 146, 284, 288–289
RPF (renal plasma flow), 79
Running, 146, 273, 312–313. *See also* Marathoners
RVBF. *See* Renal venous blood flow

S

Saline solution, 6, 10, 208. *See also* Sodium chloride
 in heat acclimation research, 125
 for heat cramps, 298
 in interstitial absorption, 125
 isotonic, 11
Saliva, volume per day, 20, 28
Salivary glands, 4
Salt. *See* Sodium chloride
Salt appetite, 9, 11, 65, 122, 189

Salt intake, 11, 192
 dietary, 264, 275
Saturation vapor pressure, 161, 169
Sauna, 284, 288, 290
Sealing strands, 101, 106
Secretin, 40, 41
Segmental perfusion, 27–28, 29, 35, 36
Seizures, 311, 313
Sensitivity, of sweating response, 149
Sepsis, 312
Serotonin, 241
Serum osmolality, 4, 68–69
Serum protein, effect of estradiol on, 238
Setpoint, of vasopressin-osmoregulatory system, 4
Shivering, 162, 166
Shock, 307, 310
Sickle cell trait, 313–314
Skin blood flow, 150, 152, 162
 changes during menstrual cycle, 239, 251
 exercise increase in, 150, 152
 during heat stroke, 304
 hypohydration reduction of, 150, 152
 in women *vs.* men, 243
Skin temperature, 162, 175, 301, 310–311
Sleep deprivation, 40, 66
Small intestine, 9, 25, 39
 necrosis of, during heat stroke, 310
 percent fluid absorbed by, 28
 sensations from the, 26
Snow, volume of fuel to melt, 172
Sodium
 absorption, 35, 39
 and body fluid homeostasis, 4
 conservation, 88
 control of total body, 88–89
 during dehydrated state, 82, 121–122
 excretion of. *See* Natriuresis
 in extracellular fluid, 119
 in glucose-electrolyte absorption, 32–34
 intake, 12. *See also* Sodium chloride, intake
 loss during sweating, 20, 54, 88
 plasma, 8, 11, 54–55, 121, 265
 during pregnancy, 242
 reabsorption
  across pulmonary epithelium, 106–107
  in heat cramps, 298
  mechanisms of decreased, 202
  by renal tubules, 190–191
  segmental tubular, 200, 202
 rejection, 200, 202

renal excretion, 190–191
renal sodium handling, 200–202
retention
  and estrogen, 237
  and oral contraceptives, 241
urinary excretion, 9, 77
in water transport, 30, 31
Sodium appetite, 9, 65, 122
Sodium chloride, 4. *See also*
  Saline solution
effect of brief osmotic pulses on, 127–128
in fluid replacement during exercise, 262, 263, 264–265, 267, 271
and heat acclimation, 124
hyperosmolar solution, 5, 8, 262
intake, 11, 192, 264, 275
and recovery during exercise, 270–272
retention, 274
salt appetite, 11, 189
sodium appetite, 9, 65, 122
supplementation, 265
in sweat, 267
Sodium-glucose cotransport, 31, 32
Sodium pump, 120
Sodium receptors, 122
Sodium-replete subjects, 200, 204, 205
Sodium-sensitive receptors, 5, 8
Solar radiation, 260
Solute load, 118
Solute-receptors, 5, 122
Solutes. *See* Electrolytes
Solute transport, role in water absorption, 29–30
Solution drag, 31, 32, 33
Somatotropin, during pregnancy, 242
SON (supraoptic nucleus), 5
Space program, 198, 210
Spironolactone, 305
Spitting, 284
Splanchnic blood flow, 127, 129
  and exercise, 34–35, 45
  during heat stroke, 304
Splanchnic nerve stimulation, 35
Splanchnic vasoconstriction, 12
Sport drinks
to avoid GI tract bleeding, 45
carbohydrates in, 21, 23
constituents of, 262–263
glucose in, 33
salt in, 265, 267
Sprint performance, 174
Starling forces, 101, 104, 109

Stomach, 9, 26, 40. *See also* Gastrointestinal tract
Stool, volume of fluid per day, 29
Stress failure, in pulmonary capillaries, 108–110
Stress of competition, 41, 44–46
Stretch receptors, 9, 120, 127
Submaximal exercise performance, 174
Substance P, 41
Sucrose, 24, 34, 270
Sudden death, in athletes with sickle cell trait, 313–314
Sulindac, 85
Superior vena cava, 9
Supraoptic nucleus (SON), 5
Surface area of body, 164, 166
Swallowing reflex, 8
Sweat gland failure, in heat stroke, 303
"Sweat-gland fatigue" (hydromeiosis), 243, 303
Sweating
and age, 305
and clothing insulation, 167
eccrine, 119
fluid loss, 54, 118
during heat stroke, 303
loss of body weight, 7, 54, 263
loss of solutes, 10, 121
in luteal phase, 244
and osmolality, 10
potassium concentration, 306
rate, 5, 20, 22, 144, 273
  and core temperature, 148
  with hyperhydration, 150, 151
  in trained vs. untrained athletes, 88
  in women, 243–244
regulation of, 148–149
salt content, 267
sensitivity to temperature, 149
in women, 243–244, 251
Swimming, 284
Sympathetic nerves (ANS), 38
effect of AVP on, 124
effect of diuresis on, 200
effect of natriuresis on, 202, 203
hormones of the, 56
peptides release by, 41
and renal function during exercise, 86–87, 191
renin release by, 64
Sympathetic tone, 11
Sympathomimetic drugs, 305
Symport (cotransport), 31, 32, 33

Index

T

Tachycardia, 299
Taste, 8, 10, 12, 121
Taurine, 300
TBW. *See* Total body water
TDEE (total daily energy expenditure), 186, 187
Temperature. *See also* Core temperature
  ambient, 187, 260, 261
  body, 146, 174, 242–243
  CNS *vs*. core, 302–303
  of drink, 8, 120–121, 273
  rectal, 8, 266, 304
  skin, 162, 175, 301
    cooling during treatment of heat stroke, 310–311
  tympanic membrane, 302
Temperature homeostasis, 4, 10, 119
Temperature regulation. *See* Thermoregulation
Terrain, type of, 171, 173
Testosterone, changes during menstrual cycle, 233–234
Thermal dehydration, 10, 11, 12
Thermal injury, 20
Thermal stimuli, and release of Substance P, 41
Thermoregulation, 8, 13, 147–150, 264. *See also* Heat balance
  biophysical factors, 161
  during cold exposure, 160–167
  effect of dehydration on, 175–176
  effect of estrogen-progesterone on, 242–243
  effect of hyperhydration on, 150–151
  effect of hypohydration on, 289
  and exercise intensity, 245–246
  heat balance, 140, 161
  loss of, with heat stroke, 302
  responses, 162
  and surface area, 164
Thiazide, 141
Third cerebral ventricle, 5
Thirst
  changes during menstrual cycle, 240–241
  control of, by osmoreceptors, 12
  definition, 260
  drives for, 54, 67
  historical background of research, 4–5, 259–260
  perception of, 305
  reduced, 122, 189–190
  role of hormones in, 55, 67

Thirst center, 4
Thirst threshold, 119
Threshold temperature, for onset of sweating, 148
Throat sensation, 4
Thrombocytopenia, 310
Tight junction, 31–32, 106
Time of day, and cold-induced diuresis, 168
Total body water (TBW), 141, 218–219
  to body weight ratio, 215, 217, 221–222, 224–227, 228–229
  effect of hypoxia on, 184–185, 189
  to height ratio, 222
  percent of FFM, 217, 221, 223
Total daily energy expenditure (TDEE), 186, 187
Track and field, 284
Trained *vs*. untrained responses
  dehydration experiments, 285
  effect of menstrual cycle on VO_2 max, 247
  renal function and water immersion, 207
  sweating rate, 88
Training, 66, 124
Trauma, mechanical, 44
Triamterine, 305
Triatheletes, 45
Triglyceride, 166
Tropomycin, 298
Tryptophan, 241
Tubular reabsorption, 76, 78, 83
Tubular secretion, 76
Tympanic membrane temperature, 302
Type I cells, 100–101, 106, 107
Type II cells, 100–101, 106, 107

U

Ultrafiltration, 103
Ultramarathoners, 45
Urea, 4, 122, 299, 306
Uric acid, 202, 299
Urinary excretion
  and blood volume, 11
  3MG, 35
  potassium, 306
  rate, 5
  sodium and water, 9
Urinary flow
  with glycerol in electrolyte beverages, 176
  during luteal phase, 246

rate during exercise, 61, 63, 80–81
during water immersion, 199
Urinary output, 6, 11, 76–77, 238
Urinary volume, 5, 265, 272
Urinary water loss, 62
Urine
  changes during heat stroke, 302
  changes in weight-controlling athletes, 287
  color, 299, 307
  production rate, 76–77
Urodilatin, 199, 205, 209
U.S. Army Extended Cold Weather Clothing System, 170

V

Vagal afferent nerves, 26
Vagus nerve, 9, 38, 40
Vapor pressure, 161, 169, 187
Vascular compliance, 11, 239
Vascular resistance, 199, 239
Vasoactive intestinal peptide (VIP), 40
Vasoconstriction, 162, 239–240
  and heat stroke, 304, 310
Vasodilation, 240, 243
Vasopressin-osmoregulatory system, 4
Vena cava, 203
Venous vascular compliance, 11
Verapamil, 128
Villi, increase in length and number of, 43
VIP (vasoactive intestinal peptide), 40
Volemic factors, 5
Volume of body fluid. See also Blood volume; Plasma volume
  effect on gastric emptying, 21–22
  homeostasis, 208
  in infancy, childhood, and adolescence, 216–223
  in young, middle-aged, and older adults, 223–228
Volume receptors, 6, 9, 12
Voluntary dehydration. See Dehydration, voluntary
Vomiting, 26, 284, 299, 310
$\dot{V}/\dot{Q}_2$ ratio, 98, 99–100

W

Water. See also Fluid
  absorption, 39, 232
  availability, 172–173, 177
  conservation, 88
  doubly-labeled, 186
  enterosystemic water cycle, 28–29
  excretion. See Diuresis
  gastric emptying, 23
  as heat stroke treatment, 311
  intake, 274
  intestinal absorption of, 28–32, 35
  loss of, 140–142. See also Dehydration; Hypohydration
    and core temperature, 147–148
    cutaneous, 187, 189
    insensible perspiration, 118
    renal, 118–119
    respiratory. See Respiratory evaporative water loss
    through extracellular space, 121
    in the lungs. See Pulmonary edema
  percent of body weight, 3, 6, 220, 224. See also Total body water, to body weight ratio
    and age, 224
    and body composition, 141, 215
    and fluid replacement, 264
  production of, metabolic, 186, 187, 188
  pure, 262–263
  reabsorption, 78–79, 119, 190, 199
  renal excretion of, 190–191
  renal water handling, 199–200
  retention, 176, 236, 237
  from snow, 172
  transport of, 30–32. See also Fluid, transport of
    in the lungs, 107–108
    maximal capacity for, 32
Water channels, 31
Water deficit. See Hypohydration
Water flux, 37
Water immersion, 9, 61, 123, 126. See also Immersion model
  as analog for weightlessness, 198, 210
  convective heat transfer during, 161
  renal, endocrine, and hemodynamic effects of, 197–210
  for volume homeostasis research, 208
Water intoxication, 90–91, 124, 313
Wedge pressure, 99
Weigh-ins, hypohydration for, 81, 82, 140, 284, 285–286, 288
Weight-bearing exercise, 249
Weight-class sports, 284
Weightlessness, water immersion as analogue for, 198, 210

Index

Weightlifting, 284, 288
Weight loss, in weight-controlling athletes, 283–294
Wind chill, 161, 163
Wind speed, 260
Women
   hormonal control of fluid balance, 231–251
   menstrual cycle, 192, 232–250
   pregnancy, 43, 232, 241–242
   premenstrual syndrome, 233, 236–237
   and thermoregulation, 165–166
Work capacity, 13, 145, 174, 285
Wrestling, 81, 284, 285–287, 288

X

Xylose, 35